THE EMOTION REGULATION SKILLS SYSTEM
FOR COGNITIVELY CHALLENGED CLIENTS

The Emotion Regulation Skills System for Cognitively Challenged Clients

A DBT-Informed Approach

JULIE F. BROWN

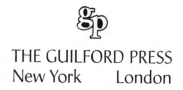

THE GUILFORD PRESS
New York   London

Published by The Guilford Press
A Division of Guilford Publications, Inc.
370 Seventh Avenue, Suite 1200, New York, NY 10001
www.guilford.com

Printed in the United States of America

This book is printed on acid-free paper.

Last digit is print number: 9   8   7   6

The author has checked with sources believed to be reliable in her efforts to provide information that is complete and generally in accord with the standards of practice that are accepted at the time of publication. However, in view of the possibility of human error or changes in behavioral, mental health, or medical sciences, neither the author, nor the editor and publisher, nor any other party who has been involved in the preparation or publication of this work warrants that the information contained herein is in every respect accurate or complete, and they are not responsible for any errors or omissions or the results obtained from the use of such information. Readers are encouraged to confirm the information contained in this book with other sources.

Library of Congress Cataloging-in-Publication Data

Brown, Julie F.
    The emotion regulation skills system for cognitively challenged clients: a DBT-informed approach / Julie F. Brown.
        pages   cm
    Includes bibliographical references and index.
    ISBN 978-1-4625-1928-6 (paperback); ISBN 978-1-4625-3364-0 (hardcover)
    1. Cognitive therapy.   2. Therapist and patient.   3. Stress management.   4. Patients—Counseling of.   I. Title.
    RC489.C63B76 2016
    616.89′1425—dc23
                                                                    2015015976

About the Author

Julie F. Brown, MSW, PhD, is Director of Program Development at Justice Resource Institute's Integrated Clinical Services in Rhode Island. She is an independent social worker who has practiced in the intellectual disabilities field for over two decades. Since 2005, Dr. Brown has been a dialectical behavior therapy (DBT) trainer with Behavioral Tech, LLC. She is a recipient of the Leadership Award from the American Association on Intellectual and Developmental Disabilities.

Acknowledgments

Many people have made this book possible. The Justice Resource Institute (JRI) provided an environment that allowed the Skills System to be developed. In particular, I would like to thank Andrew Pond for his unwavering support. My team at JRI Integrated Clinical Services (ICS), Deborah Jackson and David Damon, were central to the development of the Skills System. Their dedication to helping the individuals we treat, willingness to collaborate, and endless patience with me elicit my deep gratitude. The individuals who attended therapy at JRI ICS were key contributors and collaborators; together we created the Skills System.

The work of Marsha M. Linehan, PhD, the developer of dialectical behavior therapy (DBT), provided important foundational information for this curriculum. I would like to extend a special acknowledgment to Cynthia Sanderson, PhD, for her kindness, vision, and pivotal support. James J. Gross, PhD, editor of both editions of the *Handbook of Emotion Regulation* (2007, 2014), offered valuable feedback that improved the model. Donald Meichenbaum, PhD, Kelly Koerner, PhD, and many of the DBT trainers were also helpful and encouraging during this lengthy process. Seth Axelrod, PhD, and Kitty Moore were key influences in publication of this material by The Guilford Press. I can't thank Anna Brackett at Guilford enough for the collaboration, commitment, and creativity she demonstrated in the visual presentation of text and images in this book.

Finally, I would like to acknowledge the contribution of my family to this project. My husband's perpetual support, encouragement, and endless hours proofreading were indispensable. My mother's countless hours of editing the multiple versions of the guide were greatly appreciated. My children were wonderful teachers; they helped me better understand the human growth process and how relationships support and impede personal evolution.

I am grateful for and indebted to you all.

Preface

DEVELOPING THE SKILLS SYSTEM

The Treasure Hunt

The development of the Skills System has been a 20-year journey. This adventure began shortly after I graduated from Boston University with my MSW. I was working as a clinician in a behaviorally based 25-bed residential school for intellectually disabled, emotionally disturbed adolescent males and females in Massachusetts. One day, a youth who had a significant history of committing sexual offenses, setting fires, treating animals cruelly, and assaulting others was sitting in my office. We were discussing his latest incident of aggression toward a staff member. I posed questions, trying to elicit alternative behaviors to smashing a staff member in the head with a padlock. The young man was unable to generate useful options; thus, I suggested that he play the card game Uno instead.

In the midst of suggesting he play Uno, I experienced an epiphany. This boy had suffered numerous traumas and inflicted even more, and my solution was Uno! While pulling this suggestion out of my eclectic bag of therapeutic tricks, I suddenly became keenly aware that this isolated activity was a woefully inadequate intervention. The card game may have been a piece of a coping puzzle, yet the problem was that I did not have an adequate, synthesized framework or system to teach coping to this individual in a form that he could understand, apply, and generalize. If I did not have a comprehensive representation of a coping map, there was no way that this intellectually disabled adolescent was going to integrate my random teaching into a technically strong, yet flexible model that could help him manage the challenging internal and external factors he faced on a daily basis.

I possessed no vision about the path ahead, but the journey to find the Skills System had begun.

I spent the next 3 years immersed in treating this diverse and challenging population of youth within the residential setting. I combed the literature for insights; I found more tiny puzzle pieces but still no map: no comprehensive tools to help youth with numerous mental health diagnoses integrate the necessary skills to reduce the need for supervision; no models complex enough yet simple enough to assist individuals who struggled with effects of neglect, violent behavior, physical abuse, sexual victimization, and/or social stigmatization. I could not find a program that could help these youth reduce the need for multiple antipsychotic medications, antidepressants, mood stabilizers, and other drugs to control behavior. Although the well-structured token economy within the facility was helpful, it was not sufficient to teach these children, who had complex needs, the necessary skills to regulate their reinforced patterns of dyscontrol in settings beyond residential care. Somewhere there had to be a better solution.

During a monthly consultation in 1997, a well-regarded trauma specialist recommended I find out more about dialectical behavior therapy (DBT; Linehan, 1993a, 1993b, 2015a, 2015b). Initially, I asked myself, "How could a treatment for women with borderline personality disorder [BPD] who demonstrated suicidal and parasuicidal behaviors apply to my clients?" During my initial phases of DBT training, I discovered that although few of my clients were formally diagnosed with BPD, many experienced the BPD behavioral patterns of emotional, cognitive, and behavioral dysregulation described by Linehan. I was cautiously optimistic that DBT would prove to be a piece of the treasure map.

By 1999, I was fortunate enough to have received intensive DBT training and created Justice Resource Institute's (JRI) Integrated Clinical Services (ICS) in Rhode Island. ICS provided outpatient therapy services for adults with mild and moderate intellectual disabilities who experienced intense behavioral control problems. Standard DBT individual therapy, skills training groups, consultation team, and phone skills coaching were key ingredients of the ICS program. The comprehensive DBT treatment model was designed to help people change highly reinforced, long-term patterns of behavior associated with impaired emotion regulation. While it was clear that the DBT technology was helpful in improving self-management capacities, accommodations were necessary to allow cognitively impaired individuals to learn and generalize new adaptive coping skills. Adherence to the DBT model was paramount; our challenge was to make DBT technology accessible to cognitively impaired clients without reducing the therapeutic viability of the empirically validated treatment.

Surprisingly, the individual therapy aspects of DBT (Linehan, 1993a) required minimal adaptation for this population. While learning to do DBT individual therapy and treating cognitively impaired people is intellectually demanding for the therapist, participation in the treatment as a client is relatively straightforward. Unfortunately, the skills component (Linehan, 1993b) was a more complex problem. During the first year, we followed the standard DBT skills manual, adjusting teaching strategies to help improve comprehension of the information. The concepts contained in the mindfulness, interpersonal effectiveness, emotion regulation, and distress tolerance modules (Linehan, 1993b) were vital, yet the language and format were barriers for the clients. Despite my enthusiasm, many participants struggled to pronounce, remember, and understand several standard DBT skills terms and were therefore unable to recall and utilize the concepts within the context of life when emotionally dysregulated.

The DBT skills curriculum did not provide individuals diagnosed with intellectual disabilities, who often experience executive functioning deficits, a framework that facilitated transitions from one skill to the next within complicated contexts that required multiple skills. I continually felt that my clients' reaction to the information in skills training group was like mine when I played the game 52 Pickup as a child. As a group leader, I felt as if I were my mean older sister, who would invite me to play cards and then scream, "Fifty-two pickup!" as she squeezed the deck, gleefully sending the 52 cards into the air and all over the floor for me to pick up. Just as I had been overwhelmed by the cards strewn all over the floor, the participants seemed to stare, dazed and confused, at the divergent information, without even knowing which skill (or card) to pick up first.

While I was driven to maintain adherence to the DBT model, I had a clear sense that I needed to present the DBT concepts in a more accessible way if my clients were going to grasp the essential principles. I began creating step-by-step progressions that the participants with intellectual disabilities could learn and utilize. I knew that I had to find a simple system that offered participants a template to use skills dynamically in a self-generated way that integrated information from both the internal and external experience within each moment. While it was critical that the concepts be uncomplicated, the function had to be highly complex to synthesize these elements. The system had to help the individual be mindful of the current moment, mobilize Wise Mind (Linehan, 1993b, 2015a, 2015b) in a consistent way, cultivate effective planning, and embody both the simplicity and the sophistication required to help the person handle life's most abstract and demanding events. I spent months working and reworking these concepts to piece together this intricate puzzle.

One day, as I was driving, merging into a high-speed lane at 60 miles per hour, I noticed the core idea of the Skills System passing through my mind. It was so simple and so complicated at the same time—how dialectical! The treasure had emerged, and I was lucky enough to have noticed it careening through my mind. Fortunately, I didn't know at that moment how exciting this gift was, because I probably would have driven off the road.

The Treasure

Since that day on Route 195, my clients, team, and I have grappled with DBT concepts and emotion regulation principles to develop this version of the Skills System. Over time and through years of collaboration, the Skills System has become a simple, yet sophisticated emotion regulation road map for youth and adults. The nine skills and three System Tools provide a useful structure that helps the individual make effective choices in service of personal goals.

The Skills System Instructor's Guide: An Emotion-Regulation Skills Curriculum for All Learning Abilities was self-published in 2011. This platform allowed the material to be protected, disseminated, and improved. *The Emotion Regulation Skills System for Cognitively Challenged Clients* is the latest version, the culmination of over two decades of work.

Despite this long history, the empirical validation process is still in its infancy. In 2013, the JRI ICS pilot data were published in the *Journal of Mental Health Research in Intellectual Disabilities* (Brown, Brown, & Dibiasio, 2013). This single-group, longitudinal study examined reductions in negative behavioral outcomes of the 40 individuals with intellectual disabilities over a 4-year period who participated in DBT individual therapy and Skills System skills group. The findings indicated statistically significant reductions in low-, medium-, and high-risk challenging behaviors. Although this was not a randomized controlled trial, it is my hope that the findings encourage other professionals to explore use of the Skills System.

A DBT-INFORMED APPROACH

The Skills System is designed to be a set of skills for challenged learners. The skills are built from DBT concepts and in many places are direct adaptations of the standard DBT curriculum. DBT practitioners: Be prepared—the surgery to reconstruct and improve accessibility may seem radical. Upon reading this book, the naive DBT clinician may say, "Where are all of the

DBT terms?", while the seasoned veteran will see how certain DBT skills are deconstructed and repackaged to meet the needs of vulnerable learners. Most adaptations for people with intellectual disabilities politely add clipart and simplify through elimination. I tried that; it was insufficient and failed to meet the needs of this population adequately.

The reconstruction of the DBT skills had to be done carefully and effectively. Three key elements were integral in this process: (1) the work of James Gross, PhD, in emotion regulation; (2) cognitive load theory (Sweller, 2010); and (3) ongoing collaboration with my clients at ICS. It was necessary to keep DBT concepts intact, while simultaneously ensuring that the alternatives offered effective emotion regulation strategies in a user-friendly format consistent with DBT principles.

More specifically, the standard DBT skills modules format was replaced by a Skills List and System Tools that are used in a type of skills algorithm or dynamic formula that guides the individual to create adaptive skills chains. The Skills System framework helps the individual know which skills to choose and how many to implement given his or her level of emotion in each diverse situation. Although the nondisabled learner may be able to pick and choose skills effectively from the vast skills menu presented in the standard DBT skills manual (Linehan, 2015a), the vulnerable learner, with memory and executive functioning impairments, becomes overwhelmed. Certain DBT terms were retained, while others required adaptation. The language had to maximize recognition and recall of DBT concepts to facilitate generalization. Additionally, key skills concepts such as mindfulness (Wise Mind, Participating, and Acting Effectively), Check the Facts, Pros and Cons, and Cope Ahead had to be integrated as the base of every skills chain (Clear Picture, On-Track Thinking, and On-Track Action). An adapted DBT skills curriculum must provide functional validation to this population by presenting a maximum number of DBT concepts in ways that are accessible.

From my 26-plus years serving this population, I believe that in order to teach an individual who has moderate/mild intellectual disabilities to regulate emotions using a dialectical perspective, the skills framework must offer a structure that provides cognitive support—scaffolding—to perform high-level tasks, given that the individual has impairment in those functioning areas. Complex needs require enhanced intervention. To treat these people with more intense needs, DBT practitioners working with this population need to be bilingual, able to speak the standard DBT skills and Skills System languages.

Today I may recommend playing Uno to a given client; however, I can be confident that the individual knows several other emotion regulation skills, when to use each skill, how many skills to utilize, and how to implement the skills as a result of Skills System training. For example, recently in a skills group, one client, who was diagnosed with an intellectual disability of moderate severity, recounted a stressful situation she had managed successfully during the previous day. She described first getting a Clear Picture of the situation. She stated she was mad at a Level 4. Her staff members were not listening to what she was saying. She reported having strong urges to scream at the staff. Immediately my client stopped and stepped back. She used On-Track Thinking to reflect on whether these urges were helpful in reaching her goal. Knowing that she wanted to increase her independence and improve her relationships, she determined that screaming was not helpful. Realizing that she was too upset to use Express Myself or Problem Solving at that time (although she had urges to!), my client decided to do a Safety Plan and go to her room. She then reported doing an On-Track Action by calmly informing the staff members that she was going to her bedroom. While in her room, she did a few New-Me Activities (listening to music and drawing) that helped her think clearly, feel better, and relax. My client stated that later during the shift, she did her Clear Picture skill again and determined that she was feeling much calmer. She used On-Track Thinking to make a skills plan to talk to the staff members about the problem. Because she was calm and focused, she was able to discuss and solve the problem with the staff members.

As I listen to my clients recount detailed and effective skills usage as a part of skills training group, I periodically think of that boy with the padlock so many years ago. I think about how grateful I am to him for showing me my inadequacies. It has been a privilege working with many dedicated people—both group members and co-therapists—to improve the Skills System over the years.

THE SKILLS SYSTEM

The Emotion Regulation Skills System for Cognitively Challenged Clients provides people who wish to become skills trainers the necessary curriculum materials and enhanced teaching strategies. The term "skills trainers" refers to practitioners who teach the Skills System in individual and/or group settings. It is important to clarify that the Skills System is a "DBT-informed approach"; it is informed by DBT principles, strategies, and skills. When the Skills System is integrated as a mode of treatment in comprehensive DBT, it is an adapted delivery of DBT, provided that the practitioner is a DBT-trained clinician. When a non-DBT-trained clinician uses the Skills System, he or she is not "doing DBT." For DBT practitioners who are curious about the specific melding of DBT and the Skills System, there is a section in Chapter 3 ("Integration of DBT Concepts") that specifically addresses the adaptation process.

This book provides DBT and non-DBT practitioners with helpful background information related to emotion regulation, intellectual disabilities, cognitive load theory, enhanced teaching strategies, a 12-week Skills System curriculum, and visual aid skills that trainers need to provide effective instruction for individuals who experience learning challenges. The simplified materials and systematic teaching approach help people of all abilities surmount intellectual, emotional, and/or behavioral barriers that hinder generalization of new adaptive behaviors.

Who Can Be a Skills System Skills Trainer?

In most cases, master's- and PhD-level practitioners provide skills training. A skills trainer must fully understand the Skills System, information related to learning impairments, and enhanced teaching strategies to facilitate the transfer information effectively. The skills trainer must also be sufficiently equipped to provide specific supports to the population being instructed. For example, in the treatment of violent offenders with intellectual disabilities, the skills trainer should be an experienced professional within that specific treatment setting. Clinical knowledge may be helpful not only within the skills training session but also in addressing barriers that impede the individual's integration of skills within the context of daily life. Issues that hinder learning and the generalization of adaptive coping skills are likely to require therapeutic supports to address.

Who Can Be a Skills Coach?

Skills System coaches are people who have strong understanding of the Skills System and are available to provide supports within the context of the individual's life. Within a DBT framework, phone skills coaching is a crucial element of generalizing skills use. Additionally, parents, teachers, friends, and support staff members may be able to function as skills coaches. An individual who lives in a residential setting may have a broad array of multidisciplinary skills coaches. For example, group mates, support staff (e.g., administrative, residential, and vocational workers), housemates, roommates, and family members commonly function in the role of skills coaches. Collateral support providers, such as psychologists, nurses, physicians, and social workers, can enhance a treatment team's effectiveness by functioning as skills coaches.

Benefits for Support Providers

Residential agencies and support staff working with individuals who require supervision report that the Skills System has been helpful in at least two important ways. First, the materials help professionals provide interventions for clients who exhibit problematic behaviors. Without this knowledge base, support staff members may provide inconsistent and even unhelpful coaching advice to participants. As employees increase levels of effectiveness, job satisfaction improves. Second, professionals note that the coping strategies are personally helpful in the management of strong emotions evoked when supporting a person with emotional and behavioral problems. Rather than promoting cycles of staff ineffectiveness that trigger an individual's acting out, which can lead to staff burnout, the Skills System promotes effectiveness and improved relationships. Healthy, reciprocal, balanced relationships between the individual and support staff members can cultivate immense personal growth for both parties.

ORIENTATION TO THE EMOTION REGULATION SKILLS SYSTEM

This book provides a comprehensive set of materials to facilitate teaching the Skills System and to begin the process of implementing the model within an outpatient or residential setting. It is essential that a professional who wishes to become a skills trainer first learn the Skills System. Chapter 1 offers a brief overview of the Skills System, while Chapter 2 presents detailed descriptions of each of the skills and the System Tools to fulfill this task. It is important to note that the descriptions in both these chapters are intended to teach the skills trainer concepts and may not be in the form that individuals with intellectual deficits should learn.

Chapter 3 introduces the theoretical underpinning for the Skills System. It explores the literatures related to emotion regulation, intellectual disabilities, DBT, and cognitive load theory that all impact Skills System design and instruction. This information teaches skills trainers about key underlying principles that help them to use and teach the Skills System with diverse populations.

The Skills System's enhanced teaching strategies are an integral part of the model. Given that the concept of emotion regulation is abstract, creating fathomable learning experiences is a quintessential element of the process. Chapter 4 introduces the E-Spiral framework that organizes teaching strategies to broaden and deepen skills integration. It offers ways to manage teaching individuals who have very limited capacities for explicit learning and highlights a framework to conceptualize skills knowledge acquisition. Foundational teaching strategies that are used throughout skills training are presented in Chapter 5. Chapter 6 highlights teaching strategies that are utilized within specific phases of the E-Spiral framework.

A sample 12-week curriculum that offers a detailed, week-by-week breakdown and clear instructions is presented in Chapter 7. Depending on the group, the practitioner may choose to follow the 12-week curriculum closely or adapt the format to meet the needs of the learners. Alternatively, a less structured group format (Skills Surfing) is explained in Chapter 4.

One of the benefits of the Skills System model is that it helps to create a common, adaptive emotion regulation language within support environments. In order to maximize the impact of the Skills System, instructors need to understand how support providers can function as skills coaches. Chapter 8 outlines relevant information to being a skills coach.

The 12-week Skills System curriculum integrates numerous handouts, working examples, and worksheets; these visual aid resources are included in Appendix A. Participants will require individual copies of these materials; having a skills notebook is essential for group and home-study activities. The trainer can copy Appendix A for his or her own group to use as a skills handout notebook. A printable copy of the material is also available through The Guilford Press (*www.guilford.com/brown13-forms*) for individuals who have purchased this book. Additional information about the Skills System is available at *www.guilford.com/skills-system*.

This book also provides skills trainers with supplemental materials. Appendix B contains skills scenarios that further develop the integration of skills. These tools may be helpful when teaching clients and/or skills coaches the Skills System. Last, Appendix C is a skills test. This competency evaluation, in the form of two worksheets, may be completed by participants or support providers; it also can function as a skills worksheet. Additional quizzes, tests, and certification are currently available through the Skills System website.

It is important to note that the format of *The Emotion Regulation Skills System for Cognitively Challenged Clients* is designed to teach the reader the Skills System. Therefore, the instructor is exposed to deepening layers of skills information to broaden and expand skills knowledge throughout the reading process. While the reader may notice some repetition of points, the evolving exposure to the material will serve to improve recognition and recall.

Contents

Contents

CHAPTER 1

Introducing the Skills System

Bernice Johnson Reagon, an African American scholar and songwriter, wrote, "Life's challenges are not supposed to paralyze you—they're supposed to help you discover who you are" (cited in Lewis, 2009). Fully experiencing life's challenges and remaining present within the current moment can be excruciatingly difficult. Painful emotions and overwhelming thoughts may bombard the individual, blurring self-reflection and the course ahead. The person may not choose to be paralyzed; it is what happens when certain events occur and she* lacks effective coping skills.

While emotions may blind the individual and pose difficulties, they may also be the very vehicle of self-discovery and fulfillment. Emotions are key components of many important and joyful aspects of the human experience. Having the capacity to benefit from emotions, rather than being paralyzed by them, offers the individual the opportunity to mobilize individuality while actively learning valuable life lessons and evolving to reach personal potential. As the individual learns how to regulate emotions, thoughts, and actions, he is not paralyzed but is able to face life, relationships, and himself with courage, grace, and strength.

Developing effective emotion regulation skills is an important step toward managing life's complexities versus becoming debilitated by them. Knowing how to increase positive affect and reduce negative feelings can help the person improve his quality of life. This regulatory capacity allows the person to balance both rational and emotional aspects of situations to reach his personal goals. Regulating emotions does not mean erasing them; it means proactively and reactively making adjustments in behavior that help the individual maintain balance. This ability to balance helps the individual remain actively engaged in the process of self-discovery even when experiencing significant life challenges.

THE SKILLS SYSTEM

The Skills System is a set of nine skills and three system rules that helps the individual cope with life's challenges. This emotion regulation skills curriculum was developed to help the person

---
*I alternate between masculine and feminine pronouns throughout the book.

1

organize her internal and external experiences in ways that decrease discomfort and problematic behaviors, while increasing positive affect and goal-directed actions. This simple framework guides the person through the process of becoming aware of the current moment (mindfulness), directing attention, and activating behaviors that are in service of personal goals. The individual learns to follow steps that mobilize inner wisdom ("Wise Mind"; Linehan, 2015a) in each unique situation. As the skills and the System Tools (guidelines for assembling skills chains) are integrated into the context of the person's life, often effective coping behaviors increase. Each situation provides the person with an opportunity for self-discovery and for active participation in events. The individual is no longer paralyzed; she is a Skills Master.

User-Friendly for Individuals with Learning Challenges

Learning new, more adaptive patterns of behavior is a challenging task for anyone. This is especially difficult when the individual must manage complicating factors such as mental health issues, intellectual impairment, physical problems, or other difficult life circumstances. These life challenges may increase stress and impact the individual's ability to learn new information.

The Skills System and the curriculum contained in this book are designed to help individuals who experience learning challenges. For example, an individual who is diagnosed with an intellectual disability (ID) or mental illness may have difficulty focusing attention, remembering information, and utilizing concepts within complex situations. The Skills System itself and the teaching strategies contained in *The Emotion Regulation Skills System for Cognitively Challenged Clients* are constructed to maximize learning, integration, and ultimately generalization of the skills into life contexts. Even an individual who cannot read or write can learn and use the Skills System.

DBT Skills for the Challenged Learner

The Skills System was developed as an accessible alternative for individuals with cognitive impairment who were participating in dialectical behavior therapy (DBT; Linehan, 1993a). DBT has two main delivery modes: individual therapy and skills training group. The skills curriculum (Linehan, 2015a) is broken down into four modules. The individual learns skills in the areas of mindfulness, emotion regulation, distress tolerance, and interpersonal effectiveness in the skills group and discusses implementation of the strategies in real-life settings during individual therapy.

The standard DBT skills (Linehan, 2015a) were not specifically designed for individuals with ID. The multisyllabic terms, complex mnemonics, use of abstract language, modular teaching process, and lack of structure to facilitate integration of the divergent elements create barriers for vulnerable learners (Kalyuga, 2011; Paas & Sweller, 2012; Sweller, 1988, 2010; van Gog, Paas, & Sweller, 2010). Although the terms and format of the standard skills are challenging, the general concepts are vastly helpful for this population. The practitioner has to make an informed clinical assessment and decide whether an individual with learning challenges can comprehend essential components of the standard DBT skills through enhanced teaching strategies or if key aspects of DBT will be lost. For certain individuals with significant learning deficits, merely modifying the teaching of the standard curriculum is not sufficient to capture the essence of DBT in a way that promotes generalization of the concepts. The current studies on DBT all state that the skills curriculum requires adaptation (Brown, Brown, & DiBiasio, 2013; Inam, 2013; Sakdalan & Collier, 2012).

This DBT-informed version may not look like DBT, because semantic sacrifices were necessary to enable this population access to the essence of DBT. The Skills System utilizes DBT principles, while the language and format are adjusted to address the needs of individuals who experience comprehensive learning challenges. There may be cases when the Skills System is learned first and the standard DBT skills are added later in treatment.

The *Emotion Regulation Skills System for Cognitively Challenged Clients* manual will be used by clinicians who have DBT training and those that do not. It is essential that this book adequately address the needs of both. Conjoining DBT language with teaching the Skills System in the body of the text will add extraneous cognitive load demands on individuals who are not familiar with DBT concepts. Rather than attempting to duplicate Linehan's expert teaching, text boxes follow each description of the Skills System skills in Chapter 2. There and in the remaining chapters of this book, text boxes contain reference information for the foundational standard DBT concepts and teaching points in the *DBT Skills Training Manual, Second Edition* (Linehan, 2015a) that are relevant to the Skills System skills and/or skills training procedure. These references help the DBT practitioner better understand how DBT concepts are integrated into each element of the Skills System. The text boxes allow DBT practitioners to know where to look for related DBT information, and non-DBT clinicians can skim the information if it detracts from the learning process. If a clinician is unfamiliar with DBT, it is recommended that he do self-study of the DBT skills manuals or attend DBT trainings to deepen his knowledge about the foundations of the Skills System.

APPLICATIONS OF THE SKILLS SYSTEM

Many people have experiences or physiology that complicate learning as well as their ability to demonstrate effective emotion regulation behaviors. Each person has unique clusters of strengths and deficits, abilities and disabilities. Any individual, whether diagnosed as ID or otherwise, may be prone to overwhelming emotions, unclear thinking, or unproductive actions. All people have the capacity to make impulsive decisions that hinder the accomplishment of personal goals. Even individuals who practice adaptive coping behaviors experience overwhelming circumstances that can stress such capacities. The Skills System materials are user-friendly concepts that are accessible to learners of all abilities. The standard DBT skills manuals contain more detailed information about specific coping strategies; using those resources is preferred if the individual does not experience learning barriers.

The utilization of the Skills System is expanding. Although the Skills System was originally designed for adults participating in DBT with significant cognitive impairment, the model is often used within the context of other forms of individual therapy or with individuals not receiving these services. Similarly, although the curriculum was designed for adults, adolescent and children's programs have adopted the model. In addition, the curriculum is being used by a broad spectrum of individuals, from those with severe learning challenges to those with primarily mental health issues that impact self-regulation. The Skills System concepts and teaching strategies are constructed to facilitate learning and implementation; the ease of learning benefits all.

The Skills System model has been used in many different therapeutic settings. Hospitals, residential, vocational, corrections, and outpatient programs have implemented the Skills System groups. In these types of settings, clinicians train collateral and direct support staff to be skills coaches. Private practice clinicians are using the Skills System as a therapeutic tool with individual clients. The ancillary materials available on the Skills System website are useful for family members or other people in the client's life.

It is important to note that the Skills System is not designed as a stand-alone treatment for complex clinical cases. It is a transtheoretical treatment tool that can help vulnerable learners improve emotion regulation skills. Although it was primarily designed as a component of DBT, the Skills System can be used in conjunction with cognitive-behavioral therapy (CBT) and trauma-informed therapies. The framework can provide tangible, accessible self-regulation skills to supplement other, more comprehensive mental health treatments.

OVERVIEW OF THE SKILLS SYSTEM

There are nine skills in the Skills System; these nine skills form the Skills List. There are also three System Tools that guide utilization of the skills and assembly of skills chains. An individual who tends to become overwhelmed by emotion has difficulty focusing on thoughts that are in service of personal goals and/or reacts impulsively to urges may benefit from learning step-by-step progressions to manage these factors. A person with these issues often has difficulty transitioning successfully from one strategy to the next in traditional coping skills education that provides individual elements without offering a system to guide implementation. The unified structure assists the person in remembering strategies and moving fluidly through a multistep coping transaction, while experiencing intense emotional, cognitive, and behavioral regulation problems. As the individual learns the skills and the system, she integrates the capacity to experience successfully a full range of human emotions, practice self-determination, and acquire the means to navigate toward goals even in challenging circumstances.

The first three skills in the Skills System comprise a core progression that serves as the foundation for skills use. This sequence begins when an individual experiences a situation that prompts awareness; she begins by getting a Clear Picture (Skill 1) of the moment. Six steps lead the person to become aware of information within the current moment. This is crucial, because often individuals with self-regulation problems focus attention on the past or future rather than the present. Not only does focusing on the current moment give the person accurate information to use in making decisions, but it also allows for more in-depth processing of the experience. Mindfulness is a core DBT concept; Clear Picture leads the individual through steps of being mindfully aware in every situation.

Once the person gets a Clear Picture, he shifts to On-Track Thinking (Skill 2). In On-Track Thinking, the individual moves through a simple four-step sequence that leads her through the process of mapping out an effective coping plan. This cognitive framework serves to guide the individual's thinking patterns to promote emotion regulation and goal-directed behaviors. As the person learns the adaptive cognitive structure in the skills group, practices it within his life context, and experiences positive reinforcement, the functional thinking patterns become increasingly sophisticated and automatic over time.

On-Track Thinking requires the individual to make a Skills Plan. This component links the remaining skills together in a chain. Three simple rules (System Tools) determine which skills will be helpful and how many to use within the context of the present moment. Depending on the individual's self-reported level of emotional arousal (using the Feelings Rating Scale), she knows whether using more interactive skills (Skills 6–9) are options (using the Categories of Skills). The person learns that at high levels of emotional (and cognitive) arousal, it is necessary to choose more solitary skills (Skills 1–5) that function to reduce the sensations of uncomfortable feelings, to divert attention from problematic urges to effective actions, to minimize risks, and to improve focus. At all levels of escalation, the individual makes a plan to choose a sufficient number of skills (using the Recipe for Skills), targeting specifically the most effective skills according to the demands of the situation.

Next, the individual takes an On-Track Action (Skill 3). On-Track Actions are the behaviors the individual mobilizes to move in the direction of his goal. Therefore, the person gets a Clear Picture, does On-Track Thinking, and executes a series of On-Track Actions. If the individual is over a Level 3 emotion, he may engage in a Safety Plan (Skills 4) or New-Me Activities (Skills 5). If under a Level 3, the person can also use the Calm-Only skills, which are Problem Solving (Skill 6), Expressing Myself (Skill 7), Getting It Right (Skill 8), and Relationship Care (Skill 9). Once a cluster of skills has been completed or the circumstances change, the individual returns to do Clear Picture again to become aware of the new situation that has evolved.

Initially, the individual conceptualizes the Skills System as a series of linear events; when a sequence of skills is finished, she returns to doing Clear Picture, On-Track Thinking, On-Track Action, and so on, repeating the process in each subsequent situation. As the individual integrates the Skills System, she is more able to utilize Clear Picture and On-Track Thinking throughout the coping process in a dynamic, transactional pattern to adjust On-Track Actions. Even individuals with significant cognitive impairment gradually improve the ability to make subtle adjustments; this flexibility can enhance the person's success in reaching goals and in maintaining on-track relationships. The Skills System is a structured yet malleable framework that can help an individual reduce reliance on avoidant behaviors, bear increased responsibilities, and fully engage in the human experience. Table 1.1 lists the skills on the Skills List and the System Tools.

THE SKILLS LIST

The following section includes brief descriptions of each of the skills and System Tools. This is intended as an initial exposure to the information. These concepts are presented in greater detail in Chapter 2. This introduction serves as a skeleton on which more information will be layered in the following chapters.

Getting Started with a Clear Picture

The first skill in the Skills System is Clear Picture; the metaphor of a television represents having a clear versus fuzzy vision of a situation. Clear Picture guides the individual through steps that

TABLE 1.1. **Skills List and System Tools**	
Skills List	**System Tools**
All-the-Time Skills	A. Feelings Rating Scale
1. Clear Picture	0- to 5-point scale for rating the intensity of emotions.
2. On-Track Thinking	
3. On-Track Action	B. Categories of Skills
4. Safety Plan	Skills 1–5 are All-The-Time skills.
5. New-Me Activities	Skills 6–9 are Calm-Only skills.
Calm-Only Skills	C. Recipe for Skills
6. Problem Solving	Add one skill for every level of emotion (e.g., at a Level 2 emotion, use three skills).
7. Expressing Myself	
8. Getting It Right	
9. Relationship Care	

bring focused attention to six aspects of her present experience to gain clarity. The first of the Clear Picture Do's prompts the individual to focus on her breath. Next, she shifts attention to notice what is happening around her. Once the individual has awareness of the environment, attention is then shifted to doing a Body Check; bringing attention to the body begins a series of self-reflections that help orient the person to the realities of her internal experience. The person then labels and rates her emotions and notices thoughts and urges.

There are two important facets of this skill: (1) gaining accurate information about these important internal and external experiences in the present moment, as they are, and (2) effectively shifting attention. Some individuals who experience cognitive deficits and/or self-regulation problems have difficulty shifting attention in ways that effectively manage their level of arousal. The Clear Picture skill trains the person to see facts versus fantasies and to focus on making decisions that are in her best interest.

Using On-Track Thinking

Once the individual has a Clear Picture of his internal and external circumstances in the moment, he strategically transfers attention to Skill 2, which is On-Track Thinking. The name "On-Track" uses the metaphor of a train to represent the concept of the individual moving incrementally toward a destination or goal. Thus, the image of "off-track" communicates circumstances that are not in service of the goal.

On-Track Thinking offers the person a series of four tasks to complete to create an effective thinking process. This sequence—(1) stop and Check It, (2) Turn It Up, (3) Cheerleading, (4) Make a Skills Plan—provides an adaptive cognitive structuring template for the individual to follow in each situation. This process helps the person reflect on desired outcomes, appraise whether taking action on an urge supports his goal, generate on-track thoughts to support adaptive behavior, and create a plan to reach his goal.

Taking an On-Track Action

Once the participant gets a Clear Picture and does On-Track Thinking, she uses Skill 3, which is On-Track Action. The reuse of the word "On-Track" is designed to reinforce the concept that the person transitions from On-Track Thinking to On-Track Action. It is challenging for any person to alter problematic patterns of behavior; On-Track Actions mobilize new, adaptive actions that are directly related to personal goals. It is useful to have On-Track Thoughts, but without On-Track Actions, the individual may revert to problematic behaviors. Using Clear Picture and On-Track Thinking, and taking On-Track Actions are ways to act in "Wise Mind" (Linehan, 2015a). The combined term "123 Wise Mind" communicates that to demonstrate wisdom consistently in context, it may be helpful to be mindful (Clear Picture), generate strategic thinking (On-Track Thinking), and engage in goal-directed actions (On-Track Action).

There are five different elements of the On-Track Action skill. First, this skill includes any action that the individual takes in the direction of his goal. An action is considered on-track if the person has taken time to be self-aware within the present moment (Clear Picture) and has made an effective decision (On-Track Thinking). The remaining functions of On-Track Actions include Switching Tracks, making an On-Track Action Plan, Accepting the Situation, and/or Turn the Page. Each of these concepts give the individual tools to proactively or reactively manage off-track urges and difficult situations.

Managing Risky Situations with Safety Plans

During the process of getting a Clear Picture and doing On-Track Thinking, the person may identify possible risks that may impede her progress toward goals. In a situation such as this, the individual may take the On-Track Action to create and execute a Safety Plan. Safety Plans, the fourth skill in the Skills System, provide a framework that assists in evaluating the Level of Risk and in choosing the appropriate responses to manage the circumstances. It is important that the person be fully aware of risks, understand various options for managing the problems, and have the ability to implement actions that neither unnecessarily avoid situations nor recklessly engage in problematic ones.

Doing New-Me Activities

New-Me* Activities, the fifth skill, are activities that the person in which the person engages throughout each day. The term "New-Me" represents activities that set the person on-track to personal goals. Individuals may engage in old-me behaviors that reinforce problematic feelings,

---

*The terms "Old-Me" and "New-Me" were used by Haaven, Little, and Petre-Miller in their book *Treating Intellectually Disabled Sex Offenders* (1989). Although the term "New-Me" is used in many other forums, a special acknowledgment of these authors' contribution to the field of disabilities is warranted. I thank James Haaven for his support.

thoughts, and actions. Developing a broad array of preferred New-Me Activities can help an individual improve self-regulation and satisfaction.

New-Me Activities serve four basic functions. Focus New-Me Activities assist the client in focusing attention, while other activities promote distraction. Some activities help the person feel good; others are intended to be fun. The participant learns to evaluate what his needs are in the moment and to choose a New-Me Activity that fits best.

Problem Solving

The individual may determine that she has a problem or the urge to take action impulsively to change a situation. Problem Solving helps the person strategically evaluate when and how to solve problems, so that she reaches personal goals. The individual may have previous experiences that involved rushed, ill-planned, or extreme responses that not only fail to repair difficulties but also augment problems. Learning when to solve problems is just as important to knowing how to do it.

The Quick Fix process is used to address small problems, while a more comprehensive, multistep Problem Solving is best to use when fixing medium and large problems. During Problem Solving, the participant takes time to gain clarity about the problem, reviews multiple options for solving it, and checks the fit of the choices. The person develops Plans A, B, and C to prepare for inevitable obstacles that occur.

Expressing Myself

Expressing Myself, Skill 7, involves the individual communicating what is on his mind or in his heart. Choosing from myriad communication methods and determining when to communicate are important decisions. A person may have a habit of expressing himself while at high levels of emotional arousal. Although this may serve to purge distress, provide distraction, or mobilize the individual in challenging situations, such impulsive expression often damages relationships or causes other problems. The Expressing Myself skill helps the individual strategically and effectively utilize communication to reach personal goals. The person learns to use other skills, such as New-Me Activities, to reduce emotions at times when he is experiencing discomfort, rather than venting on others.

Getting It Right

The person may be in a situation where she needs to get something from another person. Getting It Right is used specifically for acquiring what the individual wants or needs. Getting needs met is a vital skill; unfortunately, skill deficits in this area have often contributed to cycles of ineffective behavior and high levels of dissatisfaction. When the person makes requests while at a high a level of emotional arousal, she fails to elicit help and may reduce the likelihood that her needs will be met. A person may Get It Wrong when she is unable to judge when, how, and with whom to advocate to get her needs met. It is essential to have the capacity to self-advocate and negotiate to reach personal goals.

Skill 8, Getting It Right, provides the individual with a simple framework to get what he wants from another person. The participant learns to be in the Right Mind, talk to the Right Person at the Right Time and Place, use the Right Tone, and say the Right Words. The Right Words include using Sugar (being polite), Explaining the Situation, Asking for What You Want, Listening, and Seal a Deal (SEALS).

Relationship Care

Each of us experiences countless urges each day that potentially harm our relationships. Relationship Care is designed to help the individual effectively assess relationship situations so that he can make personal decisions that improve his quality of life. Many life problems are fueled by ill-timed and impulsive relationship behaviors. While it is challenging to manage all of the changing forces that are continually transacting as part of the human experience, the individual increases mastery within relationships when he gains the ability to use this and the other skills effectively.

The ninth skill, Relationship Care, assists the person in managing her self-relationship and interactions with other people. Building On-Track Relationships, Balancing On-Track Relationships, and Changing Off-Track Relationships are the essential components. As the individual becomes more aware of her personal needs and learns how various actions either enhance personal connections or lead to creating distance between people, she is better able to actively manage interactions with others.

SYSTEM TOOLS

A person who has coping skills deficits and self-regulation problems may have difficulty accurately evaluating internal and external experiences. Additionally, the person may not have the ability to monitor his levels of self-regulation strategically to choose behaviors that achieve desired outcomes. The Skills System is designed to help an individual develop coping tools and also the ability to use the skills to get his needs met. The System Tools are simple concepts that guide the participant's use of the nine skills on the Skills List. There are three System Tools: the Feelings Rating Scale, the Categories of Skills, and the Recipe for Skills.

Feelings Rating Scale

The Feelings Rating Scale is a simple 0- to 5-point scale that the individual uses to rate the intensity of sensations she is feeling. It is an important tool to help the person be aware of and organize her current experiences. The scale concretizes the abstract experience of emotions, which is particularly important for an individual who has intellectual impairments.

Through the skills training experience, the participant learns to differentiate emotional experiences and categorize the feelings rating. A feeling rated 0 means that the person is not experiencing sensations related to the emotion. A feeling rated 1 means the person is experiencing a tiny amount of the sensation from the emotion. A feeling is rated 2 when the individual has a small amount of sensation. An emotion is rated 3 when a medium level of emotion is felt. Generally, the individual's ability to focus and control behavior is intact when emotions are rated between 0 and 3; above a 3, the person's cognitive and behavioral control abilities may be compromised. A feeling rated 4 is a strong emotion; often some kind of behavioral dyscontrol or urge to have off-track actions is present. A feeling is rated 5 when the individual becomes overwhelmed and exhibits behavior that harms self, others, or property.

The scale serves a dual purpose: (1) The Feelings Rating Scale helps the person get a Clear Picture of the current moment, and (2) the individual also uses the rating to determine which (Categories of Skills) and how many skills to use in the situation (Recipe for Skills) in On-Track Thinking. The person learns that at lower levels of arousal, she has the capacity to think clearly and interact effectively; therefore, it is possible to use interactive skills at that time. Conversely, a higher rating communicates to the individual that she will have more difficulty thinking clearly and interacting effectively with other people. At high-rated levels of feelings, more skills are indicated to manage the experience, and the goal at that point is to reduce arousal. The Feelings Rating Scale helps the individual build the capacity to manage impulses and productively wait until she is in the proper mindset to utilize interactive skills.

Categories of Skills

Many behavioral problems result when an individual engages in interactive skills at high levels of emotion. While it is natural to experience strong urges to take action to fix situations, express feelings, demand that needs be met, and exert control over people, acting on these urges often fails to help the individual reach long-term personal goals. The Categories of Skills help the individual know which skills are effective at given levels of arousal.

There are two Categories of Skills. Skills 1–5 (Clear Picture, On-Track Thinking, On-Track Action, Safety Plan, and New-Me Activities) are called All-the-Time skills. All-the-Time skills can be used at any level of emotion, from 0 to 5. The other Category of Skills is called Calm-Only skills. The person can use Skills 6–9 (Problem Solving, Expressing Myself, Getting It Right, and Relationship Care) only when he is at or below a Level 3 emotion. Therefore, the person can utilize all nine skills if he is at or below a Level 3 emotion and just Skills 1–5 if he is over a Level 3 emotion.

Recipe for Skills

Another common pitfall is when a person does not chain together a sufficient number of skills within a situation. When high levels of emotions trigger body sensations, the effects can be uncomfortable and long-lasting. It is essential that the person chain together multiple skills to use multiple strategies to span the extended duration of the feeling experience.

The Recipe for Skills calls for using at least one more skill than the level of emotion. For example, if an individual is at a Level 2 emotion, at least three skills must be used. If the individual is at a Level 5 emotion, at least six skills are needed. In this case, since the person is over a Level 3 emotion, it is necessary for the person to use an extra All-the-Time skill (e.g., using two On-Track Actions or two New-Me Activities), rather than having the sixth skill be from the Calm-Only category.

The goal of the Recipe for Skills is to ensure that the person plans and executes a sufficient number of skills. The number of skills changes relative to the severity of the situation;

the intensity of the event is calibrated through the emotional impact the circumstance has on the individual. It is not uncommon for individuals with emotion regulation problems to rush through insufficient strategies that do not adequately address the multiple components of complex internal and external situations. The Recipe for Skills is intended to teach the person to maximize skill use.

PUTTING IT ALL TOGETHER

When a participant begins learning the Skills System, her ability to recall all of the concepts and terms is expectedly inconsistent. Group teaching strategies continually expose participant to the Skills List and the System Tools within the contexts of their lives. This revolving approach allows the individual to cobble together comprehension over time. Suggestions for structuring skills instruction, teaching strategies, and implementing a 12-week curriculum are presented in Chapters 4–7.

Relatively early in skills training, the participant learns to be increasingly mindful of the present moment. The individual becomes able to take a quick snapshot of internal and external factors using the Clear Picture Do's. With practice, the person increases his speed and accuracy in these tasks.

The information gathered during the Clear Picture Do's is used to help the person generate On-Track Thinking. For example, the feelings rating score (e.g., Level 4, Angry) guides the individual to choose which Category of Skills will be helpful at his current level of emotion. The person learns that All-the-Time skills (1–5) may be utilized at any level of emotion, while Calm-Only skills (6–9) are only used when the individual is below a Level 3 emotion. In the previous example, at a Level 4 emotion, the participant would engage only in All-the-Time skills and not utilize Calm-Only skills. All-the-Time skills allow the individual to reregulate prior to engaging in the more interactive Calm-Only skills. Additionally, the individual learns to use ample skills for the situation. The Recipe for Skills sets guidelines for the minimum number of skills. Quickly the person learns the adage: The more skills, the better.

On-Track Thinking is a relatively complex skill; mastery is slow and builds over time. The participant may initially have primitive self-dialogue. Often, as skills capacities develop, more sophistication evolves. For example, the person may initially self-reflect and think, "I feel angry at Level 4; I need to go to my room." As self-awareness continues to evolve, self-statements become more elaborated: "I am at Level 4 anger; I have to use my All-the-Time skills. I have the urge to use Expressing Myself skills, but I must wait until I am below a Level 3 emotion. If I do it now, I will yell. Instead I will do a Safety Plan and New-Me Activities. I have to use my skills, because I want to reach my goals. I can do this."

Throughout the skills training experience, the individual often becomes aware of (and committed to) taking On-Track versus Off-Track Actions. The individual may have the ability to notice an urge and move away rather than being aggressive. Over time, with more group discussions and practice, the chains are elaborated. The mindfulness (Clear Picture) training paired with the cognitive structuring (On-Track Thinking) offers the participant a framework that guides him toward taking effective, self-determined On-Track Actions (123 Wise Mind). The participant may become increasingly able to strategically intertwine various combinations of skills to manage oscillating internal and external needs. The nine skills and three System Tools are repeated, practiced, and reinforced so that the adaptive coping patterns become default settings.

Integration within Living and Learning Environments

The Skills System may provide a therapeutic language base and adaptive coping skills model for many different environments. The Skills System can be helpful in residential, outpatient, classroom, and/or home settings. Parents can partner with their children to learn and use the material together. The preliminary research is currently limited, yet the opportunities for future study and exploration are broad.

The visual nature of the Skills System can promote integration within environments. The visual aid materials can provide visual cues that prompt skill use for participants and skills coaches. Programs mount skills posters and personalized decorations throughout the site. When the model becomes immersed in the Skills System, many creative programmatic, group, and individualized interventions are possible.

There are many benefits of integrating the Skills System into group settings. The Skills System provides common language and a framework of information related to managing emotions, thoughts, and actions. This shared framework and language facilitate learning. When participants and support providers both actively engage in positive relating behaviors, opportunities for adaptive learning and relating increase. For example, there are multiple benefits for participants and staff who take part in peer skills tutoring activities. Ideally, participants and support providers learn how to cope effectively and are able to engage in positive social behaviors that are mutually beneficial and reciprocal.

CHAPTER 2

Learning the Skills System

The first portion of this chapter is designed to provide the skills trainer with specific information about each of the nine skills and the System Tools that guide the utilization of the skills. While the Skills System is a structured model, it is not a prescriptive formula. Rather, it is a revolving process that shifts to respond to the dynamic perceptions and needs of each person within each changing moment. Knowing all of the elements of the Skills System helps trainers, coaches, and, ultimately, the individual make and execute self-determined, finely-tuned Skills Plans.

Skills coaches may also find utility in reading this chapter. It will give the support person a strong understanding of the skills and how the system functions. Specific techniques for providing skills coaching are presented in Chapter 8.

Chapter 2 may also serve as home study material for the skills group participant. If an individual has difficulty reading or comprehending the language, support providers can read and/or review the material with him. The general information can help expand the participant's knowledge about the skills and System Tools. Home study, peer tutoring, and engaging in skills review with support staff can be useful techniques to enhance mastery. Learning concepts in individual or group training sessions, participating in home study, and applying the Skills System within daily living broaden and deepen each person's understanding of emotion regulation skills.

References to sections in the *DBT Skills Training Manual, Second Edition* (Linehan, 2015a) citing relevant foundational DBT concepts and standard DBT teaching points are provided in boxes that follow each of the skills descriptions in this chapter.

THE SKILLS LIST

Clear Picture

Clear Picture is the first skill in the Skills System, and it is an All-the-Time skill. This means that Clear Picture can be used at any level of feeling, 0–5. There are six steps, which collectively are referred to as the Clear Picture Do's. The purpose of Clear Picture is to help the person become aware of and accept what is happening inside and outside herself in the current moment. This systematic progression leads the individual through steps to be mindful in each situation. The individual reviews the Clear Picture Do's when she notices a situation changing or when she is having a new reaction.

The word "clear" helps the individual understand that it is important to see the present moment *as it is* and to have an accurate perception of the facts. The alternative is a fuzzy picture. A fuzzy picture occurs when an individual is experiencing cognitive dysregulation, is disoriented, or is not perceiving actualities within the situation. When the person has a fuzzy picture, she may be in Emotional Mind (Linehan, 2015a), when her emotions are in the driver's seat, Off-Track Thinking prevails, and effective coping is impeded by the lack of clarity. Clear Picture is the first skill for a reason: It must be done first in every situation. It is always the first link in a skills chain. The following steps help the individual become aware of internal and external factors that are currently happening.

Notice the Breath

The first step in Clear Picture is to Notice the Breath. As the individual takes a few breaths, it is important to bring attention to the physical sensations of breathing. Noticing the air going in and out of the nose, feeling the chest expand, and observing the snugness of his waistband as he brings the air into his belly area are common focal points during breathing.

It is important that the individual notice the breath *as it is* versus needing to do a particular type of breathing. Accepting the breath *as it is* is an important step toward the individual seeing himself and the situation clearly. Often, one of the other Clear Picture Do's comes into awareness first, and the breath is one of the first conscious emotion regulation actions the person takes to have a skillful response. Taking a breath begins the process of gaining intentional awareness that is free of distortions and avoidance. Being oriented helps him "Check the Facts" (Linehan, 2015a, p. 319) in the situation. Simultaneously, this concrete action of breathing can bring the individual into awareness of the intangible aspects of the current moment. Having clarity about the realities of the present, the person is more capable of planning and executing impactful behaviors. Additionally, when the person brings 100% of his attention to the breath, attention shifts from the escalating emotions and cognitions, and only the breath is in awareness. Managing this one moment becomes more possible.

Teaching awareness of breath is a simple first step that triggers Skills System usage. Not only is the skill construct linked to this one simple step but the individual also has the breath with him at all times, in all contexts. Learning, practicing, and reinforcing the linkages between taking a breath, completing the Clear Picture Do's, and executing other skills helps to promote integration and automation of skills use in the person's life.

Notice Surroundings

It is important for the person to Notice Surroundings, the second step in Clear Picture. She must take a moment to look around to gain a clear understanding of what is happening outside of herself *right now*. This scan includes noticing aspects of the physical environment and of the relationships that are present. Awareness of surroundings may reflect immediate tangible experiences, as well as macro-level realities (e.g., societal norms, legal ramifications). Seeing the situations, relationships, and environmental factors *as they are* is crucial. When the individual's emotions escalate, it is not uncommon for her to blur factors; inconsistencies between the realities of the situation and the perceptions of the individual can impede effective skills utilization. For example, focusing on what happened in the past, what might happen in the future, or what *should* be happening in the present hinders clarity in the present moment. Gathering accurate information, based on the facts in the current situation, helps the individual to handle the situation effectively. Noticing Surroundings is a particularly important step if there are risks that must be managed.

As the person develops an understanding that it is easier to manage one clear moment in time, he is more likely to evaluate situations accurately. The individual learns that clarity, although potentially uncomfortable for the moment, allows effective coping and the accomplishment of personal goals. The individual may use fewer avoidant strategies as he experiences them as less effective and more problematic in the long term.

Body Check

Body Check, the third step in Clear Picture, is noticing that sensations that are happening inside *right now* gives the individual important information. Noticing physical sensations such as heart rate, breathing, aches, and tension can help the individual to understand emotional responses. Noticing body sensations can help the individual accurately label and rate feelings. Not only is having clarity within the present moment vital, but as the person continually monitors her physical being, she also learns that sensations come and go through the natural course of each day. This mindful awareness helps her understand the concept of "this too shall pass." Understanding that painful experiences come and go naturally helps the individual tolerate being present in the moment. The awareness that painful feelings will abate in time helps the individual be present in, tolerate, and manage discomfort.

Label and Rate Feelings

The fourth step in Clear Picture is to Label and Rate Feelings. The person notices and describes emotions, such as fear, anger, disgust, envy, jealousy, love, sadness, shame, and guilt (Linehan, 2015a). Other sensations, such as hunger and fatigue, can be labeled and rated as well. The term "feeling" versus "emotion" is more inclusive of myriad physiological experiences that impact functioning. Once the person labels the feeling, it is important to rate it using the Feelings Rating Scale (0– to 5-level scale). For example, the individual could label and rate an experience as a 3, Sad. The act of labeling and rating an emotion can serve to reduce ambiguity and improve emotion regulation (Lieberman, Inagaki, Tabibnia, & Crockett, 2011; Zaki & Williams, 2013). In addition, the monitoring teaches the individual that emotions rise and fall, come and go. The image of the television screen also exemplifies the concept that feelings may flash across the screen and then pass. This awareness helps the person believe that painful states are transient and that emotions are survivable. As skills develop further, the individual begins to become aware that it is possible to decrease painful experiences, while increasing pleasant ones. With practice, the individual can notice, accept, and allow challenging emotions to pass without taking impulsive action or retriggering more painful feelings.

Notice Thoughts

The fifth step in Clear Picture is Notice Thoughts. The individual learns to pay attention to thoughts as they pass through his mind *right now*. The thoughts "I hate him" or "If I punch him, I will get arrested" are examples of thoughts that may pass through the individual's mind. By noticing thoughts, the person learns that thoughts continually come and go; being aware of this flow helps the individual see that it is possible not to react automatically to thoughts. The participant learns that thoughts are like city buses. The individual watches as the buses (thoughts) go by, ultimately using On-Track Thinking to sort which thoughts will take him to his preferred destination. During the Clear Picture skill, the individual becomes aware of thoughts. This mindful observation and description are essential first steps toward exerting attentional control and generating goal-directed, On-Track Thinking in the next skill.

Notice Urges

The sixth step in Clear Picture is to Notice Urges. Becoming aware of action urges that are associated with various emotions and thoughts is a crucial aspect of managing behaviors effectively. Fight and flight are examples of action urges—for example, "I want to punch him in the face" or "I gotta get out of here." Urges, much like sensations, emotions, and thoughts, naturally come and go, they flash across our screens. Impulsively reacting to urges usually creates diminished levels of effectiveness when compared to taking a few moments to reflect on personal goals, situational options, and likely outcomes. Not only is Notice Urges a key aspect of getting a Clear Picture, but it is also the transition point to utilizing the other skills in the Skills System. Once the individual notices her urge, she shifts attention to On-Track Thinking.

If an individual does not have the capacity to learn all six Clear Picture Do's, it is helpful to focus on a portion of the skill. Noticing the breath is a useful cue that enhances focus and begins the skill utilization process. It is also very important to complete the process of labeling and rating an emotion using the Feelings Rating Scale. Establishing the rating level helps the person decide which Category of Skills to use (Calm-Only and/or All-the-Time); this is significant, because the person has to understand when he is too upset to interact with others. Last, Notice Urges is a critical step. Becoming aware of the action urge gives the individual an opportunity to stop and Check It and progress through the microtransitions in On-Track Thinking. Noticing the Breath, Label and Rate Feelings, and Notice Urges are the key aspects of Clear Picture that facilitate transitions through the skills chaining process.

Clear Picture:
Foundational DBT Concepts and Teaching Points (Linehan, 2015a)

- Mindfulness Skills (pp. 151–230)
- What Emotions Do for You (pp. 326–332)
- A Model of Emotions (pp. 335–345)
- Observing, Describing, and Naming Emotions (pp. 345–349)

- Check the Facts (pp. 350–359)
- Mindfulness of Current Emotions (pp. 403–407)
- Paired Muscle Relaxation (pp. 436–439)
- Self-Soothing with a Body Scan Meditation (pp. 444–445)
- Allowing the Mind: Mindfulness of Current Thoughts (pp. 473–476)

On-Track Thinking

On-Track Thinking, the second skill in the Skills System, is an All-the-Time skill, so it can be used at any level of emotion, 0–5. On-Track Thinking is the second skill because it is always used directly after getting a Clear Picture. All skills chains begin with Clear Picture (1) and On-Track Thinking (2); this chain is represented in numbers as "12." These four steps of On-Track Thinking help individuals appraise and navigate their internal and external experiences.

Stop and Check It

First, the person is required to Check It. In this task the individual pauses to reflect and evaluate the utility of the urge in relation to his goal. Check It implicitly asks the person to step back and think about what he wants. The individual gives a thumbs up if acting on the urge will help him reach his goal. A thumbs down is given if the action would be off-track to the goal. The thumbs-up and -down signs are useful visual aids that give tangible representations to intangible thoughts. Using the phrase "Check It" with a simple hand signal can prompt a participant to check the urge. Urges, like thoughts, are like city buses. Some urges take us to where we want to go and others do not.

Sometimes people have trouble knowing exactly where they want to go. Sorting urges into helpful (thumbs up) and not helpful (thumbs down) can be a clear process at times or one that requires more in-depth reflection at others. Urges, wants, needs, short-term goals, long-term goals, and priorities can support each other or be in conflict. Similarly, potential outcomes of actions can be obvious at times and unclear at others. Check It offers the individual an appraisal process through which she takes time to reflect on the internal and external factors happening in the moment; this opportunity is designed to help her make flexible and informed personal decisions. It may be beneficial for the individual to seek consultation from people she trusts to help her clarify murky situations. It is important to validate dialectical tensions that exist within the human experience that complicate coping efforts.

The individual's abilities to Check It may become more elaborate over time. The individual also may increase capacities to communicate about the Check It process (e.g., disclosing needs, goals, and concerns) as his comfort with participants in group and his Skills System knowledge expands. As the individual gains mastery, it can be helpful to introduce factors such as short- and long-term consequences for actions, as well as, short- and long-term goals. Discussions and exercises that review these expanded elements may improve appraisal capacities. Learning adaptive coping skills is a lengthy process in which a person discovers evolving personal preferences, goals, means to reach goals, and knowledge about how life tends to work.

Turn It Up

If the thoughts and urges are off-track, it is important to Check It and then Turn It Up. Turn It Up is reappraisal. It counteracts an appraisal and prompts the generation of on-track thoughts. This thumbs-up thought motivates the individual be on-track. For example, if the individual thinks, "I feel like hitting him," and evaluates it as a thumbs down for herself, she may Turn It by thinking, "If I hit him, I will be on restriction or get arrested." Turn It Up thoughts often highlight an undesirable outcome if the individual takes action on the urge. It also could be on-track self-instruction or coaching about a more on-track alternative or perspective: "I don't want to hit people anymore."

Cheerleading

When the person Checks It and finds that the urge is on-track or he successfully has turned it up, it is important to generate Cheerleading thoughts throughout the skills chain. Cheerleading occurs when the person cultivates several helpful, on-track coaching self-statements that guide him to have an on-track mindset and behavior. Off-track thinking can be persistent. Countering with multiple, pervasive on-track cheerleading thoughts can help sustain goal-directed actions. For example, "Hitting him is off-track"; "If I do that I will be disappointed in myself"; "I don't want to be an aggressive person"; "I want to get my own apartment"; "I think my family will be upset with me"; "I want to move ahead"; "I can make myself feel better"; "I can do this"; and "I need to take an On-Track Action" are **Cheerleading** thoughts.

Prior to skills training, the individual's self-talk often consists of self-devaluing, self-invalidating internal dialogue that undermines motivation and self-efficacy (e.g., "I can't do this"; "I am stupid"; "I don't care"). The individual may need to improve capacities to generate self-encouraging statements that help motivate him to continue skills use and endure challenging states without reverting to problematic patterns. Cheering himself on with self-talk such as "I can do this" and "I can stay on track" is useful throughout the entire situation and promotes self-efficacy, a more positive mood, and efficient skills implementation. On-Track Thinking is used throughout the entire skills chain to help the person transition effectively from one skill to the next.

Make a Skills Plan

Once the individual has Checked It, Turned It Up, if necessary, and done **Cheerleading**, she makes a Skills Plan. Choosing which skills and how many to chain together are key aspects of this process. Initially, the person may need to go through concrete steps to learn how to formulate an effective Skills Plan. As the individual becomes familiar with concepts, the process happens more intuitively.

Choosing Category of Skills

Deciding whether the individual can use Calm-Only skills (Skills 6–9) is important. If the individual is over a 3-level emotion, All-the-Time skills (Skills 1–5) should be used. Using

Calm-Only skills when over a 3 level often causes problems for the individual. It may be helpful to validate the individual's urge to solve the problem, express emotions, try to get needs met, or settle relationship conflicts immediately, but using the All-the-Time skills first to reduce arousal is generally more effective.

Recipe for Skills

The Recipe for Skills tells the person the minimum number of skills to use in the skills chain. It is necessary to use at least one skill for every level of feeling, including 0. Therefore, at Level 1, two skills are the minimum. At Level 2, at least three are needed. At Level 4, five skills are necessary. At Level 5 feeling, six skills are recommended. Since it is not possible to use Calm-Only skills over a Level 3, doubling up on one of the All-the-Time skills is necessary at a Level 5.

The Recipe helps teach about the basic construction of skills chains: Clear Picture (Skill 1) and On-Track Thinking (Skill 2) determine the On-Track Actions (Skill 3). This "123" chain of skills is a core progression of emotion regulation skills. For example, if a person's On-Track Action was to do a Safety Plan and move away from the risk, that skills chain would be a "1234." When the individual does a New-Me Activity after leaving the risky area, it turns into a "12345" chain. The "123" foundation become rote as the individual learns how to add on skills to better manage situations. The base of "123" helps the individual act with Wise Mind (Linehan, 2015a).

The Recipe for Skills conveys in simple terms the more complex idea of assembling skills into progressions to facilitate effective microtransitions through a situation. Cobbling together enough small steps to span an event effectively is like stretching a walking bridge across a ravine. Without knowing discrete steps to take in highly emotional situations, the person may have a polarized response and avoid the experience or fall off-track into the ravine. The Recipe for Skills guards against having insufficient links in the chain that will not bridge an intense emotional experience. Additionally, in skills coaching situations, coaches can ask the participant to calculate the Recipe for Skills to shift attention from Off-Track to On-Track Thinking and to improve focus.

Choosing the Best Skills for the Situation

Making a Skills Plan is a preliminary step toward charting a course of action to reach personal goals. When the individual Copes Ahead (Linehan, 2015a) the individual thinks about outcomes and possible skills that will help him to achieve the desired effect. For example, the individual may often choose to chain together Clear Picture, On-Track Thinking, On-Track Action, Safety Plan, and New-Me Activities in a risky situation. When the individual has a problem (and is under a Level 3 feeling) doing Clear Picture, On-Track Thinking, On-Track Action, and Problem Solving may be effective. This is a "1236" chain. As the individual becomes more familiar with the Skills List through skills training and experience, he accumulates more viable options for proactive behaviors. The Skills System Handout 2 ("How Our Skills Help Us," p. 200) is a brief summary of the functions of each skill; learning this information can aid recall related to which skills to use in various situations.

On-Track Thinking:
Foundational DBT Concepts and Teaching Points (Linehan, 2015a)

- Cheerleading Strategies (p. 90)
- Mindfulness "How" Skills: Nonjudgmentally (pp. 199–208)
- Mindfulness "How" Skills: One-Mindfully (pp. 208–210)
- Mindfulness "How" Skills: Effectively (pp. 210–213)
- Skillful Means: Balancing Doing Mind and Being Mind (pp. 222–225)
- Wise Mind: Walking the Middle Path (pp. 225–227)
- Factors Reducing Interpersonal Effectiveness (pp. 237–241)
- Clarifying Goals in Interpersonal Situations (pp. 242–248)
- Evaluating Your Options: How Intensely to Ask or Say No (pp. 263–266)
- Troubleshooting Interpersonal Effectiveness Skills (pp. 266–270)
- Dialectics (pp. 286–294)
- Validation Skills (pp. 294–295)
- Recovering from Invalidation (pp. 302–306)
- Cope Ahead (pp. 393–396)
- Troubleshooting Emotion Regulation Skills (pp. 409–410)
- STOP Problematic Behavior Immediately (pp. 424–427)
- Pros and Cons As a Way to Make Behavioral Decisions (pp. 427–431)
- Improving the Moment (pp. 445–450)

On-Track Action

On-Track Action is the third skill in the Skills System. It is an All-the-Time skill; thus, it can be used at any level of emotion, 0–5. On-Track Actions are skillful actions the person takes. As a general rule, the individual is not advised to take an action unless it is an On-Track Action! Doing Clear Picture and On-Track Thinking before taking an action increases the chances that it will be on-track rather than off-track. There are five types of On-Track Actions in the Skills System.

The first type of On-Track Action is when the individual Takes a Step toward My Goal. For example, if the person is trying to lose weight, reaching for the bag of carrots when preparing lunch may be an On-Track Action. Reaching for a bag of chips may be an Off-Track Action. An On-Track Action occurs when the individual does something that helps her reach a personal goal in a situation. Quickly reacting while hoping that an action is on-track may work, yet it may not incorporate the totality of available information and may not have maximum positive impact.

It is essential to understand that *only the individual, in that moment,* can decide whether an action is on-track or off-track. For example, perhaps an individual who has lost 10 pounds is at a holiday party. Perhaps having a few chips as a treat may still be an On-Track Action. The personal decision-making process is a vital opportunity for self-determination and activation of inner wisdom, or Wise Mind (Linehan, 2015a). The goal is to help the person engage in a skills process prior to taking actions versus leading him to particular choices.

Skills trainers and coaches have to balance the role of being supportive to the individual while encouraging autonomy. For example, the support provider can offer reflections about her own choices in similar situations and the effectiveness of those decisions in terms of reaching personal goals. She can also highlight possible outcomes for certain actions, so that the individual is oriented to the results of decisions prior to making a choice. It is generally not helpful for trainers and coaches to dictate whether an action is on-track or off-track for the person unless it is a high-risk situation.

Switch Tracks

On-Track Action—Switch Tracks is when the person does something to shift from off-track (or heading off-track) to on-track. For example, if a person is engaging in Getting It Right, he is meeting resistance, and his feelings escalate to over a Level 3. "Turning the Mind" (Linehan, 2015a, p. 417) or Switching Tracks to accepting the situation diverts off-track actions. The situation changed, so he quickly gets a Clear Picture, uses On-Track Thinking, and Switch Tracks to use All-the-Time skills instead.

Switch Tracks is helpful when the individual is experiencing off-track urges or behavior. Shifting tracks as soon as possible after going off-track is beneficial; the longer a person waits, the more challenging the task of getting back on-track may be. For example, if I am sitting down watching a TV show during my normal exercise time, it might be helpful to Shift Tracks and go put on workout clothes. The longer I watch, the less likely I am to workout. Shifting behavior to do several On-Track Actions helps the individual be securely on the road to his goals. For example, changing into shorts, putting on running shoes, getting my music player, and filling my bottle of water would increase the likelihood that I would exercise.

There are times when the individual continues to trigger uncomfortable emotions and/or ruminates about certain thoughts and urges; these behaviors may serve to increase painful emotions and hinder movement toward goals. *Jumping in with Both Feet* to On-Track Actions is important. If one foot is on-track and one is off-track, the individual is still engaging in off-track patterns.

Taking an "Opposite Action" (Linehan, 2015a, p. 359), is another way to Switch Tracks. Doing the opposite of off-track urges can (1) initiate on-track behaviors and (2) reduce cues to avoid, because the individual approaches the task. Doing the Opposite Action of the off-track urges may decrease cues that perpetuate problematic patterns. For example, if the urge was to be rude, being polite would be its opposite. It is important that Opposite Action be done with 100% effort and focus. For example, being neutral to someone may not be rude, but it is an Opposite Action. "Opposite" means that the individual goes all the way to the other end of the spectrum and is clearly polite. Clinicians should review pages 359–372 in the *DBT Skills Training Manual, Second Edition* (Linehan, 2015a) to gain a complete understanding of Opposite Action.

On-Track Action Plans

On-Track Action Plans are activities that are part of the individual's daily routines that help balance his mind, body, and spirit. When the individual proactively manages his body, it helps him manage his mind. For example, the individual may have an exercise schedule, eat healthy food, take proper medications, get suitable amounts of sleep, and talk to friends as part of an On-Track Action Plan each day. Doing written Safety Plans before medium- and high-risk events may be part of an On-Track Action Plan. When balancing various aspects of daily living, the person may be better prepared to mitigate and manage stressful situations that arise.

Accept the Situation

When the person has done what she can to manage a situation, it may be helpful to do On-Track Action—Accept the Situation to wait for the situation to change. There are many times when it is not possible to solve problems right away, and waiting is necessary. When the person engages in Calm-Only skills and does not experience cooperation, feelings can escalate. On-Track Action—Accept the Situation can help the person withdraw, wait, and regroup rather than making the situation worse. When the person has to do things that she would prefer not to do, Accepting the Situation can increase "willingness" (Linehan, 2015a, p. 468). When there is nothing that can be done to change a situation or it is not possible to control the outcome, On-Track Action—Accept the Situation may be the best option for the moment. It is important for the person to use other skills, such as New-Me Activities, to help her tolerate the discomfort that On-Track Action—Accepting the Situation causes. Practicing the DBT skills of "Half-Smiling" and "Willing Hands" (Linehan, 2015a, pp. 471–473) offer tangible acceptance-based actions that can be used in context. It may be important for the individual to engage in Problem Solving at a later time to address underlying issues that may have led to the situation.

Turn the Page

It may be helpful to do On-Track Action—Turn the Page when the individual has difficulty shifting attention away from thoughts, feeling, or urges that increase emotions. For example, if he continues to focus on an ex-partner and this attention increases affect and off-track urges, On-Track Action—Turn the Page may be help him turn his mind away from a situation that exacerbates emotions toward one that either reduces affect or is in service of his new-me goals. The individual may want to Turn the Page on certain worries, memories, painful emotions, or urges that are leading him off-track. It is important to refocus attention on On-Track Thinking and demonstrate one or more on-track skills. Turn the Page is both a cognitive process of letting go and a behavioral process of taking an On-Track Action that seals the deal. A "123" skills chain helps the individual know when to Turn the Page and to what he should shift his attention.

On-Track Action:
Foundational DBT Concepts and Teaching Points (Linehan, 2015a)

- Mindfulness "What" Skills: Participate (pp. 192–199)
- Mindfulness "How" Skills: Effectively (pp. 210–213)
- Build Mastery (pp. 392–393)

- Taking Care of Your Mind by Taking Care of Your Body (pp. 396–398)
- Sleep Hygiene Protocol (pp. 400–402)
- Radical Acceptance (pp. 451–466)
- Turning the Mind (pp. 466–468)
- Willingness (pp. 468–471)
- Half-Smile and Willing Hands (pp. 471–473)

Safety Plan

Safety Plan, the fourth skill in the Skills System, is an All-the-Time skill. This means that Safety Plan can be used at any level of emotion, 0–5. If the individual determines, after doing Clear Picture and On-Track Thinking, that some kind of risk exists, a Safety Plan is often an On-Track Action. The person must decide what level the risk is, what kind of Safety Plan to use, and what actions are necessary to manage the current level of risk. Safety Plan offers a structure to Cope Ahead (Linehan, 2015a) in risky situations.

Levels of Risk

The first step in a Safety Plan is to get a Clear Picture of the risk. There are Inside Risks, such as off-track Thoughts, Urges, Feelings, and Fantasies (TUFFs). There are also Outside Risks (people, places, and things), including people who upset the individual, places that are dangerous, and objects that trigger off-track thoughts. The person handles Inside- and Outside Risks before larger problems develop.

There are three Levels of Risk: low, medium, and high. In a *low*-risk situation, the problem is far away and/or the contact may cause stress. For example, if the individual's neighbors are having a loud argument in their house, the danger is far away and there is little potential for her to be hurt. In a *medium*-risk situation, the danger is in the area and/or contact may cause problems. If the neighbor walked over to the individual's fence and started screaming at her, the risk is closer and the contact with the neighbor may increase problems. In *high*-risk situations, the danger is close and/or contact may cause serious damage. The irate neighbor might come over and starts banging on the individual's door, threatening to break it down. This is high risk because the risk is close and the threat of harm is immediate.

It is important not to overrate or underrate risks. Overrating risk means that the individual rates the risk as high, when it is low. This may cause the individual to avoid activities that are helpful. For example, if the person rates going to work on the first day as high risk because he is anxious, he may not go to work. In this case, it may be better to do an On-Track Action and Jump in with Both Feet on the first day of a new job! Underrating risk is when the individual rates a risk that is high as being low. This can lead to danger and harm, because his efforts to manage the risk are insufficient (e.g., if he drives a car after having four drinks and thinks it is fine). If the individual is not thinking clearly, it is important that he seeks support from someone to discuss options for managing the risk (Talking Safety Plan). Once the individual has a Clear Picture of the risk, it is necessary to choose the type of Safety Plan to use.

Types of Safety Plans

There are three types of Safety Plans: Thinking, Talking, and Written. In a Thinking Safety Plan, the person thinks about how to manage the risk safely. For example, if the individual hears the neighbors fighting, she may make the decision to watch through the window to see if the couple's fight escalates to a higher level of risk or turn up her TV so that they do not bother her as much. A Thinking Safety Plan is often used in low-risk situations.

In a Talking Safety Plan, the individual decides to tell someone about the risk to elicit support. It is generally helpful to use Talking Safety Plans in medium- and high-risk situations. For example, the individual may approach a skills coach and say, "I am having TUFFs right now. Could you help me make a good Safety Plan?" It is important to note that if the person's emotion level is over a 3, the focus of the communication during a Talking Safety Plan is strictly on tactics to manage the risk versus encouraging lengthy and detailed discussions about the content of the situation.

It is important that the individual understand the difference between a Talking Safety Plan and Expressing Myself. In a Talking Safety Plan, the discussion is related to the risk or strong emotions and how to manage the situation effectively. Expressing Myself, which is a Calm-Only skill, would communicate the individual's thoughts, concerns, needs, feeling, likes–dislikes, and hopes/dreams. Delving into Expressing Myself, especially related to the risk, increases levels of feelings (and in turn risk). It may be important for the individual to express feelings about the issues, but it is essential to choose the best time to do that.

In a Written Safety Plan, the individual, with or without assistance, writes down the possible risk and dangers, either prior to, during, or after risky events. The person writes or completes an individualized form that highlights possible problems and strategies to manage difficulties that arise. Written Safety Plans are particularly important in high-risk situations. The individual may choose to share the written plan with a trusted friend who can assist him in following it.

Ways to Manage Risk

There are three ways to manage risks: Focus on New-Me Activities, Move Away, and Leave the Area. The first, least invasive way of managing risk is to Focus on a New-Me Activity. New-Me Activities are various positive tasks that the individual does throughout the day. For example, if the person notices a low risk while at work, she may choose to focus on the work task she is doing—sweeping the floor, for instance. If she is not engaged in an activity, participating in one may help her remain safe, focused, and on-track. Focusing on a New-Me Activity prompts the individual to take a positive action versus merely ignoring the risk, which does not guide her toward an On-Track Action. It is important to give full attention to the activity, yet be alert to any changes in the environment and risk level of the situation.

For example, Jim is at work. He hears his coworker raising his voice in the next room. He decides to do a "1234" skills chain. When he is thinks about what kind of Safety Plan to do, he knows that the coworker is merely venting and no significant danger exists. Jim also feels that he is at a safe distance from the trouble and therefore assesses the situation as low risk. He thinks about what he should do to handle the situation. Jim decides to stay where he is and focus on his work task.

The second way to manage risk is to Move Away. This means that the individual moves to a safer area and gets distance from the problem. Once the person has Moved Away, she may want to refocus on a New-Me Activity to stay on track. It is often necessary to Move Away in medium-risk situations when either the problem is nearby or there is the possibility that contact will cause problems. Continuing to have a Clear Picture and doing On-Track Thinking will help the person use other skills to manage the situation effectively. For example, Jim is in the break room at work. His coworker comes in complaining about the boss. Jim does a "1234" skills chain. He realizes that this situation could cause him problems, so he moves to the other end of the break room.

The third and most invasive way to manage risk is to Leave the Area completely. In high-risk situations where there is serious danger, it may be necessary to leave the area. Under these circumstances, the individual may need to go where she cannot hear, see, talk to, or touch the risk. Similarly, if the individual engages in self-injurious behaviors, it is important to remove all objects that may be used to inflict harm. Doing a Talking Safety Plan and letting another person know about the danger can help ensure that the individual remains a safe distance from perpetrators, potential victims, and possible weapons that are creating high Levels of Risk. If there is imminent danger, it is crucial to seek support. Additionally, after Leaving the Area, it may be helpful to refocus on a New-Me Activity. For example, Jim is in the break room. His coworker starts yelling and swearing about the company. The man throws a fire extinguisher and breaks a chair. Jim quickly does a "1234" skills chain and leaves the area because of the high level of danger. He tells the security guard and returns to his work area on the other side of the building.

Safety Plan:
Foundational DBT Concepts and Teaching Points (Linehan, 2015a)

- Cope Ahead (pp. 393–396)
- Taking Care of Your Mind by Taking Care of Your Body (pp. 396–398)

New-Me Activity

The New-Me Activity, the fifth skill in the Skills System, is an All-the-Time skill. This means that the individual can use New-Me Activities at any level of emotion, 0–5. New-Me Activities are the on-track activities that the individual does during each day. New-Me Activities are a useful emotion regulation strategy to increase positive emotions and decrease negative ones. It is important to note that different New-Me Activities affect people in various ways, and situations require different tactics. There are four types: Focus, Feel Good, Distraction, and Fun New-Me Activities.

Focus New-Me Activities

Focus activities improve attention and focus in the moment. When the individual engages in activities that involve sorting, organizing, following step-by-step instructions, and/or counting, his mind becomes more focused. Examples of Focus New-Me Activities are sorting cards, playing solitaire, word searches, cooking with a recipe, counting money, folding clothes, cleaning, reading, and playing video games. Activities can be made into Focus New-Me Activities by adding counting or patterns. For example, counting a certain number of times while dribbling a basketball with the right hand and then switching to do the same number with the left would be adding counting and a pattern. Just playing basketball may be a Fun New-Me Activity instead.

When a person is highly emotional and not thinking clearly, it can be helpful to do a simple card-sorting activity. First, the individual separates the deck into two piles, with the red cards in one pile and the black ones in another. The person should try to keep the cards in organized, tidy piles rather than allow the cards to slide all over the table. Even this rudimentary task is challenging when a person is in an escalated state. Once that is complete, the person separates the deck by suits—hearts, diamonds, clubs, and spades—each in its own pile. Finally, the individual takes each pile containing one suit and puts it in order, either from the highest card down or the lowest card up. The goal is to perform a task that does not increase cognitive load demands and frustration significantly but rather helps the individual focus attention. If the person is unable to do one of the tasks, it may be useful to return to a simpler version of the sorting activity. Other sorting games can be created, such as separating the deck by the numbers on the cards (placing all four of the aces together, etc.).

Feel Good New-Me Activities

Feel Good New-Me Activities help the individual feel comfortable and soothed. The individual may engage in Soothing the Senses (Linehan, 2015a) activities that help her engage in nurturing self-care. It is important to note that each individual must have an opportunity to define what she finds soothing. Each person's experience of activities and preferences vary. Engaging in activities that trigger memories, problematic thoughts, or painful emotions may not function to help the individual feel good. The following items are self-soothing activities that involve each of the senses.

- *Sight.* The individual may look at pleasant sights to increase positive feelings and experiences. For example, sitting and looking at a beautiful view, taking a walk in nature, and/ or looking at attractive pictures may make the individual feel better.
- *Hearing.* The person may listen to things that increase joy. For example, putting on music, listening to birds sing, or hearing water in a stream can be soothing.
- *Smell.* Experiencing pleasant aromas can help a person feel good. Smelling cookies baking, burning scented candles, and using fragrant hand lotion are examples of Feel Good New-Me Activities.
- *Touch.* Various types of touching can sooth an individual. Putting on cozy slippers, taking a warm bath, and petting an animal are common ways to experience comfort through touch.
- *Taste.* Eating and drinking things that have a pleasant taste can provide pleasure and make people feel good. Having a nice meal, sipping hot tea, eating a piece of chocolate, or drinking ice-cold lemonade on a hot day are examples of some Feel Good New-Me Activities.

Distraction New-Me Activities

Distraction New-Me Activities help the individual to Switch Tracks and focus on something different than the event that prompts challenging emotions or off-track behaviors. Distraction can not only avert emotional escalation, but it can also alter aspects of the emotional response (Linehan, 2015a). Some strategies are used to Distract My Mind, whereas others are used to Distract My Body. Distract My Mind activities help me get my mind off one thing and onto something else that is more pleasant. Activities such as watching TV or movies, playing video games, reading, or helping other people can help the individual focus his mind on a positive alternative. For example, if the individual is waiting for a ride home from the doctor's office, staring at the clock may increase discomfort. Instead, the individual can look at a magazine.

Distracting My Body activities can help when an individual is experiencing uncomfortable sensations or circumstances that cannot be changed. For example, rigorous physical activity helps the individual Switch Tracks from focusing on factors that may increase emotions to focusing on his body. Although, this is a type of Focus New-Me Activity, it also functions to distract the person from factors that are driving affect up. Activities that get the individual's heart pumping, such as walking, jogging, yoga, and use of a workout DVD, distract through exercise. Using ice cubes/packs can distract with temperature. Spicy food, sour candies, and cinnamon gum are ways to distract through taste.

It is important to note that using Distraction New-Me Activities may be most helpful when the person has done everything possible to manage the situation and she just needs to relax or wait. For example, if the person needs to be picked up at the doctor's office, it is important to call to arrange a ride prior to reading a magazine.

Fun New-Me Activities

Fun New-Me Activities make the individual feel happiness and joy. It is important that the person has the ability to do many different Pleasant Events (Linehan, 2015a) that help him increase positive emotions within the context of daily life. Exploring new activities can help the person improve emotion regulation abilities by providing beneficial alternatives to experiences that tend to elicit problematic emotions and behaviors. Each person finds joy in different ways: Drawing, playing sports, video games, working, cooking, cleaning, reading, watching TV, listening to music, talking to friends, going out, and studying skills are just a few Fun New-Me Activities. Creating On-Track Action Plans that include a variety of these types of activities (that fit into his budget) can help a person maintain balance within his life.

Choosing the Best New-Me Activity

Each kind of New-Me Activity has a different function; choosing the proper New-Me Activity in a situation can help the individual reach personal goals. For example, if the person is becoming upset or confused, choosing a Focus New-Me Activity will help promote clear thinking. If the person is feeling tense or stressed, a Feel Good New-Me Activity may increase relaxation and comfort. If the individual has to wait for a few hours and does not want continually to trigger the emotion of boredom, doing a Distraction New-Me Activity may be a beneficial choice.

If the individual wants to feel good about life and experience connection with others, doing a Fun New-Me Activity would be helpful.

Some New-Me Activities serve more than one function. For example, video games may help the person focus, distract him from worries, and provide entertainment. Similarly, a phone call to a friend may make the individual feel better and be fun at the same time. The individual uses Clear Picture and On-Track Thinking to determine which New-Me Activities is the best On-Track Action for each different situation. It can be challenging to try new New-Me Activities. It may be necessary for the individual to do an On-Track Action to reach out of her current comfort zone to expand capacities.

New-Me Activities: Foundational DBT Concepts and Teaching Points (Linehan, 2015a)

- Pleasant Events List (pp. 382–391)
- TIP Skills for Managing Extreme Arousal (pp. 431–439)
- Distracting with Wise Mind Accepts (pp. 439–442)
- Self-Soothing (pp. 442–445)
- Improving the Moment (pp. 445–450)

Problem Solving

Problem Solving, the sixth skill in the Skills System, is a Calm-Only skill. This means that the individual can use Problem Solving *only* when below a Level 3 emotion. To attempt Problem Solving when over a Level 3 emotion generally creates more rather than fewer problems. Rushing through Problem Solving may lead the individual to miss effective options and choose alternatives that may feel good in the short term, yet not be helpful in the long term. Problem Solving when a person has over a Level 3 emotion tends to be impulsive and is therefore less likely to aid the individual in reaching personal goals. If the individual is interacting with other people during Problem Solving, it is important that all involved are below a Level 3 emotion. When anyone is escalated in the situation, it may hinder the Problem Solving effort; waiting may be beneficial.

Labeling the size of the problem helps the person appraise a commensurate emotional response and ample resources to fix it. A small problem can cause annoyance rather than serious issues; it usually leads to Level 2 or 3 emotions. Small problems can trigger higher level emotions, but often the individual can reappraise the situation to have a more regulated response. An example of a small problem would be losing my favorite hat. It makes me Level 2, Sad, but it would not really cause other harm. Small problems usually get fixed with a few simple steps; I can go to the bank, take out $15, and buy another hat. Medium-size problems generally cause higher emotions (Levels 3 to 4) and take more steps and time to fix. For example, if I lose my car keys, I have to call a taxi, be late for work, miss my meeting, find out how to get a new key, and get a ride to get a new key. Large or overwhelming problems are very serious: for example, if I lose my job or if someone I love passes away. Large problems often cause me to have Level 4 or 5 feelings, may take weeks–months–years to fix, and may change my life in serious ways.

Quick Fix

The Quick Fix worksheet (Problem Solving Worksheet 1, p. 297) may help to solve small problems. Using the worksheet to examine the problem, the solutions, and barriers to the fix can help the individual make a simple problem-solving plan. Additionally, there is a question that asks the individual to reflect on whether he wants to follow through on fixing it, Make Lemonade (change how he thinks about the problem), Accept the Situation (as it is), or suffer (do nothing). This review helps the individual understand his different options when he has a problem. If the problem is more complex, this worksheet will be inadequate.

Problem Solving

Solving medium-size and large problems is a more complicated, multistep progression. Gaining mastery in Problem Solving is a long-term learning process. The following steps find solutions to more serious or confusing situations:

1. Getting a Clear Picture of the problem. The individual has to determine what she wants in a situation, what the problem is, and what the barriers are to reaching the goal. Rating the size of the problem helps her gauge the amount of resources necessary to fix it.

2. Checking All Options. During this step, the person brainstorms about many different options. He "fast forwards" each option to see what the outcomes may be and weighs the "pros" (thumbs up) and "cons" (thumbs down) of each choice. He chooses an option that best fits his goal.

3. Creating Plan A, Plan B, and Plan C. The individual creates multiple plans to ensure some level of success.

Getting a Clear Picture of the Problem

The first step in doing successful Problem Solving is for the individual to get a Clear Picture of what he wants and to clarify what is getting in the way of that goal. Clarifying goals and barriers may be simple or complex, depending on the situation. The person may need to take time to self-reflect or contact a skills coach to illuminate the issues. An example of a relatively simple situation would be Joseph finding out that he has a basketball game in 3 days. He wants to play in the game, but realizes that he does not have sneakers that fit him. Wanting to play in the game is Joseph's goal, and not having the proper shoes is the problem. Once Joseph understands the problem, he can Check All Options and make a Plan A, B, or C to get new sneakers.

Sometimes the individual is unclear about personal goals; a situation can also be confusing or require multiple steps to solve the problem. Additionally, there may be environmental challenges and/or power differentials that make it difficult for a person with significant learning challenges to solve problems within complex social systems. Dissatisfaction in relationships, family conflicts, and vocational problems are examples of multifaceted problems. It may be necessary for the person to address components of a problem as part of a larger Problem Solving effort. The individual may benefit from seeking consultation from skills coaches, professionals who support the individual, and trusted friends, to get a Clear Picture of her goals and address complex problems. Feedback can be useful during the problem-solving process to assess what can be changed in a situation and what needs to be accepted.

Checking All Options

Once the person has clarified what she wants and what is in the way of these goals, it is time to Check All Options. The person begins by generating possible solutions to the problem. She then reviews the pros (positive outcomes) and cons (negative outcomes) for each option. The metaphor of fast-forwarding to see the end teaches the concept that reflecting on consequences of action can be helpful. The individual checks the fit of each option to determine whether the action would be on-track (thumbs up) or off-track (thumbs down) to the goal. As the individual sifts through, checking options, she begins to develop a series of Problem Solving plans. Plans may be simple and have a single step or be more challenging, requiring multiple skills. It is often necessary to use Clear Picture, On-Track Thinking, On-Track Actions, Expressing Myself, Getting It Right, and Relationship Care to execute Problem Solving. Once multiple options are reviewed, the individual chooses the option that best fits her goal.

Making Plans A, B, and C

Plan A is the plan that the individual believes will work best to fix the problem. Plan A best fits the needs of the person and has the highest likelihood of solving the problem in an effective way. Consulting with skills coaches or supportive friends prior to taking action, thinking about what to say, and rehearsing tactics can strengthen a plan.

It is sometimes necessary to negotiate with people while doing Problem Solving. It is therefore helpful to have other alternatives in mind when engaging in discussions with people. A secondary plan, called Plan B, is the backup plan if Plan A does not work. Plan B is usually a second alternative or the strategy to reevaluate the situation.

There are times when Plan A and Plan B are not possible. Rather than getting in a negative situation that drives emotions up, the individual makes Plan C, or a fall-back position. Plan C usually is either a third, less desirable option that is acceptable or a plan to tolerate the distress of losing preferred options. Not getting problems solved and/or encountering resistance can elicit heightened emotional responses. The individual will need to get a Clear Picture, use On-Track Thinking, and implement On-Track Actions to deal with the new situation.

Problem Solving:
Foundational DBT Concepts and Teaching Points (Linehan, 2015a)

- Options for Solving Any Problem (pp. 129–131)
- Preparing for Opposite Action and Problem Solving (pp. 359–361)
- Problem Solving (pp. 372–381)

Expressing Myself

Expressing Myself, the seventh skill in the Skills System, is a Calm-Only skill. This means an individual can use Expressing Myself *only* when he is below a Level 3 emotion. If the individual is using Expressing Myself with other people, it is helpful that all involved be below a Level 3 to reduce the likelihood of an off-track interaction.

What Is Expressing Myself?

Expressing Myself is when the individual communicates what is On My Mind and In My Heart. Thoughts, concerns, and needs are a few things that are On My Mind. Feelings, likes, dislikes, hopes, and dreams are a few things that are In My Heart. The person can communicate by talking face-to-face, on the phone, through video, and by sign language. Letters, e-mails, social media, and texts are ways to Expressing Myself through writing. If the individual has difficulty reading and writing, eliciting help from others may be necessary. Pictures, drawings, other art forms, and photos are also forms of visual communication. The individual expresses through New-Me Activities such as singing, dancing, playing a musical instrument, drawing, and acting. The individual can use body language to Expressing Myself. Expression through frowning, smiling, eye rolling, sighing, crossed arms, and eye contact send messages to other people. Communicating through body language is often less clear than verbal or written forms of expression.

Why Do We Use Expressing Myself?

Sharing what is On My Mind and In My Heart can increase emotions. Being strategic about what emotions are being increased helps a person know when Expressing Myself is helpful. Expressing Myself is often used in conjunction with other Calm-Only skills. Use of Expressing Myself when the individual has small issues, concerns, and needs may keep them from growing into larger problems. Expressing Myself is an important tool in solving problems and in Getting It Right—Right Words (SEALS). The individual communicates respect by using Sugar, describes the situation with Explain, Asks for what he wants, Listens to the other person, and Seals the Deal with Expressing Myself. Expressing Myself is a vital part of two-way-street relationships, Finding Middle Ground, and taking the Steps of Responsibility in Relationship Care.

How Do We Use Expressing Myself?

Talking is one way to communicate. There are pros and cons with talking. Some of the pros are that talking can be a quick, easy, and clear way to make a point. The cons include miscommunication, if the individual does not choose her words carefully. Speech and language difference between people can make it more difficult for them to understand each other. Communicating through writing also has pros and cons. One pro is that when the individual writes, she can make her whole point without interruption. When writing, it is possible to communicate things that are hard to say face-to-face. A con for writing is the fact that the person may show it to other people. It is important to consider what the person may do with the communication when deciding what to write. Utilizing body language to communicate can be unreliable. Being a mind reader, or thinking someone can read minds, decreases clarity of the messages.

When Do We Use Expressing Myself?

Expressing Myself is a Calm-Only skill, which means that it is more effective to express when both the individual who is doing the communicating and the person she is communicating with are below a Level 3 feeling. Gross and Thompson (2009), in the *Handbook of Emotion Regulation*, explain that "emotion-expressive behavior slightly increases the feeling of that emotion" (p. 15). In light of this trend, it may be helpful to use Expressing Myself at emotion Levels 0–2, because the process of expression may naturally bring the individual to a Level 3 or higher emotion. If the individual begins Expressing Myself at a Level 3 emotion and the result is increased arousal to a Level 4, it is important for the person to get a Clear Picture and use On-Track Thinking to determine what On-Track Actions and other All-the-Time skills would be best in the situation.

An individual may inhibit expression as a strategy to regulate emotion. Gross and Thompson (2009, p. 15) explain further that "interestingly, decreasing emotion-expressive behavior seems to have mixed effects on the emotion experience (decreasing positive but not negative emotion experience)." Overall, Gross and Thompson conclude that an individual appears to regulate emotions more effectively when he finds "ways of expressing them in adaptive rather than maladaptive ways" (p. 15). Although venting emotions is a type of Expressing Myself, Gross and Thompson highlight that there may be increased benefits to communication that promote "problem solving and interpersonal understanding" (p. 15).

When the individual is over a Level 3 emotion, there is a strong possibility that she will experience urges to engage in emotion expression. Getting a Clear Picture and using On-Track Thinking can help the individual allow these urges to pass and focus on more helpful thoughts. At higher levels of emotion, it may be more difficult to focus and perform complex interactive skills. Ultimately, the person must gauge whether the expression is going to be an On-Track or an Off-Track Action. Over a Level 3 emotion, it is more likely that communication can morph from effective Expressing Myself to venting, blaming, ranting, demanding, yelling, and swearing. Unfortunately, in situations where the individual is trying to gain cooperation, these tactics cause the other party to recoil, disengage, and even retaliate. Although these strategies may be effective in specific situations, as a general rule, when an individual is experiencing an emotion that ranks over a Level 3, it is difficult for her to coordinate all the necessary skills to reach personal goals successfully. Additionally, the individual may feel guilty and experience self-directed frustration after expressing emotion over Level 3. Waiting for the proper time to use Expressing Myself helps the individual maintain positive relationships with herself and other people.

Expressing Myself:
Foundational DBT Concepts and Teaching Points (Linehan, 2015a)

- Objectives Effectiveness Skills: DEARMAN (pp. 248–255)
- Relationship Effectiveness Skills: GIVE (pp. 255–260)

Getting It Right

Getting It Right, Skill 8, is a series of tactics that the individual considers when attempting to get something that he wants from another person. This eighth skill in the Skills System is a Calm-Only skill, which means that the individual can use Getting It Right *only* when below a Level 3 emotion. It is important to note that the other person also needs to be below a Level 3. If either person in the interaction is above a Level 3, it may be best to wait until a later time, when both individuals' emotions are less escalated. To acquire things successfully, the person must be in the Right Mind and talk to the Right Person at the Right Time and Place, using the Right Tone and the Right Words.

Right Mind

Being in the Right Mind to use Getting It Right means that the person has a Clear Picture and has used On-Track Thinking to make a plan related to the best tactics to get what is desired. The individual must be acting in Wise Mind; she should be prepared, focused, below a Level 3 on the Feelings Rating Scale, and be ready to do what works. As with Expressing Myself, it is common for emotions to rise prior to and during use of Getting It Right. It is important for the individual to self-monitor her emotional status. To become demanding, to act as though she is right and the other person is incorrect, or to use intimidation are signs that the person is starting to get it wrong.

Approaching another person to make requests can increase emotional responses. It is vital that the individual continue to use all necessary skills to manage the situation. Creating a Getting It Right Plan (see Getting It Right Worked Example 1, p. 322) can help the individual be organized; rehearsing and practicing can increase effectiveness as well. Planning ahead can help the individual remain effective even if he unexpectedly experiences cognitive overloaded in the moment. If the person has a fuzzy picture or engages in Off-Track Thinking, Getting It Right will quickly turn into getting it wrong. Therefore, if either person's emotions begin to escalate to the Level 4 or 5 range, it is best to retreat, returning to Clear Picture and On-Track Thinking to make another Skills Plan.

Right Person

When making a Getting It Right Plan, it is important to talk to the Right Person. This is the person who can and will help the individual get his needs met. For example, the individual may want to discuss a raise with his employer rather than his coworker. In complex situations, it may be challenging to know who is best. For example, if the person lives in a residential program, he may either talk to a supervisor, program manager, or psychologist regarding a clarification about his individual service plan. Seeking consultation from skills coaches to make these choices may be beneficial. Additionally, if the Right Person is not readily available, it may be necessary to set up a specific time to talk. There may be delays that are frustrating. It is important to use other skills while waiting to talk to the Right Person. Getting a Clear Picture, using On-Track Thinking, and doing On-Track Actions, such as New-Me Activities, may help him wait and remain in the Right Mind

Right Time and Place

Choosing the Right Time and Place is important. The individual will want to choose an opportunity when the Right Person is able to give full attention to the interaction. The circumstances have to be conducive to the Right Person helping the individual. The individual may want to rush to use Getting It Right at a time that is not convenient for the Right Person. It is often more effective to adjust the Getting It Right plan and wait, rather than have emotions dictate the timing of this process.

Right Tone

Using the Right Tone is critically important. The individual must get a Clear Picture and do On-Track Thinking to gauge what tone will work best. Usually being too passive or wimpy makes the Right Person not take the individual seriously. Often, being demanding makes the Right Person pull away, stop listening, and think that the individual is not able to handle the situation. When the individual utilizes an aggressive tone, it may stress the relationship so much that the Right Person will not want to help again, and it may make the circumstances more difficult.

Right Words

SEALS represents the Right Words or tasks in Getting It Right. Sugar, Explaining the Situation, Asking for What I Want, Listening, and Seal a Deal are the Right Words in Getting It Right.

Sugar

Using Sugar represents adding sweetness to the situation. This means that the individual is respectful and polite to the Right Person to create a positive relationship environment—for example, "Excuse me, Mr. Smith, may I speak to you for a moment?" Sugar is an ingredient that makes the Right Person want to help the individual get what she needs. Throughout the interaction, the individual responds to the Right Person's needs (showing strong Relationship Care) while advocating for her own agenda: "Mr. Smith, I know you run a business that helps many people. I would really appreciate your help at this time." If the individual remains positive, the Right Person may want to return the favor.

Explaining the Situation

Next, the individual Explains the situation. The individual highlights why it is important that the Right Person help him: "Mr. Smith, as you know, there was a huge flood in Nepal last year. The homes of over 60,000 villagers were destroyed. Many people are still homeless there." Explaining the situation helps the Right Person become motivated to do whatever it takes to help the individual. The individual wants the Right Person to feel good about contributing. Rushing to make the request before using ample Sugar and fully Explaining the situation can fail to mobilize the Right Person's motivation to help.

Asking for What I Want

After using Sugar and Explaining the Situation, the individual Asks for what she wants: "Mr. Smith, my organization is collecting donations of money and supplies to send to Nepal to help build homes for families whose houses were destroyed in the flood." It is helpful to be specific, so that the Right Person clearly understands the request. "If you could either donate $100 or send tools to our organization to ship there, it would benefit many people. A donation of $300 builds one temporary home for a family." Asking in a clear and direct way helps the Right Person reflect on her ability to help and to make a decision about how to proceed.

Listening

Throughout the entire process of Getting It Right, it is important to listen to the Right Person's opinions and feedback. For example, the answer from the Right Person may be "no." In this case the individual listens to the reasons and tries to negotiate; perhaps only a portion of the request can be fulfilled. Right Person might say, "I'm sorry, Ms. Brown, but our company already made donations to the floor survivors." The individual may say, "Mr. Smith, is there any way your company could donate used tools to our efforts?" or thank him for his time. Finding the balance between being assertive enough to maximize the likelihood of success and still being respectful and maintaining the relationship is important. Sprinkling Sugar throughout the interaction can help the individual reach the goal and facilitate future success.

Despite setbacks, it is vital that the individual stay on track. In all cases, the individual uses Clear Picture and On-Track Thinking to remain focused and to do On-Track Actions that work. It is possible that the individual may find out the person really is not the Right Person, and changes in tactics may be necessary. Listening carefully is an essential step toward being able to Seal a Deal.

Seal a Deal

Finally, the individual tries to Seal a Deal with the Right Person—for example, "Ms. Brown, I am going to give $500 and send three tool boxes to your organization." The individual then seals the deal by saying, "Thank you, Mr. Smith, for your generosity. The check is made out to Helping Homes. The check and tools can be sent to 22 Main Street in Harrisville. I really appreciate this; do you have a sense of when you will be able to make this donation?" It is very important to pin down the details as part of Seal a Deal. It is great when the Right Person agrees to help, but it is vital to ensure the execution of the plan.

Getting It Right:
Foundational DBT Concepts and Teaching Points (Linehan, 2015a)

- Objectives Effectiveness Skills: DEARMAN (pp. 248–255)
- Relationship Effectiveness Skills: GIVE (pp. 255–260)

Relationship Care

Relationship Care, the ninth skill in the Skills System, is a Calm-Only skill. Managing relationships is a complex task that may require using other Calm-Only skills, such as Problem Solving, Expressing Myself, and Getting It Right. Just as with the other Calm-Only skills, it is helpful to use Relationship Care when all involved are below a Level 3. If the individual is in a conversation with someone who shifts to over a Level 3, he needs to get a Clear Picture and do On-Track Thinking to plan how to handle the situation.

There are multiple elements of Relationship Care. Building On-Track Relationships, Balancing On-Track Relationships, and Changing Off-Track Relationships are a few aspects of the skill. Healthy, balanced, fulfillment of On-Track Relationships with the self and other people can significantly add to the individual's quality of life.

Building an On-Track Relationship with Myself

The concept of the Core Self helps the individual understand what it means to have a strong self-relationship. There are four elements of the Core Self: self-awareness, self-acceptance, self-value, and self-trust.

Self-Awareness

Clear Picture teaches the individual steps that foster self-awareness. In addition, On-Track Thinking prompts the individual to reflect on goals. When the individual is clear about goals, it is much more likely that she will implement effective strategies to reach her goal in a situation. As the person understands that it is beneficial to see the moment *as is,* in order to manage the circumstance effectively, self-awareness grows.

Self-Acceptance

When the individual is able to be present in the moment, he begins the process of self-acceptance. Seeing himself *as is,* is more possible when he has the capacities to manage the awareness and realities of the situation. Unfortunately, seeing the self *as is* may generate painful emotions. Factors such as medical issues, physical disabilities, obesity, diagnosis of ID, mental health problems, trauma, and chronic behavioral dysregulation are a few examples of challenges that can significantly complicate the person's self-acceptance efforts.

The process of strengthening the Core Self often continues as the person improves self-awareness and self-acceptance to include increased self-value. Practicing Clear Picture, demonstrating On-Track Thinking, and taking On-Track Actions helps the person accomplish mastery. Experiencing success in more challenging situations leads the person have a positive self-experience versus self-avoidance. The Skills System is built to continually mobilize the person's inner wisdom and guide him to engage actively in adaptive behaviors. Over time, the person discovers self-capacities and in turn develops the ability to self-value.

Self-Trust

Each of the previous elements of the Core Self serves to improve the individual's self-trust. The person sees situations clearly, accepts the realities, remains positive in the face of challenges, and makes skillful decisions that help her move toward personal goals. Experiencing these abilities gives the person the knowledge that she can not only survive but also get what she needs. Previous patterns of overdoing and underdoing are replaced by skillful self-management and, ultimately, improved self-trust.

Building Relationships with Others

Developing capacities of self-awareness, self-acceptance, self-value, and self-trust may positively impact the individual's functioning relationships with others. For example, the individual's ability to be aware of other people may allow him to be more aware of what other people are experiencing. Being more aware of the other person can help the individual be more responsive and empathetic. Similarly, as the individual self-accepts, he may become more accepting of other people. Likewise, valuing and trusting other people may offer the individual opportunities for richer relationships. Having the ability to be aware of, accept, value, and trust other people potentially improves relationships and enhances the individual's ability to reach personal goals.

Balancing On-Track Relationships with Others

It is the right and responsibility of each individual to make personal decisions related to her level of participation in relationships on an ongoing basis. The person uses Clear Picture and On-Track Thinking to balance her changing needs and the needs of other people. For example, if a housemate has a brain injury, the person may choose to accept that her housemate repeats statements frequently. Conversely, there may be a situation in which the individual seeks to move from the home, because the housemate's behavior is unacceptable. Thus, Relationship Care is not prescriptive but is a process of using skills to make adjustments within each moment that reflect her Wise Mind. Balancing relationships is a dynamic process that requires the individual to use many tools throughout each day.

Types of Relationships

Each individual has many different types of relationships in his life, and these relationship may change through time. For example, the person who has an intellectual disability may need to relate with residential agencies, employers, job coaches, support staff, housemates, friends, organization members, state social workers, family, and significant others. It is important that the individual learn about the socially effective ways to manage each different type of relationship. As the person ages, his individual role and the role of other people may transform. Developing and maintaining effective relationships with all the different people in the individual's life requires utilization of all of the skills in the Skills System on an ongoing basis.

Relationship Behaviors

The individual uses Clear Picture and On-Track Thinking to make decisions about on-track relationship behaviors. The person continually assesses and balances actions that reflect her personal preferences, values, and goals within the moment. It is vital to use Clear Picture, On-Track Thinking, and On-Track Actions with Relationship Care to manage the multiple changing internal and external factors that transact in relationships. The process of caring for relationships is dynamic. It is necessary to enact a sequence of actions that serve to maintain self-respect and respect for other people as the individual changes, as other people change, and as life changes. Because there are no Relationship Care prescriptions, it is important to use various relationship tools to make adjustments in each moment.

To manage the variability within relationship environments, it is helpful to understand what factors tend to affect relationships so that the person can make adjustments within the current moment. For example, certain Relationship Care behaviors tend to increase positive feelings between people: acting like the person is important, responding with thoughtful comments, calling people and making plans, using appropriate touch, giving gifts, paying compliments, doing activities together, being flexible, and so on.

The person may have important people and relationships in his life. It may be helpful for the person to incorporate Relationship Care behaviors into On-Track Action plans that proactively maintain relationships. Using tools that enhance connection, communication, and support from the individual to those significant friends, family members, or support providers can help the relationships stay on track.

Conversely, certain behaviors tend to increase distance between people in relationships. Keeping conversations short, avoiding disclosing personal information, avoiding making plans, and setting clear personal limits are examples of how to create distance in relationships. Awareness of these tools can help the individual understand the impact of such actions, so that relationship behaviors can be strategically utilized to meet personal goals. For example, if the individual has gone out on a date with someone she is not interested in seeing again, she may discuss her lack of interest directly or she may use Relationship Care behaviors that add distance. As she becomes more mindful of these diverse tools, increased self-determination and active Relationship Care can improve the quality of her life.

It is important to know how to build new relationships. Finding New Friends (based on the DBT worksheet Finding and Getting People to Like You; Linehan, 2015b) can offer tangible ideas about how to expand social connections. Stretching personal limits and hurdling barriers often requires taking an On-Track Action and jumping in with both feet.

Two-Way-Street Relationships

One goal of the Skills System is to give the individual proper tools to participate in Two-Way-Street Relationships. Although the individual cannot control the behavior of the other person, Relationship Care teaches him to act in a way that allows a Two-Way-Street Relationship to happen. A Two-Way-Street Relationship is a reciprocal relationship in which there is mutual respect and communication. The individual must learn to participate actively, both as a giver and receiver, in a Two-Way-Street Relationship. For example, the individual must talk and listen to the other person. He clarifies his points of view and prompts the other person to use Expressing Myself. Within a Two-Way-Street Relationship, participants are able to be present, discuss, negotiate, and collaborate. Working together creates a synthesis and a heightened development of each person and the relationship.

One-Way-Street Relationships

One-Way-Street Relationships occur (1) when the individual does relationship behaviors that add distance in the relationship or (2) when she experiences the other person not reciprocating. There are times when the person may evaluate a One-Way-Street Relationship as out of balance and do Problem Solving to make a plan to address the relationship problem. In that case, she may decide to increase Relationship Care behaviors that improve connections or use Finding Middle Ground to assess and change the off-track relationship. At other times, the individual may want to create a One-Way-Street Relationship, if she is using relationship behaviors intended to keep distance.

Changing Off-Track Relationships

When the individual's self-relationship becomes off track, it can impede reaching personal goals. For example, off-track thinking that is self-devaluing may undermine the person's abilities to function to his potential. Another common problem is when the individual has a fuzzy picture about goals and is therefore unable to make and execute effective Skills Plans. Additionally, certain behavior patterns may be hindering him from reaching goals. Changing off-track habits, such as smoking, alcoholism, drug use, overeating, undereating, and medication inconsistency, may improve the individual's self-relationship and help him be on track. It is challenging to change any kind of off-track habit. Therefore, it is necessary to use all of the skills in the Skills System to manage off-track urges and create new behavior patterns.

Changing Relationships with Others: Finding Middle Ground

Addressing relationship problems often requires using all of the Calm-Only skills. For example, the first step to change an off-track relationship may be to do Problem Solving to get a clear picture of the relationship problem. If the individual determines that meeting and discussing the issue with the other person is Plan A, she then chooses the best means of Expressing Myself. She decides whether talking face-to-face, on the phone, or writing a letter or e-mail is the best tactic. If she wants the other person to change his behavior, she will have to use Getting It Right. The individual will have to be in the Right Mind, choose the Right Time and Place, and use the Right Tone and the Right Words. Finding Middle Ground expands Getting It Right to be a collaborative process in which both the individual talk and listen to hear both sides. Through this Two-Way-Street process there is a give and take and search for a win–win solution to the relationship problem. When they can negotiate a resolution that benefits both, the pair Finds Middle Ground that creates a new level of balance in the relationship.

There are times when the individual's best efforts to Finding Middle Ground do not fix the relationship problems. If the other person is not responsive, chooses not to engage in the collaboration, and does not make accommodations for the individual, then ending the relationship may need to be considered. Revisiting Clear Picture, On-Track Thinking, and Problem Solving may be necessary to determine the next On-Track Action.

Steps of Responsibility

When the individual feels that he has created a relationship problem, it may be helpful to repair the relationship by doing the Steps of Responsibility. This process involves (1) clearly admitting the problem and the impact the behaviors had on the other person, (2) apologizing for what the individual regrets, (3) committing to change his behavior, and (4) taking an On-Track Action. It is not easy to take responsibility, because the individual may feel shame, have the urge to be stubborn, blame the other person, or insist that he is right. Although doing the Steps of Responsibility may cause discomfort, the process can ultimately strengthen the individual's self-relationship and the relationship with the other person.

Ending Relationships with Others

There may be instances when the individual has made efforts to repair the relationship but relationship problems still exist. The individual may determine that a relationship is off track. For example, if the other person is continually demonstrating poor Relationship Care behaviors or encouraging the individual to make off-track choices, perhaps the relationship needs to be ended. The individual can begin to use One-Way Street behaviors that increase the distance in the relationship or she can formally end the relationship. The individual uses Clear Picture, On-Track Thinking, On-Track Action, and Problem Solving to determine how best to stop an off-track relationship. Living with problematic relationships can lead her to be off track, out of balance, and miserable.

Individuals must also learn to deal with relationships changing or ending through no actions of their own. For example, staff leaving, romantic partners breaking up, people moving away, and people dying are common reasons for disruptions in relationships. It may be necessary for the individual to use many skills to cope effectively with relationships that are ending. Although these are often painful experiences, the individual can remain on track toward her goals while managing loss and grief.

Relationship Care:
Foundational DBT Concepts and Teaching Points (Linehan, 2015a)

- Mindfulness Practice: A Spiritual Perspective (pp. 214–218)
- Wise Mind: A Spiritual Perspective (pp. 218–219)
- Practicing Loving Kindness (pp. 219–222)
- Walking the Middle Path (pp. 233–234)
- Factors Reducing Interpersonal Effectiveness (pp. 237–241)
- Skills for Finding Potential Friends (pp. 270–276)
- Mindfulness of Others (pp. 276–280)
- How to End Relationships (pp. 280–285)
- Validation Skills (pp. 294–306)

SYSTEM TOOLS

There are three System Tools within the Skills System. The Feelings Rating Scale, Categories of Skills, and the Recipe for Skills help the individual organize his current experiences and execute a series of behaviors intended to reach personal goals. The System Tools are designed to help the individual create effective skills chains.

Feelings Rating Scale

The Feelings Rating Scale is a 0- to 5-level self-report scale used to rate the intensity of emotions, feelings, and/or sensory experiences during a situation that are happening in the moment. The more intense the sensations and impact on thinking, the higher the rating. The term "feeling" is generally used in the Skills System because it is the broadest term and the simplest to pronounce. The Feelings Rating Scale is used to rate both uncomfortable and more pleasurable experiences.

Emotions impact the individual's capacity to focus. The Feeling Rating Scale can also be conceptualized as a focus rating scale. At the lower levels of emotion, focus is often sharper. At higher levels of feeling, focus is more variable, fuzzier. The individual learns to do more interacting at lower levels of feeling when focus is intact.

The Feelings Rating Scale serves a dual purpose in the Skills System. First, the individual learns to continually rate her feelings rating as part of getting a Clear Picture. The scale is a tool that provides a simple framework that promotes self-awareness and internal organization. Second, the Feelings Rating Scale is utilized during On-Track Thinking. The person uses the Feelings Rating Scale to determine which skills and how many skills would be helpful in a particular situation (Categories of Skills). If the individual is below a Level 3 emotion, it is possible to use all nine skills in the Skills System. If the rating is over a Level 3 emotion, only the All-the-Time skills are used.

Each person rates feelings differently. The same experience may elicit a Level 1 emotion from one person and a Level 3 from someone else. Discussions about ratings and the similarities and differences in peoples' perspectives in skills group can help individuals become aware of how their ratings align with others. For example, if an individual becomes aware the he has high-level reactions in a situation in which others consistently have low-level reactions, then he has an opportunity to explore different, enhanced skills options to address the strong responses.

Feelings ratings adjust as a person gains emotion regulation capacities. The individual is able to experience stronger emotions, enact skills chains, and remain emotionally, cognitively, and behaviorally regulated in increasingly challenging situations. For example, a situation that would have previously elicited a Level 4 emotion may only produce a Level 3 emotion as more effective skills chains are used earlier in the escalation process. When this shift happens, the person is more able to handle stressful, demanding, and increasingly tenuous interactions in on-track ways. For example, the person may gain the ability to do on-track Expressing Myself, talking and listening in situations that would have previously elicited a Level 4 feeling, precluding the use of a Calm-Only skill.

A *Level 0 feelings rating* means that no feeling is being experienced. For example, Level 0 anger means that the person is not experiencing anger at that moment. Skills trainers may find that some participants display patterns of underrating feelings at Level 0. As the person develops the capacity to regulate experiences, the accuracy of rating generally increases as well.

A *Level 1 feelings rating* is a tiny reaction to something that is just noticeable, a twinge. For example, if the individual sees a nice car driving by, he may feel Level 1 envy. He may notice a twinge of the emotion and fleeting thoughts about how nice that car is and how he would like to have one like that. If he allows the emotions and thoughts to pass, the feeling dissipates; if he perseverates about what a piece of junk his own car is, the feeling will increase.

A Level 1 feelings rating may be as high as the emotion goes, or a stronger feeling might be forming. Conversely, the individual might have reduced arousal from a stronger emotion. It is crucial that the individual learn to become aware of Level 1 feelings, because it can help him maintain awareness and effective coping throughout the situation.

At a Level 1 feeling, the person is likely able to think clearly; thus, he can use any of the nine skills on the Skills List. Because of the individual's capacity to cognitively regulate, he is able to use Calm-Only skills. The slight sensations and minimal cognitive disruption contribute to the relative ease of managing urges, impulses, and actions at a Level 1 emotion.

A *Level 2 feelings rating* is a small feeling. The sensations of a Level 2 feeling are noticeable, yet they do not generally cause disruptions that negatively impact the individual's capacities to be on track. For example, at Level 2 anger the individual may feel her heart beating faster and notice her muscles tightening. Although, there may be discomfort at Level 2, she is able to use all nine of the skills on the Skills List. This may be a good time to use skills that involve Expressing Myself, rather than at a Level 3 or above feeling. Optimally, the person is able to experience the situation fully and move strategically toward personal goals.

A *Level 3 feelings rating* is a medium-size feeling. This level of emotion will cause noticeable and possibly multiple body sensations. Sweaty hands, stomachache, racing heart rate, and pacing are a few examples. At Level 3, "negative" feelings such as sadness, fear, anger, guilt, or jealousy, may be uncomfortable for the individual. Although, he may notice more off-track thoughts and urges at Level 3, he is able to focus attention and be on-track relative to his goals.

He is able to talk and listen in ways that preserve his relationship to himself and the other person. At Level 3, the individual can use Calm-Only skills; careful self-monitoring through Clear Picture and On-Track Thinking are necessary to ensure that he engages in On-Track versus Off-Track Actions. If the person begins to use the more interactive Calm-Only skills (Problem Solving, Expressing Myself, Getting It Right, and Relationship Care) and notices that emotions are increasing or the strategies are not working effectively, it is best to return to using the All-the-Time skills (Clear Picture, On-Track Thinking, On-Track Action, Safety Plan, and New-Me Activities) until he is more regulated. If the individual rates the feeling as 3.5, it is over a Level 3, and Calm-Only skills are not recommended.

A *Level 4 feelings rating* is a strong feeling. At a Level 4 feeling, it is likely that the individual is experiencing sustained, intense emotions and body sensations. For example, she may cry, tremble, breathe quickly, sweat profusely, or feel nauseated. Thought processes are disrupted. For example, her thoughts may be racing, disorganized, or nonexistent (blank).

At a Level 4 feelings rating, the individual may be having strong off-track urges to say or do things that will harm his relationship with himself or with another person. He is unable to talk and listen effectively at a Level 4. Using Calm-Only skills, such as Problem Solving and Expressing Myself, can be a desperate attempt to reduce emotional discomfort that unfortunately leave goals unmet and creates collateral damage that makes situations worse. Interactive, Calm-Only skills are not recommended at a Level 4 feeling because of the high level of emotional, cognitive, and behavioral instability.

A *Level 5 feelings rating* is an out-of-control feeling that results in the individual harming himself, others, or property. Often, either a Level 5 is a catastrophe or it is a Level 4 situation that escalates to Level 5 due to a lack of skills use. In the latter case, the actual sensations of a Level 5 may or may not be different than a Level 4, but the individual is overwhelmed and unable to contain his behaviors.

Each individual's appraisal of what out-of-control behaviors or what harming self, others, or property means may be different. One person may rate her anger at Level 5 when she yells at someone (hurting the person emotionally and injuring the relationship), while someone else may view behaviors such as slamming doors, storming around, and/or yelling as not directly causing harm, and may therefore rate them at Level 4. Just as each person's perceptions of what is on track and off track are individualized, feelings rating is a personal process.

At Level 5, All-the-Time skills are necessary. Clear Picture, On-Track Thinking, On-Track Action, Safety Plan, and multiple New-Me Activities generally are necessary to help the individual reduce high-level feelings. These skills help the individual regain the control and capacity to function safely. The situation may require Problem Solving, Expressing Myself, Getting It Right, and/or Relationship Care at a later point, but the individual must utilize other skills to reduce the level of escalation prior to engaging in these interactive skills.

Categories of Skills

There are two Categories of Skills. The first five skills (Clear Picture, On-Track Thinking, On-Track Action, Safety Plan, and New-Me Activities) are All-the-Time skills that can be used at any level of emotion, 0–5. When a person is over a Level 3, it is imperative that All-the-Time skills are used. All-the-Time skills are designed to help the person self-regulate internal factors.

Knowing how and when to step back and self-regulate emotions through All-the-Time skills is crucial to reaching personal goals. Table 2.1 lists the All-the-Time and Calm-Only skills.

The second Category of Skills is Calm-Only skills. The last four skills (Problem Solving, Expressing Myself, Getting It Right, and Relationship Care) often require interaction with other people and should therefore be used *only* when an individual is calm. If a person is even a tiny bit higher than a Level 3 feeling, All-the-Time skills should be used first.

Calm-Only skills are essential in helping the individual manage social relationships. Interacting with others and getting personal needs met is a challenging, ever-changing, ongoing process. Calm-Only skills are more complex, multistep, and take longer to complete than All-the-Time skills. The individual must continually use skills chains (e.g., "1236," "1237," "1238," "1239") to remain on track during these experiences. When doing Problem Solving, Expressing Myself, Getting It Right, and Relationship Care, there are more variables and more opportunities for the environment to drive the individual's feelings up.

Despite the increased risks, it is essential that the individual engage in Calm-Only skills to manage her life. A key factor is knowing when she is able to do them effectively given her level of feeling. Avoidance of Calm-Only skills can be associated with patterns of off-track behavior. For example, if the individual avoids Problem Solving, problems grow, become overwhelming, and lead to off-track actions.

The Category of Skills is used during On-Track Thinking—Making a Skills Plan. At that point, the person reflects on his current level of emotion (via Clear Picture) and determines which skills can be used. If the level is over a 3, All-the-Time skills are the only option for the moment. If 0–3, then both All-the-Time and Calm-Only skills can be used.

Recipe for Skills

The Recipe for Skills is a System Tool that helps calculate the minimum number of skills are necessary in any situation. It is intended generally to guide the individual to use more skills at higher levels of feeling. Medium, strong, and overwhelming feelings have higher intensity and last longer. Spanning a skills chain across those events increases the likelihood of getting through it successfully.

The Recipe for Skills is a conceptual framework that offers guiding principles about assem-

TABLE 2.1. **Categories of Skills**	
All-the-Time Skills **(Level 0–5 emotions)**	**Calm-Only Skills** **(Level 0–3 emotions)**
1. Clear Picture	6. Problem Solving
2. On-Track Thinking	7. Expressing Myself
3. On-Track Action	8. Getting It Right
4. Safety Plan	9. Relationship Care
5. New-Me Activities	

bling skills chains. It is not a prescription about the number of skills that must be linked; it highlights minimum requirements. A Skills Master learns quickly that using longer chains of All-the-Time and Calm-Only skills at low levels of emotion (0–3) is more effective than following the Recipe for Skills minimum recommendations. The Recipe is useful during the skills planning process (e.g., at Level 4, five All-the-Time skill are needed) and to help the individual look back on experiences to see whether ample skills were used. For example, if an individual is reflecting on an off-track incident, he may be able to see that he used no skills at a Level 4, when at least Level 5 skills were needed.

Each individual may use the Recipe for Skills differently. During the initial skills learning phases the Recipe for Skills may be used more consciously; as building skills chains becomes more automatic, checking the Recipe is less necessary. The cognitive demands of the Recipe for Skills may impact individuals differently at different times. For example, if the individual has difficulty with simple math concepts, the Recipe for Skills could trigger emotional reactions that reduce cognitive functioning rather than improve focus. Conversely, for other people, reflecting on what skills have been used and doing the simple math computation can improve focus in the moment. The Recipe for Skills is a general guideline rather than a complex math equation or strict rules to overengineer skills plans.

The Recipe for Skills recommends that the individual use *at least* one skill for every level of feeling, including Level 0.

- At Level 0, the person should continue to have a Clear Picture of the current moment, although there may not be a prompting event that evokes any responses.
- At Level 1, at least two skills are needed. When the individual feels a twinge of feeling, it is helpful to use Clear Picture and On-Track Thinking. This is a "12" skills chain. It is likely that the individual will surpass this requirement and take various On-Track Actions that include the other All-the Time and Calm-Only skills.
- At Level 2, at least three skills are necessary. Doing Clear Picture, On-Track Thinking, and On-Track Action would often be recommended.
- At Level 3, at least four skills are needed. Any number of skills chains can be created at this level (e.g., "1234," "1235," "1236," "1237," "1238," "1239"). If there is risk, a "1234" (Safety Plan) may be best, or if the individual is bored, a "1235" (New-Me Activity). If the individual has a problem to be solved, "1236" may work well. If he wants to express something, "1237" may be a good option. If he needs something from someone, "1238" may be useful. If he wants to sort out a Relationship Care issue, a "1239" may work. Longer chains that combine multiple All-the-Time and/or Calm-Only skills may be even more effective (e.g., "12345," "123455," "12367," "12378," "12379") .
- At Level 4, at least four skills are needed. Because the individual is over a Level 3, the five skills must be All-the-Time skills. A common skills chain for when the individual is at Level 4 is "12345." At Level 4, when there may be off-track urges and off-track actions, doing a Safety Plan helps the individual manage the risk, and engaging in New-Me Activities can focus attention.
- At Level 5, at least six skills are needed. Since there are only five All-the-Time skills, it is necessary to double up on one of the All-the-Time skills. For example, the individual may use multiple New-Me Activities. In that case, he would get a Clear Picture, use On-Track Thinking,

take an On-Track Action, do a Safety Plan, and engage in two New-Me Activities (e.g., playing a video game and listen to music in his room). The individual could choose to double up on On-Track Actions such as Accept the Situation or Turn the Page.

TRANSITION TO CHAPTER 3

Chapter 3 introduces the multiple models that create the theoretical foundation for the Skills System. This information teaches the skills trainer about emotion regulation, the development of the Skills System as a DBT-based curriculum, and cognitive load theory. These frameworks not only help the reader better understand the Skills System but they also expand the practitioner's capacities to teach the material to individuals who experience complex learning and mental health issues.

CHAPTER 3

Theoretical Underpinning of the Skills System

This chapter begins with an exploration of the "modal model" of emotion generation (Gross & Thompson, 2009, p. 5; Gross, 2014a), as well as the "process model" of emotion regulation (p. 10). Next, the chapter reviews cognitive factors associated with the diagnosis of ID that may impact emotion regulation capacity and skills integration. Additional behavioral, environmental, and mental health factors that commonly transact to impact the individual's emotional functioning are introduced. This foundational information helps the clinician to better understand the multitude of complex internal and environmental factors that are relevant when teaching emotion regulation skills.

The second half of the chapter delves into the design of the Skills System, which triangulates three theoretical frameworks as the underpinning of the model. Emotion regulation strategies (Gross & Thompson, 2009; Gross, 2014a), principles of DBT, and cognitive load theory are integrated as the basis for the Skills System. DBT is a comprehensive cognitive-behavioral method designed to treat emotional, cognitive, and behavioral regulation problems. This population's multiple vulnerability factors create the need for DBT treatment, yet simultaneously hinder accessibility to the DBT model. This chapter explains how cognitive load theory (CLT) guided the transformation of emotion regulation and DBT skills concepts into an accessible curriculum. CLT principles impact the design of the Skills System and influence the instruction strategies.

> The biosocial theory, the theoretical underpinning of DBT, is presented as it relates to skills training in the Introduction (pp. 5–11) and later in the Teaching Notes (pp. 138–143) of the *DBT Skills Training Manual, Second Edition* (Linehan, 2015a).

EMOTIONS AND EMOTION REGULATION

The Skills System is designed to help an individual modulate emotions, cognitions, and actions, which are foundational skills for improving quality of life and reaching personal goals. This section of the chapter provides for the skills trainer basic information about emotions and emotion regulation strategies. The "modal model" of emotion generation and the "process model" of emotion regulation are two constructs that can give the trainer a basic understanding of elements that improve self-regulation capacities (Gross & Thompson, 2009).

The facts that emotions trigger quickly and an individual with ID often lacks the meta-cognitive awareness and mastery of adaptive coping strategies, contribute to challenges transitioning effectively through the phases of an emotion. Gross's modal model breaks an emotion into component parts that allows the individual to build capacities in each of the stages. Task analysis approaches are commonly used in the disabilities field to ensure that an individual has discrete skills that can be integrated into more complex chains. Without capacities in each area, assembly of adaptive coping chains is less likely. An individual with severe learning challenges not only needs the capacities to "be in the moment," as in standard DBT, but she must develop skills to "be in the second" to navigate the entire process of an emotion. The Skills System offers supports for all stages of an emotion, so that the generalization of skills is more possible.

The Modal Model of Emotion

Gross and Thompson (2009) describe a "modal model" of emotion generation as a four-part sequence: situation–attention–appraisal–response. The individual first experiences a *situation*. He brings *attention* to the situation because it is relevant to his goals. The relevance or meaning of the situation elicits the emotion. The individual then makes an *appraisal* or assessment about the situation or the emotion that leads to an emotional *response*. Emotional responses involve experiential, behavioral, and neurobiological systems.

Emotions can be of utility to an individual but may also impede progress toward personal goals. Cultivating helpful emotions and managing those that are detrimental are key aspects of emotion regulation (Gross, 2013). Gross explains that most people want to increase positive emotions (e.g., happiness, love, and joy) and decrease negative emotions (e.g., sadness, fear, and anger).

There are different types of emotion regulation. For example, "intrinsic" emotion regulation occurs when the individual initiates strategies to regulate herself, and an "extrinsic" process occurs when someone outside helps regulate her emotion (Gross, 2013, p. 359). Similarly, implicit emotion regulation strategies are not implemented consciously (e.g., one may look away quickly to avoid seeing something unpleasant) and other techniques are explicit. Explicit emotion regulation techniques are used when the individual engages in behaviors to manage an emotion (Gross, 2013).

The Skills System utilizes each of these four types of emotion regulation strategies. Although the Skills System is built to increase intrinsic emotion regulation capacities, it also provides a common language for *in vivo* skills coaches to offer extrinsic emotion regulation support (specific skills coaching techniques are presented in Chapter 8). Additionally, the Skills System structure has implicit emotion regulation strategies built into the design and explicit elements (Skills and System Tools) to manage emotions.

It is important for skills trainers to understand how basic strategies function to up- and down-regulate emotions. Sheppes et al. (2014) explain that different emotion regulation techniques have different impacts in various contexts. For example, the use of distraction has benefits and costs. Distracting oneself requires minimal cognitive capacity and can be an effective strategy in certain situations to reduce reactions to high-emotion information, yet "motivationally it does not allow processing, evaluating, and remembering emotional information, which are crucial for one's long term goals and adaptation" (p. 165). Conversely, "reappraisal" (altering the situation's meaning to change its impact; Gross & Thompson, 2009), may increase the intensity of a response and be a more complex cognitive task, yet it allows emotional engagement with the information that supports reaching long-term goals (Sheppes et al., 2014). "Suppression" is a behaviorally oriented strategy in which the individual restricts emotion-expressive behavior (Gross, 2014a). Suppression has been shown to decrease positive emotional experiences, but it does not reduce negative ones. In fact, suppression increases arousal levels, reduces memory function, and creates stress within relationships (Gross & Thompson, 2009; Gross, 2014a). These various functions and outcomes highlight the advantage of having a broad set of skills that can strategically up- or down-regulate emotions in ways that respond to each moment in a flexible way depending on the individual's needs.

Regulating emotions relies on many factors that are changeable; therefore, it is common for misregulation to occur (Gross, 2013). Gross explains that when an individual does not regulate emotions, it may be due to "simple tracking failures" related to inaccurately anticipating outcomes of certain responses (p. 362). The individual may also choose a strategy that does not function to reach the intended goal (e.g., choosing suppression to increase positive emotions).

Understanding Stimulus and Response Selection

These types of miscalculations may be related to how the individual is processing an experience. Hübner, Steinhauser, and Lehle (2010) present a "dual-stage two-phase process model" for attention selection that can help the trainer better understand the different stages of processing and how responding at these different stages can impact a strategy's effectiveness. A warning is that this model may create high cognitive load for the reader.

According to the dual-stage two-phase process model, there are two stages in the process of creating an emotional response: stimulus selection and response selection (Hübner et al., 2010). There are two stages of stimulus selection: an "early" and a "late" stage (p. 761). In the early stage of stimulus selection, the individual utilizes "perceptual filtering" to process a broad array of information; the individual is aware of both useful and extraneous information without discriminating (p. 761). In the late stage, the individual focuses attention on one stimulus or target. Initiating emotion regulation strategies with the information provided during the early stage is considered to be the "first phase" of stimulus response. These first-phase responses that rely on nondiscriminated information of the early stage are often rapid, inaccurate responses, and do not allow for processing, evaluating, and remembering emotional information (Hübner et al., 2010; Sheppes et al., 2014).

Conversely, "second-phase" responses happen during late-stage stimulus selection; these are focused and targeted. Second-phase responses may be slower (due to the more elaborated processing), yet they are more accurate and reliable. These second-phase responses also allow individuals to process, evaluate, and remember emotional information that is essential for learning, adapting, and reaching long-term goals (Sheppes et al., 2014).

Expanding and Structuring Processing

As an individual has increased awareness and learned multiple strategies to regulate emotions, options beyond reactivity become available. The Skills System offers strategies and a structure to support this process. For example, the six Clear Picture Do's guide the individual through the process of focusing attention. On-Track Thinking offers four steps that lead the individual through the appraisal process. On-Track Actions (which include all of the skills) are options for effective responses. The System Tools help integrate and organize these processes to address stimuli in different situations. Figure 3.1 illustrates how the Skills System cognitive framework provides schemata that help the individual navigate through late-stage second-phase emotion regulation coping responses. Although, both first- and second-phase responses are important at different times; having a spectrum of capacities reduces undifferentiated reactivity and gives the individual ample tools to be effective in diverse situations.

The Process Model of Emotion Regulation and the Skills System

It is helpful for the skills trainer to understand principles of emotion regulation. Gross (2013) describes five "families" of emotion regulation strategies that align an emotion regulation response to each of the steps of the emotion-generative cycle (e.g., situation–attention–appraisal–response; p. 360). These emotion regulation response categories are "situation selection, situation modification, attentional deployment, cognitive change, and response modulation" (Gross, 2014a, p. 7; see also Gross 2013; Gross & Thompson, 2009). These five functions are embedded within the Skills System design. The following sections define each of the families and highlight how the emotion regulation strategies are integrated into the Skills System process.

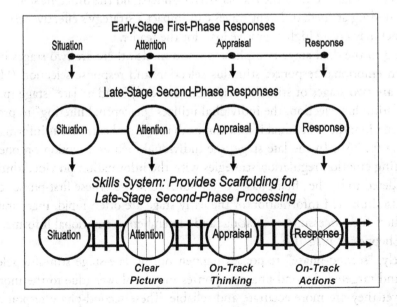

FIGURE 3.1. Scaffolding for late-stage processing.

Situation Selection

Situation selection occurs when one "takes actions that make it more (or less) likely that the individual will end up in a situation we expect will give rise to desirable (or undesirable) emotions" (Gross, 2014a, p. 9). A situation selection response anticipates outcomes and chooses a course of action that facilitates a desired goal. The accuracy of both reflections of the past and perceptions about the future regarding anticipated levels of emotion is less reliable than the awareness in the current moment; therefore, anticipating the impact of an event can be biased (Gross & Thompson, 2009).

The Skills System's first three skills (Clear Picture, On-Track Thinking, and On-Track Action—skills chain "123") provide a structure or path that leads the individual to understand the situation, focus attention, make an appraisal, and execute a response. First, Clear Picture helps her focus and understand the current moment. Second, On-Track Thinking guides her to reflect on potential outcomes, appraise current options, and make a situation selection plan. Third, On-Track Action is a goal-directed response.

Other skills can be used in situation selection. For example, Safety Plans can be used proactively to select safe, and avoid risky, situations. Choosing to do New-Me Activities can increase positive emotions.

Situation Modification

Gross (2014a) describes situation modification as "efforts to directly modify the situation so as to alter its emotional impact" (p. 9). Situation modification can include the efforts the individual makes to control his external environment. Additionally, the environment can offer emotion regulation support that modifies the individual's situation; collateral supporters can offer verbal praise and coping support as extrinsic forms of situation modification.

Several Skills System skills are used in situation modification. For example, Safety Plans are a way to reactively (and proactively) manage risky situations. The Calm-Only skills (Problem Solving, Expressing Myself, Getting It Right, and Relationship Care) are means to make adjustments and be engaged in situations. Problem Solving helps the individual change problematic circumstances; Expressing Myself can communicate needs to others; Getting It Right can facilitate the individual getting what she wants from the environment; and Relationship Care can build, balance, and change relationships. Gross explains that situation modification creates a new situation and opportunity for situation selection (Gross, 2014a). The Skills System is built to reflect this pattern; as the individual completes a skills chain she returns to Clear Picture to begin another skills chain in the new situation.

Attentional Deployment

Attentional deployment is how the individual "directs attention within a given situation in order to influence one's emotions" (Gross, 2014a, p. 10). When the individual shifts attention toward or away from a situation, emotions may be altered. "Distraction" is one form of attentional deployment. Shifting external or internal attention away from something, or to a different part of it, can serve to alter emotion intensity. "Concentration" is an attentional deployment strategy that involves increasing focus on a situation or feature of it. "Ruminating" occurs when the individual repeatedly focuses on the emotion and consequences. Ruminating on sad events may increase depressed moods. Ruminating on threats in the future may create low-level anxiety but ultimately reduce the intensity of strong negative responses (Gross & Thompson, 2009). With attentional deployment, the individual is selecting what to focus on; it is like an internal version of situation selection (Gross & Thompson, 2009).

Individuals diagnosed with ID experience conceptual deficits (outlined in the next section) that may impact the individual's capacities to manage attention strategically. The Skills System provides both implicit and explicit emotion regulation strategies to help maximize the individual's ability to deploy attention strategically. For example, if an individual has impaired executive functioning, she may not have the capacity to sustain attention to solve a complex problem. Therefore, the Skills System's implicit structure and explicit skills (stored in long-term memory) are designed to guide attentional deployment through the complex multistep process of Problem Solving.

Individuals diagnosed with ID have difficulties with attentional transitions. Factors such as uncertainty about the unknown, low self-efficacy, and fight–flight responses are factors that hinder effective progression through coping processes. The Skills System infrastructure reduces the fear of the unknown because the nine skills and System Tools offer learned options that encourage activation rather than trigger avoidance of novel stimuli. Additionally, individuals diagnosed with ID may experience receptive and expressive language deficits that impact emotion regulation capacities. Gross and Thompson (2009) explain that language facilitates the understanding, communication of, reflection on, and modulating of emotions. The Skills System skills and tools provide language to help the individual generate intrinsic emotion regulation strategies and receive accessible extrinsic support to modulate emotions.

Situations that elicit strong emotions are often complex and multidimensional. It can be difficult to focus attention and appraise overwhelming experiences. Breaking down complicated situations in fathomable/manageable steps facilitates effective completion of the general emotion regulation task. The Skills System breaks down an experience into chunks of information that facilitate and sustain attentional deployment.

Each skill and its component parts are small, understandable chunks of information. The individual learns to navigate through a series of these elements, making *microtransitions* across the span of an emotion. For example, the Clear Picture skill has six parts (breathe, notice surroundings, body check, label and rate feeling, notice thoughts, and notice urges), each elaborating information about the current moment. As the individual deploys attention to these different aspects of her internal and external moment, later-stage second-phase responses can occur. Similarly, the individual deploys attention to the microtransitions within On-Track Thinking. By doing the sequence Check It, Turn It Up, Cheerleading, and making a Skills Plan in a situation, the individual shifts attention through a structured, yet flexible, appraisal process. As the individual becomes increasingly able to selectively control attention, she is better able to modulate internal and external experiences. Shifting attention through multiple microtransitions from one task to another within a skill, and from one skill to another, allows the individual to focus in the moment and be able to execute goal-directed behavior. Additionally, having capacities to regulate effectively through all parts of an emotion event may increase the individual's abilities to be present in the moment as it is, reduce polarizing reactions, increase opportunities for synthesis of conflicting points, and facilitate understanding of abstract concepts.

Attentional deployment is a foundational part of On-Track Action—Switch Tracks. In a difficult situation, the individual may use On-Track Thinking to appraise and plan a response, deciding it is important to shift thinking and actions from off-track to on-track. In this case, she does On-Track Action—Switch Tracks to generate thoughts and execute behaviors that head her in the direction of her goals.

New-Me Activities also involve the emotion regulation skill of attentional deployment. Focus New-Me Activities can increase concentration on an organizing activity to counteract the disorganizing impact of cognitive dysregulation. Distraction New-Me Activities can assist the individual in diverting attention from triggers that may increase emotions.

Cognitive Change

Cognitive change is when the individual modifies "how one appraises a situation so as to alter its emotional significance, either by changing how one thinks about the situation or about one's capacities to manage the demands it poses" (Gross, 2014a, p. 10). The individual can change self-perceptions or adjust thoughts about external factors. Reappraisal (e.g., making lemonade out of lemons) is an important emotion regulation strategy. Individual who use reappraisal tend to experience increased positive emotions and fewer negative ones (Gross, 2013; Nezlek & Kuppens, 2008). Additionally, they have better memory capacities and social relationships (Gross, 2013).

On-Track Thinking is the primary cognitive skill in the Skills System. The Check It portion serves as appraisal function, whereas Turn It Up is a cognitive change strategy. For example, if the individual notices experiencing urges to yell at his boss, he would use Check It to determine whether action urges are going to get him to his goal. If the urge is given a "thumbs down," Turn It Up follows, prompting the individual to generate thoughts that are in service of the goal. Cheerleading and other goal-directed thoughts can mobilize goal-directed actions.

Response Modulation

Response modulation strategies, "occur late in the emotion-generation process, after response tendencies have already been initiated, and refers to directly influencing experiential, behavioral, or physiological components of emotional response" of an emotion (Gross, 2014a, p. 10). Actions such as exercise and relaxation can reduce the physiological impact of emotions (Gross & Thompson, 2009). Emotion-expressive behaviors are often used to modulate responses, but can slightly increase the intensity of emotions. Inhibiting emotion expression reduces positive emotions but not negative ones; it also increases "sympathetic activation" (p. 15). Gross and Thompson highlight that effectiveness of emotions regulation depends on the "availability of adaptive response alternative for expressing emotion, such as to provoke problem solving or interpersonal understanding, rather than simply venting" (p. 15).

New-Me Activities are commonly used as response modulation strategies. Focus New-Me

Activities can be done to engage attention while arousal levels decrease. Progressive relaxation and patterned breathing exercises can help the individual focus attention and relax. Feel Good New-Me Activities are designed to help the individual self-soothe by engaging in pleasant sensory experiences to help her tolerate the distress. Distraction and Fun New-Me Activities can be useful as response modulation strategies.

The next section of this chapter shifts from a focus on emotions to exploration of cognitive factors that impact emotion regulation of individuals diagnosed with ID. Affective and cognitive systems interact; therefore, it is crucial for a skills trainer to understand cognitive deficits that impact (1) emotion regulation, (2) skills acquisition, and (3) skills instruction.

COGNITIVE FACTORS

The fields of emotion regulation and neuroscience research are evolving rapidly; therefore, practitioners working in the ID field should stay current with the fast-emerging literature. Unfortunately, research is limited in many important areas associated with disabled compared to non-disabled populations (Forte, Jahoda, & Dagnan, 2011; Reilly & Holland, 2011; Sappok et al., 2013). The heterogeneous nature of this population and lack of rigorous research designs used with individuals diagnosed with ID further complicates access to and utility of the available resources (Forte et al., 2011; Reilly & Holland, 2011; Sappok et al., 2013).

DSM-5 (American Psychiatric Association, 2013) provides criteria for diagnosing individuals with intellectual developmental disorder, which I refer to simply as "intellectual disability," or ID. Although the information is general, it does define deficits in conceptual, social, and practical factors commonly associated with individuals diagnosed with ID. By understanding the nature of cognitive impairments associated with a diagnosis of ID, skills trainers can better understand how cognitive functioning capacities impact emotion regulation, adaptive functioning, and ultimately effective design/instruction of interventions.

Many DSM-5 diagnoses include criteria that highlight impaired cognitive functioning of different kinds. Although the Skills System is utilized with different populations, it was designed to accommodate the pervasive cognitive impairment that individuals with ID experience. Because this model is built to address these intense learning needs, it may increase accessibility for other individuals who experience less significant learning challenges. High emotion degrades cognitive processing abilities for people, so one might argue that the simplified model could promote recall and adaptive functioning in high-stress situations for nondisabled individuals as well.

It is important that skills trainers working with individuals diagnosed with ID have a strengths-based mindset. Simultaneously, it is helpful to be realistic about barriers the individuals may have. By understanding deficits, it is possible to maximize existing cognitive resources and mobilize strengths.

DSM-5 criteria do not highlight strengths; they define deficits. Although the DSM-5 framework potentially fuels stereotypes and marginalization of this population, it is used here to define what capacities may require enhanced supports. To be able to mobilize intact capacities and strengths (e.g., tacit knowledge), it is necessary to understand better both internal and external factors that influence an individual's capacity to process information and engage in explicit learning.

DSM-5 Criteria for ID

Criterion A highlights the conceptual deficits an individual diagnosed with ID commonly experiences. It states that the individual has difficulty with "reasoning, problem solving, planning, abstract thinking, judgment, academic learning, and learning from experience" (American Psychiatric Association, 2013, p. 33). In the clarification of diagnostic features it states that capacities such as "verbal comprehension, working memory, perceptual reasoning, and quantitative reasoning" (p. 33) are impaired.

A table in DSM-5 highlights factors associated with the four severity levels of ID (mild, moderate, severe, and profound). It explains that school-age individuals with mild-severity ID experience difficulties mastering academic tasks such as reading, writing, arithmetic, money skills, and understanding concepts of time. These youth reportedly utilize more concrete problem-solving strategies than do their agemates. The adults diagnosed with mild severity have impaired "abstract thinking, executive function (i.e., planning, strategizing, priority setting, and cognitive flexibility), short-term memory, as well as functional use of academic skills" (American Psychiatric Association, 2013, p. 34). Although preschool youth with mild ID may not show significant conceptual differences from nondisabled agemates, those with moderate-severity ID show clear delays. Adults diagnosed with moderate severity progress to elementary academic levels and require ongoing daily living supports.

Criterion B defines impairments that impact adaptive functioning, impede development, and hinder the individual's capacities for independent social functioning. More specifically, the criterion states that deficits limit functioning in at least one area of daily living (communication, social participation, independent living skills) across residential, vocational, and educational settings. In the social domain for individuals diagnosed with mild ID, it states that there may be difficulties with emotion and behavioral regulation. Criterion C states that the onset of the impairments that span conceptual, social, and practical domains is during the developmental period (American Psychiatric Association, 2013, p. 33). Table 3.1 provides brief definitions from the *APA Dictionary of Psychology* (American Psychological Association, 2007) of the deficits outlined in DSM-5 diagnostic criteria.

Emotion regulation and cognitive capacities impact each other. Cognitive deficits impede the execution of effective emotion regulation strategies. Similarly, emotions reduce cognitive processing capacities. A multitude of other vulnerability factors transact to impact the individual's abilities to regulate emotions. For example, individuals diagnosed with ID experience behavioral dysregulation, environmental stress, and mental health issues. It is important that skills trainers understand (1) the impact these factors have on the individual's abilities and (2) the natural environment within which the individual will need to generalize skills.

BEHAVIORAL FACTORS

Although the source of an individual's behavioral regulation difficulties may be related to a combination of emotional, cognitive, environmental, and mental health issues, often individuals are referred for mental health services to address behavioral problems (Bhaumik, Tyrer, McGrother, & Ganghadaran, 2008; Hurley, 2008; Russell, Hahn, & Hayward, 2011). The

TABLE 3.1. Commonly Occurring Psychological Terms in DSM-5 Diagnostic Criteria and Their Definitions

Terms	Definitions
Verbal comprehension	Ability to understand the language used by others that is impacted by receptive vocabulary and language skills (p. 979).
Short-term memory	The capacity to perform reproduction, recognition, and recall of a limited amount of information after approximately 10–30 seconds (p. 850).
Working memory	The model of short-term memory that consists of the phonological loop (verbal information), visuospatial scratchpad (visual information), and the central executive that coordinates attention between them (p. 1003).
Learning from experience	Gaining new knowledge, behavior patterns, or abilities as a result of practice, study, or experience (p. 529).
Academic learning	Learning with theoretical and conventional study in educational settings (p. 5).
Abstract thinking	Thinking that uses abstraction. Abstraction involves the capacity to understand intangible concepts (p. 4).
Quantitative reasoning	Reasoning uses logic through a process of deduction and induction to draw conclusions (p. 774). The term "quantitative" is associated with utilizing numbers (p. 763).
Perceptual reasoning	Perception is awareness of objects, events, and relationships via sensory stimuli; it is associated with observing, recognizing, and discriminating (p. 638).
Problem solving	The process of planning and action that overcomes barriers to goals that often requires mental functions such as reasoning and creativity (p. 735).
Priority setting	The ability to determine that something or someone is more important and dealing with that first (*www.merriamwebster.com/dictionary/priority*).
Planning	The process of creating a mental representation of an intended action that potentially guides the individual to initiate the action (p. 705).
Strategizing	The process of developing a plan of action designed to reach a goal (p. 897).
Cognitive flexibility	The ability to make appraisals and take actions that demonstrate adaptability, objectivity, and fair-mindedness (p. 189).
Judgment	The ability to be awareness of relationships, draw conclusions from the information, and make critical evaluation of the people and situations (p. 509).

Note. Unless otherwise indicated, page numbers refer to the *APA Dictionary of Psychology* (American Psychological Association, 2007).

term "challenging behaviors" is frequently used in the disabilities' literature to describe behaviors at a level of intensity, duration, and frequency that places the individual or others at risk for physical harm that limits the use of ordinary community facilities (Emerson et al., 2001). Some common forms of challenging behaviors include aggression, pica, self-injury, property destruction, and sexual offending (Brown et al., 2013; Matson, Neal, & Kozlowski, 2012).

There is variability in the prevalence rates of challenging behavior. For example, the rates are as low as 10–15% (Emerson et al., 2001; Lowe et al., 2007; Tyrer et al., 2006) to 85% of institutionalized adults with profound intellectual and multiple disabilities engaged in self-injurious behaviors (Poppes, van der Putten, & Vlaskamp, 2010). Grey, Pollard, McClean, MacAuley, and Hastings (2010) found that 45% of a sample (N = 159) of individuals diagnosed with mild to moderate ID living in a community-based setting had challenging behaviors. Although there is variability within these findings, there is a consensus that behavioral problems impact the lives of many individuals diagnosed with ID and create significant challenges for support providers.

The Skills System offers a framework that teaches behavioral regulation skills to individuals diagnosed with ID. Common responses to challenging behaviors (e.g., behavioral treatment planning, environmental supports, and staff supervision) do not offer a comprehensive system of self-regulation strategies that address the core regulation deficits. Traditional interventions may be important elements of an integrated plan (as shown in Brown et al., 2013); adding Skills System training and DBT individual therapy may offer an enhanced level of treatment necessary to address reinforced patterns of emotional, cognitive, and behavioral dysregulation.

ENVIRONMENTAL FACTORS

The literature has described several transacting factors that contribute to challenging behaviors, a prominent one of which is environmental factors. For example, relationships with support providers are associated with individuals diagnosed with ID exhibiting behavioral dyscontrol (McGrath, 2013; Phillips & Rose, 2010). Experiences such as residing in congregate living situations and receiving staff supervision can increase stress; high frustration paired with inadequate coping skills may result in behavioral impulsivity (Crocker, Mercier, Allaire, & Roy, 2007; Janssen, Schuengel, & Stolk, 2002; Matson et al., 2012). Additionally, challenging social environments and insufficient emotion regulation skills, combined with insecure attachments, may be associated with prevalence of challenging behaviors (Janssen et al., 2002).

Heightened social stigma is a force that impacts individuals on multiple levels. The manifestations and impact of social stigma (e.g., biases devaluing individuals with ID; limited residential and vocational resources) may worsen problematic social transactions that maintain behavioral dysregulation (Crocker et al., 2007). Stigmatization can lower self-efficacy, exacerbate mental health issues, and reduce access to adequate health and mental health services (Ali et al., 2013; Ditchman et al., 2013).

MENTAL HEALTH FACTORS

Individuals with ID experience higher rates of co-occurring mental illness than the general population (Bhaumik et al., 2008; Weiss, 2012). It is difficult to understand prevalence, because diagnosis of mental health disorders is complicated by the impact of diagnostic overshadowing and expressive–receptive language deficits (Mevissen, Lievegoed, Seubert, & De Jongh, 2011). Additionally, individuals with ID and co-occurring mental health diagnoses may exhibit different symptoms than people without ID (Hurley, 2008; Mevissen et al., 2011).

Individuals with ID also experience more traumatic experiences (e.g., neglect, physical abuse, witnessing violence, and sexual abuse) than nondisabled people (Beadle-Brown, Mansell, Cambridge, Milne, & Whelton, 2010; Horner-Johnson & Drum, 2006). Despite these higher rates, there are limited assessment tools and treatment options for individuals with ID who exhibit symptoms of posttraumatic stress disorder (PTSD; Mevissen et al., 2011; Mitchell, Clegg, & Furniss, 2006; Turk, Robbins, & Woodhead, 2005). Trauma impacts emotional and cognitive functioning; individuals with ID and histories of trauma may exhibit challenging behaviors, increase anxiety, sleep disturbances, and irritability that are not necessarily attributed to PTSD (Turk, Robbins, & Woodhead, 2005).

It is useful to conceptualize challenging behaviors as a symptom of a mental health issue rather than the primary problem (Glaesser & Perkins, 2013; Hurley, 2008). Because of the tendency to utilize psychotropic medications to treat challenging behaviors, it is vital to assess mental health issues separately from behavioral problems (Matson et al., 2012). Utilizing psychopharmacology to manage behaviors versus treating specific mental health diagnoses may lead to polypharmacy and problematic side effects of medications (Hess et al., 2010; Matson, Rivet, & Fodstad, 2010).

Emotion regulation capacities of individuals diagnosed with ID are impacted by a broad array of cognitive, behavioral, environmental, and mental health factors. McClure, Halpern, Wolper, and Donahue (2009) reported that although research related to emotion regulation in the general population is expanding rapidly, there is still minimal information regarding emotion regulation, associated factors, or treatment for people with ID. Given the lack of options for individuals diagnosed with ID, exploring the use of DBT (which is an empirically validated treatment for nondisabled individuals who have co-occurring mental health diagnoses and problems associated with emotional dysregulation) is justified.

DIALECTICAL BEHAVIOR THERAPY

DBT is a comprehensive cognitive-behavioral model developed by Linehan (1993a, 1993b, 2015a, 2015b) to treat individuals with borderline personality disorder (BPD). To date, several published randomized controlled trials have highlighted the efficacy of DBT with clients with BPD (Feigenbaum et al., 2011; Hill, Craighead, & Safer, 2011; Harned, Jackson, Comtois, & Linehan, 2010; Neacsiu, Rizvi, & Linehan, 2010; Linehan, Armstrong, Suarez, Allmon, & Heard, 1991; Linehan et al., 2006; Priebe et al., 2012; van den Bosch, Verheul, Schippers, & van den Brink, 2002; van den Bosch, Koeter, Verheul, & van den Brink, 2005); Verheul et al., 2003). The application of DBT has been expanded to treat other populations of clients with various types of mental illnesses and who experience intense levels of dysregulation. Randomized controlled studies empirically support the efficacy of DBT in treating populations with substance abuse (Linehan et al., 1999, 2002), those with eating disorders (Safer & Joyce, 2011; Telch, Agras, & Linehan, 2001; Safer, Robinson, & Joyce, 2010; Safer, Telch, & Agras, 2001), female veterans with BPD symptoms (Koons et al., 2001), and older adults with depression (Lynch, Morse, Mendelson, & Robins, 2003). The expanding validation for using DBT with diverse populations supports exploring the utilization of DBT with individuals with ID.

There is an emerging literature exploring the use of DBT with individuals with ID. Most are case studies and small-n nonexperimental designs. All of the published efficacy studies utilized modified versions of the standard DBT skills curriculum versus standard skills manuals (Brown et al., 2013; Inam Ul, 2013; Lew, Matta, Tripp-Tebo, & Watts, 2006; Sakdalan & Collier, 2009; Sakdalan & Collier, 2012). Modifications include simplification of the language, use of visual aid materials, reorganization of the modules, and adjusted treatment timelines (Brown et al., 2013; Inam Ul, 2013; Sakdalan & Collier, 2012).

Increasing the Accessibility of DBT

DBT is an evidence-based treatment; adapting it invalidates this empirical support. Given the spectrum of challenges this population experiences, it is justified to make accommodations to improve accessibility to DBT principles. The Skills System design integrates elements of CLT (Sweller, 1988, 2010) to create a DBT-based emotion regulation skills curriculum that can be learned and generalized by individuals diagnosed with ID. The following section introduces CLT principles.

Cognitive Load Theory

The Skills System is a treatment tool that integrates (1) DBT principles and skills (Linehan, 1993a, 1993b, 2015a, 2015b) and (2) emotion regulation strategies (presented in the first section of this chapter). CLT was used to reorganize the DBT and emotion regulation models to address the needs of individuals diagnosed with ID. CLT impacts the design of the Skills System, as well as the theoretical underpinning for skills instruction.

CLT is a learning and instruction theory (Ayres & Paas, 2012; Paas & Sweller, 2012; Paas, Van Gog, & Sweller, 2010; Sweller, 1988, 2010; Sweller, van Merrienboer, & Paas, 1998; Van Gog, Paas, & Sweller, 2010) that is used to design instruction of complex tasks to maximize cognitive functioning capacities and learning. Managing cognitive load is crucial because of the complex nature of emotion regulation and the cognitive challenges this population experiences. CLT works to design interventions in ways that utilize the large resources of long-term memory and limited capacities of working memory (Kalyuga, 2011).

Intrinsic Cognitive Load

The term "cognitive load" represents the amount of mental resources a particular thinking or reasoning task demands (American Psychological Association, 2007, p. 189). There are three types of cognitive load in CLT: intrinsic, extraneous, and germane. Intrinsic cognitive load is the fixed "natural complexity" of information that must be understood (separate from instructional issues); this internal complexity can only be changed by altering the nature of the information or by changing the knowledge level of the learner (Sweller, 2010). High element interactivity increases cognitive load demands, and low interactivity reduces it. "Low interactivity" means that information is presented in discrete components (Sweller, 2010). For example, dividing Clear Picture into six parts that are learned one at a time requires lower cognitive load than a broader concept of mindfulness. Breaking complex, multistep emotion regulation tasks into component parts decreases cognitive load demands. On-Track Thinking schemata consolidate adaptive, goal-directed thinking into four steps (Check It, Turn It Up, Cheerleading, Make a Skills Plan). As these schemata are stored and elaborated in long-term memory, demands on working memory are reduced. Conversely, the standard DBT skills do not describe an explicit thinking process or schemata but instead rely on the learner's ability to consolidate information effectively (while under duress) from the four separate modules.

Connectivity that links discrete bits of information facilitates recall (Kalyuga, 2011). Without an organizing system of parts, retrieval of divergent, unlinked chunks creates high cognitive demand. To address this function, the System Tools (Feelings Rating Scale, Categories of Skills, and Recipe for Skills) guide the assembly of the component skills into skills chains. The DBT skills (Linehan, 1993b, 2015a, 2015b) do not have instructions integrated into the modules to guide skills usage. This type of "search-and-match" design creates cognitive load demands (Kulyuga, 2011, p. 2).

Extraneous Cognitive Load

Sweller (2010) explains that extraneous cognitive load is associated with "nonoptimal instructional procedures" that impede learning. CLT is primarily concerned with techniques designed to reduce extraneous cognitive load (Sweller, 2010). Cognitive overload impairs schema acquisition, which results in a lower performance (Sweller, 1988). The threat of cognitive overload derailing skills acquisition and retrieval is a concern for individuals diagnosed with ID.

Instruction design can increase cognitive load. For example, simultaneous process increases cognitive load demands. If information is introduced at different times or in different areas, it increases demand on working memory. The Skills System instruction strategies introduce the basic elements (nine skills and System Tools) early in the curriculum to begin the process of storing information in long-term memory. Conversely, the standard DBT skills are broken down into four modules that are taught over a series of months; this deconstruction impedes retrieval of skills concepts. When the individual diagnosed with ID is in her natural environment, CL demands are higher and the impact of extraneous cognitive load is more pronounced.

It is important to use terms that do not waste cognitive load resources. Terms that are intrinsic to the task create lower cognitive load demands than does unassociated jargon. For example, the term "On-Track Thinking" contains the concept of being oriented to a goal through the use of the term "on-track"; it is also linked to the term "thinking," which communicates the concepts of goal-directed thinking. This schema draws on existing knowledge stored in long-term memory and creates a relatively low cognitive load demand in relation to the complexity of the concepts that are being retrieved.

Germane Cognitive Load

"Germane cognitive load" refers to the working memory resources the learner devotes to the process (Sweller, 2010). If the extraneous cognitive load is high, germane cognitive load is reduced, because there is more demand on the working memory. If the design of interventions is thoughtful, it is possible to maximize germane cognitive load. Individuals diagnosed with ID have cognitive impairments that impact germane cognitive load levels. Consequently, interventions need to be efficiently designed to minimize cognitive load and maximize cognitive functioning and learning. CLT brings attention to extraneous processing that impedes efficient integration of information.

Factors That Impede Cognitive Functioning

The following five factors impede cognitive functioning (Sweller, 1988).

Simultaneous Processing of Information

Simultaneous processing is required when integrating movement, visual stimuli, and auditory information at the same time. For example, when an individual is playing a board game, the activity may require him to manage visual, auditory, and kinesthetic information to play the game. The activity may tax long-term and working-memory capacities, as well as involve processing information related to the social relationships and context.

High Volume and Interactivity of Information

Cognitive load increases when an individual is asked to (1) recall or manage large amounts of interactive information, (2) assess subtle differences and similarities between elements, and (3) understand intricate relationships between different parts of a whole (especially when there is a deficit of general knowledge about the topic). The Skills System Calm-Only skills are the most interactive tasks; for this reason, it is recommended that the individual be at a low level of emotion to maximize resources.

Retrieval of Divergent Information

Information is "divergent" when it is learned at different times and perhaps within different contexts. For example, if the person learns a piece of information in group and associates that information with specific elements of that experience, it may be challenging to recall the information in a work setting. Multiple cues may be necessary to help the person link the information in divergent contexts.

Rapid Shifts without Transition from One Topic to Another

Quick movement from topic to topic or context to context increases cognitive load. Individuals diagnosed with ID often have difficulty transitioning from one event, location, activity, and relationship to another. For example, the person may experience difficulties during shift change or during a transition to and from a vocational site. Cognitive resources are required to manage shifting contexts. Orienting the individual to changes helps reduce the cognitive load of transitions. Continually reviewing and repeating the construction/execution of Skills System chains process facilitates movement through microtransitions. The familiarity reduces cognitive load demands and allows mastery to develop.

Strong Emotional Responses to Information or While Processing Information

If the individual experiences strong emotional responses while processing information, cognitive demands increase. For example, if the comment, question, or teaching point in skills group discussions address "hot" topics (e.g., living with impairments, victimization, losses, and/or processing past behavioral problems), strong emotions that increase cognitive load may result.

ADAPTING STANDARD DBT FOR ID

An essential DBT principle is to teach the client to "do what works." That same tenet impacted the evolution of the Skills System as a treatment tool for individuals with ID. Although the Skills System retained several standard DBT terms, many DBT concepts had to be repackaged to allow for comprehension and facilitate generalization. The following section will describe the adaptation process.

Directly after I was intensively trained in DBT in 1999, I was dedicated to using the standard DBT skills curriculum (Linehan, 1993b) as written. Very quickly it was clear that modifications were necessary to meet the mandate of skills acquisition, strengthening, and generalization. Wanting to make the least invasive changes, I spent over a year making accommodations through implementing enhanced teaching strategies rather than adapting the standard DBT terms and format. One tactic was to teach a limited number of skills from each module. Key concepts were then sacrificed. Given that DBT is an evidence-based treatment, I was hesitant to omit elements. In order to retain complex or abstract terms (e.g., nonjudgmental, rational, reinforce), I tried breaking skills down into component parts, teaching the meaning of each term in greater depth. This task analysis process simplified individual concepts, but produced large amounts of divergent information that increased cognitive load and hindered generalization. To make the maximum number of DBT concepts available to people with IQs in the range of 45–70, I had to extract and repackage global concepts.

There is precedent for adapting great works to improve access for the masses. For example, children being raised in a Christian tradition often read a children's version of the Bible or stories that contain certain terms so that youth can access and repackage more abstract religious concepts to promote maximum learning. Much of the unfamiliar language and magnitude of information in the King James version would otherwise be barriers to what parents might feel are vital foundational principles. Not dissimilar to the Bible, the DBT concepts are more essential than semantics. People with ID who experience emotional, cognitive, and/or behavioral regulation challenges deserve and need access to core DBT technology.

The Skills System has come full circle. The first versions of the model contained many key DBT terms integrated with several modified ones. There were conflicts in getting copyright permission to disseminate the standard terms, which led to the total extraction of all DBT terms and reliance on DBT concepts alone. In 2014, the collaboration with The Guilford Press allowed me to reintegrate DBT terms that augment the functioning of the Skills System. Happily, many were brought back in; others that were not are there in spirit!

The copyright restrictions, although devastating at the time, were ultimately vital to the functionality of the Skills System. The form had to follow function versus function following a prescribed form. It was necessary to extract essential DBT concepts and reassemble them in a way that facilitated learning and recall. CLT was used to guide the creation of the terms and the framework or "systems" approach. Terms had to be simplified and needed to refer directly to common knowledge language to reduce cognitive load demands on working memory. The number of total concepts had to be reduced and linked conceptually. It had to be a layered system, so that individuals with moderate ID could gain essential DBT concepts through learning just the skills names. Structured emotion regulation progressions were necessary to buttress inconsistent executive functioning capacities, and the framework had to conversely stimulate response flexibility. The abstract concept of dialectics had to be embedded implicitly in the content, process, and teaching, so that individuals diagnosed with ID would learn to adopt a dialectical perspective without needing to explicitly understand the intangible concept.

INTEGRATION OF DBT CONCEPTS

More specifically, the mindfulness skills of "observe," "describe," and "participate" (Linehan, 2015a, p. 166) had to be taken from a principle-driven model and transformed into tangible steps that were integrated into every skills chain. Terms such as "nonjudgmentally" and "one-mindfully" (Linehan, 2015a, p. 166) had to be taught implicitly due to their complexity. Guiding the individual through a sequential progression that encourages targeting attention to systematic use of Checks the Facts in a step-by-step progression leads the individual to act one-mindfully and nonjudgmentally. The Skills System's overarching theme is to help the individual act "effectively," yet that three syllable, abstract term is not directly used due to the extraneous cognitive load demands. Regarding the "states of mind" (Linehan, 2015a, p. 166), the term "emotion mind" is useful, yet the other two terms and the three integrating circles are abstract. Given that "Wise Mind" (Linehan, 2015a, p. 167) is a critical DBT concept, it needed to be woven implicitly into each skills chain. The sequence of Clear Picture, On-Track Thinking, and On-Track Action was designed to facilitate acting in Wise Mind, as well as to integrate a dialectical perspective by creating concrete steps that lead the individual through an acceptance and change process. The six Clear Picture Do's conjoined mindfulness with elements of the "model for describing emotions" (Linehan, 2015a, p. 335) to ensure the individual became aware of important processes that are foundational to effective coping.

The Skills System needed to consolidate adaptive thinking into each skills chain that represented DBT principles. Examples of a "DBT perspective" run throughout the standard DBT skills modules (Linehan, 2015a). For example, worksheet topics such as "effectively," "Wise Mind," "objectives effectiveness," "relationship effectiveness," "self-respect effectiveness," "cheer-leading statements," "options for whether or how intensely to ask for something or say no," "clarifying goals in interpersonal situations," "model for describing emotions," "accumulating positive emotions," "mindfulness of your current moment—letting go of emotional suffering," "observing and describing emotions," "steps for reducing painful emotions," "pros and cons," "cope ahead," and "turning the mind" all address adaptive cognitive processes. The individual with ID is unable to extract concepts from a vast number of divergent sources; therefore, it was necessary to create an adaptive cognitive framework (On-Track Thinking) that consolidated "DBT thinking" into a simple progression that was used in each situation. It was also vital to help individuals with ID understand the difference between skills that require them to be regulated (Calm-Only skills), and ones that can be used effectively at higher levels of emotion (All-the-Time skills). The terms "Wise Mind," "Cheerleading," "Opposite Action," "Problem Solving," "Pros and Cons," "Cope Ahead," and "Turning the Mind" are integrated into the Skills System teaching.

Individuals with ID often have challenges associated with behavioral activation, due to a myriad of factors (e.g., self-invalidation, low self-efficacy, anticipating negative emotions). Activation of effective behaviors and practicing willingness versus avoiding challenging experiences are important elements of DBT that need to be embedded in each skills chain to improve generalization (On-Track Action). The On-Track Action skill also integrates the DBT concepts of "radical acceptance," "opposite action," "PLEASE," and "letting go of emotional suffering" (Linehan, 2015a).

Clearly defining techniques to manage risky situations in effective ways is important given the high rate of behavioral dyscontrol of this population. Safety Plan needs to increase the individual's understanding of the situation and offer a dynamic process that guides her to balance the multiple internal and external factors to reach long-term personal goals. For example, Safety Plan promotes evaluating levels of risk accurately to ensure the individual does not overrate danger, reinforcing avoiding situations that are in her best interest to approach (informal exposure).

Activities are an important component of building a life worth living. New-Me Activities combine elements of emotion regulation and distress tolerance in DBT. New-Me Activities categorize "Pleasant Events" (Linehan, 2015a) by their regulatory function to encourage strategic choices that increase effectiveness. New-Me Activities also integrate aspects of the distress tolerance skills such as "Wise Mind ACCEPTS" and "Self-Soothing" (Linehan, 2015a). The "Reality Acceptance" skills (Linehan, 2015a) would be addressed both in Clear Picture (Notice the Breath) and in New-Me Activity, where the individual engages in action that increases focus. Because New-Me Activity is used in a "1235" chain, it teaches the individual that full attention and mindfulness are essential components of On-Track Actions.

Problem solving is a core DBT strategy that has multiple steps and places high cognitive load demands on even nondisabled individuals. The Problem Solving skill in the Skills System provides a simple framework that breaks down this process into component parts. It also integrates concepts related to balance, flexibility, and effectiveness.

Self-expression is a foundational component within multiple DBT interpersonal effectiveness skills (e.g., "DEAR MAN," "GIVE," "FAST") (Linehan, 2015a). Individuals diagnosed with ID need basic training to develop and improve capacities to communicate (Expressing Myself). In addition, individuals with ID often struggle to get what they need from people. Cognitive deficits, communication challenges, and power differentials in relationships often negatively impact people's needs being met. The language in DEAR MAN is too complex for individuals with ID to articulate and recall. Getting It Right was a derivative that provided tangible information in a user-friendly form. The Skills System tries to build interpersonal effectiveness concepts such as identity, reciprocity, roles, self-respect, and gauging intensity into Relationship Care (and other Calm-Only skills) in ways that are pertinent for this population.

TRANSITION TO CHAPTER 4

This chapter has explored concepts associated with emotion regulation, DBT, and CLT to help the skills trainer understand Skills System design. The upcoming chapters offer the trainer instruction options. Chapter 4 presents ideas about structuring a skills group, logistics related to skills group, the E-Spiral framework, and a 12-week curriculum. Two less structured approaches to instruction are introduced, as well as ways to conceptualize skills knowledge acquisition.

Structuring Skills System Instruction

Treating individuals with complex learning challenges requires careful attention to all aspects of instruction. There are many similarities between standard DBT and Skills System teaching principles, yet differences exist. For example, the change from the four modules in standard DBT skills training to the nine Skills System skills and three System Tools approach altered the basic format of skills training. Similarly, teaching individuals with ID requires the Skills System instructor to teach consistently in ways that maximize memory functioning. This chapter introduces structural factors within Skills System instruction that are foundational for teaching individuals with significant cognitive impairments.

The first section of this chapter presents information to which a trainer can refer when structuring individual and group skills training. Next, three elements of the Skills System teaching model are presented: the E-Spiral framework, Skills System session format, and 12-week-cycle curriculum. Two additional instruction strategies, Skills Surfing and an experiential approach, are introduced as alternatives to structured approaches. The last section of this chapter presents a knowledge acquisition framework designed to help trainers better understand how an individual may build Skills System knowledge and competency.

Chapter 3: Structuring Skills Training Sessions in the *DBT Skills Training Manual, Second Edition* (Linehan, 2015a), provides useful information for the DBT practitioner about pretreatment procedures, the organization of skills training sessions, and observing limits. Having an understanding of both the standard structure and the modification for individuals with ID offered here helps the Skills System trainer adapt skills training for the specific needs of the population in ways that are principally characteristic of DBT.

INDIVIDUAL AND GROUP SKILLS TRAINING

If the Skills System is being used within a DBT treatment model, then following the specific standard DBT group rules and procedures presented in the *DBT Skills Training Manual, Second Edition* (Linehan, 2015a) as closely as possible is recommended. If the Skills System is being used with other treatments or as a stand-alone tool, it may be helpful for skills trainers to meet with group participants prior to joining a skills group to discuss the concept of commitment to learning skills, as is done in standard DBT. This preliminary meeting (or meetings) is an opportunity to orient the individual to the group, review informed consent, discuss treatment goals, elicit commitment, address logistics, and review the basic group rules.

The rules for Skills System groups are similar to those for standard DBT groups. The individual agrees to be supportive and not harm him- or herself, others, or property during group. Relationship Care behaviors such as calling ahead for nonattendance and lateness are expected. Coming to group impaired by alcohol/drugs is not allowed. For the individual who is at risk for these behaviors, it may be helpful to complete a written Safety Plan that highlights risks and ways the individual will handle them. Additionally, the participant must agree that if he becomes romantically involved with another person in group, one of the participants will shift to a different group. It is important to note that due to the poverty of social relationships that many individuals with significant learning challenges face, it is not uncommon for group members to form friendships. The impact of relationships in group must be monitored to ensure that group process is not adversely affected.

If the individual receives staff supervision, it is necessary to be mindful of the trainer–staff relationship. The individual is the client and should be consulted about the therapist contact with the staff. For example, if the trainer would like to discuss transportation with the staff, the trainer may consider asking the individual for permission to do so. The DBT "Consultation to the Patient" strategies are very helpful (Linehan, 1993a, pp. 410–411) to guide trainer–staff contacts. If the individual has a behavioral treatment plan, it is important to discuss how behaviors will be managed in group.

If the skills trainer assesses that a participant is unable to manage the social environment of group and learn information, it may be necessary for the person to have individual skills training first. With the provision of foundational informational skills on an individual basis, the person may be better able to develop basic self-regulation skills that enable him to learn in the group setting. Skills training dyads and triads can be useful and shape the individual to be able to manage a larger group. Although some participants may benefit from beginning in individual skills training, the ultimate goal may be to help the person engage in a group setting. Skills groups provide learning experiences that aid in the generalization of skills into the social environment.

The main goal of group is to help participants build adaptive coping skills. This mission can be used as a guide for maintaining a positive group culture. For example, behaviors that support learning skills are helpful, while actions that actively work against learning experiences need to be addressed. Helpful hints about ways to discuss problematic behaviors can be found on page 86 within the Contingency Management section in Chapter 5.

Group Makeup

The Skills System groups do not need to have a specific number of participants. It may be ideal to have multiple options for group sizes to suit the needs of the individuals. Small groups of two to four participants offer more individualized training and coaching. Groups of four to seven people allow for individual participation and opportunities for social interaction. Larger groups (seven to 10 participants) allow the individual to practice skills in a more complex social setting. Less individual sharing and practice may be possible in larger groups. Unfortunately, logistics and resources can dictate group size; by understanding factors that impact learning, the skills trainer can advocate for groups that optimize learning. It may be particularly helpful to have instructors co-lead larger groups.

DBT groups have co-leaders, which is also optimal for Skills System groups. The primary leader focuses on teaching content, and the other is available to assess and support individuals who are experiencing difficulty. Staff and/or family members may ask to attend group. It is important for individuals to be able to talk openly about challenging situations to assemble effective skills chains; having family or staff in group can inhibit the exploration of factors that are essential to manage in these relationships. Rather than inconsistently inviting outsiders in, the format should be clear, as in DBT for adolescents' multifamily groups (Miller, Rathus, & Linehan, 2006). Parallel versus integrated skills training for collateral support providers may be a useful option.

Time Frames of Group Sessions

Group sessions generally meet for 1 hour per week. Group skills training places high cognitive and emotional demands on participants and skills trainers. Fatigue is a legitimate concern as time frames lengthen. In residential settings, it may be useful to run multiple 1-hour skills groups per week. Meeting more than once per week may create opportunity for heightened integration of the Skills System concepts. This exposure may foster improved generalization of skills. Shortening groups to less than 1 hour (and increasing the frequency) may be workable. Having a general group once per week and then shorter ones on topics such as Problem Solving, Getting It Right, or New-Me Activities can offer opportunities for practice. It is important to design groups so that there is sufficient time for all aspects of the E-Spiral learning process to occur.

Participants Revolve Multiple Times through the 12-Week-Cycle Curriculum

The pace at which the group and individuals progress through Skills System materials is variable. Generally, the basic Skills System material cannot be integrated by individuals with cognitive challenges within a single 12-week cycle through group. Individuals with cognitive impairment require repetition of the Skills System curriculum to learn and generalize the information. Thus, it is recommended that an individual with significant learning challenges participate in the Skills System for a minimum of 1 year. During the course of a year, the person cycles through the material four times. This format allows ample time to introduce the basic Skills System concepts and offers opportunity for repetition.

It may be beneficial for the individual to remain in a skills group on an ongoing basis. As people increase capacities, often they accept more personal responsibilities. For example, the person may move from working in a vocational site to being employed in the community. Skills group continually helps the participant develop improved coping skills as she is participating in more demanding tasks. Each accomplishment brings new challenges; group helps the individual to face transitions and continually progress toward personal goals. Perhaps attending monthly or biweekly could address these needs.

Open Versus Closed Groups

Skills System groups can be either open or closed groups. There is often variability in attendance; due to logistical factors, participants may frequently miss sessions or drop out of skills training. These factors dictate that group be constructed in a way that allows an individual to miss a group meeting and not experience a significant gap in learning. Additionally, it may be important to invite new members into the group. Instruction needs to be adjusted to accommodate this flow, but generally it does not negatively impact the skills training process.

If a new member is joining the group, then it may be helpful to give the person a skills handout notebook and Skills System CD prior to going to group. The trainer could also offer basic skills instruction during the pretreatment session. Showing the individual the Skills System website (*www.guilford.com/skills-system*) could help him become more aware of the materials.

The design of the Skills System session format and the 12-week-cycle curriculum build in opportunities for review of materials. When a new person joins group, the skills trainer facilitates a discussion during the review phase that serves to orient the person to the basic concepts of the Skills System. The skills trainer must be able to address the learning needs of the new person, as well as the participant who has been studying skills for 5 years. Often more seasoned participants enjoy teaching and coaching newer members.

Homogeneous versus Heterogeneous Groups

The skills trainer must decide whether the group is going to be heterogeneous or homogeneous. Frequently, participants have commonalities in one area, while being diverse in others. For example, at my clinic, groups were homogeneous, in that participants were all diagnosed with some form of ID. The groups were heterogeneous in that within each group, participants have a wide range of mental health diagnoses, intellectual capacities, and academic levels. The individual therapist, skills trainer, and individual collaborate to evaluate whether the individual is in the proper group. Given the unique presentations of each person, it is important to individualize rather than generalize regarding group makeup decisions. Unfortunately, there may not be multiple options for this population due to limited clinical resources.

There may be benefits to grouping participants by academic functioning level. This distribution may allow individuals with more cognitive capacities to move through material at a faster rate and in greater depth. While reading and writing are not prerequisite skills for participating in the curriculum, clustering individuals who can read and write may increase options for instructors to utilize activities that integrate these media. For example, skills trainers may create written individual or group homework assignments that reinforce topics addressed in group.

Dividing group by gender may also be helpful. If participants have high levels of emotional, cognitive, and behavioral dysregulation, then a mixed-gender group can create interpersonal dynamics that impede learning. For example, in groups of individuals with ID, it is not uncommon for victims of sexual abuse to be in group with perpetrators of abuse. The transaction between a participant with unresolved trauma issues and one who has unmanaged deviant sexual arousal can amount to a dangerous exchange. There are programs that run specific women's and men's skills groups that target specific gender-based needs. A combination of gender-mixed and -specific groups would address a broad spectrum of needs.

THE SKILLS SYSTEM TEACHING MODEL: THE E-SPIRAL FRAMEWORK

The E-Spiral is a teaching framework that guides Skills System curriculum teaching practices. It serves only as a general guide and framework to help practitioners remember the multiple steps within the learning process. Four phases of the E-Spiral are addressed during a group (or individual) training session: Exploring Existing Knowledge Base, Encoding, Elaboration, and Efficacy.

In Phase 1, Exploring Existing Knowledge Base, the group reviews past learning related to the topic that is introduced. Active discussion activates recall of past learning that primes individuals to undergo new learning. The goal is to create a relevant context for learning.

In Phase 2, Encoding, individuals participate in direct instruction and multimodal activities to learn the skill topic. The aim is to teach new information.

In Phase 3, Elaboration, individuals engage in practice exercises and discussions that expand and link new information to their existing knowledge base. The elaboration process is a vital yet fun step toward deepening understandings about skills. Thus, the purpose is to link and expand knowledge to enhance retention.

In Phase 4, Efficacy, participants continue to build mastery and confidence through contextual learning activities that promote skills integration in real-life contexts. Activities such as role play, *in vivo* practice, addressing commitment, and troubleshooting challenges facilitate generalization. It is critical that individuals with intellectual impairment experience a sense of self-efficacy as part of the learning process. The E-Spiral is designed to provide contextual learning opportunities that maximize retention and generalization of skills.

The 12-week Skills System curriculum (presented in Chapter 7) provides lesson plans that are broken down to address each of the E-Spiral steps. As learners move through these phases and activities, their knowledge about the topic is broadened and deepened. This learning process guides people through steps that naturally transition skills information from short-term to long-term memory. Building skills knowledge in long-term memory can reduce cognitive load demands and increase the individual's abilities to recall skills in high stress situations. The E-Spiral multilayered learning experience helps intellectually impaired individuals gain mastery that promotes generalization of skills.

The E-Spiral functions as a guide for teaching practices. While issues and time constraints commonly force the skills trainer to make adjustments, the E-Spiral serves as a template for organizing effective teaching strategies. Even when time frames are limited, skills trainers learn how to quickly review past learning, teach a new concept, practice it, and make a bridge to real-life contexts. Organizing teaching in this looping progression that layers old and new information, deepens learning, enhances retention, and improves recall. Being mindful of these principles helps skills trainers avoid truncating the teaching process, which may jeopardize the integration of concepts.

Benefits of the Skills System Teaching Model

The 12-week cycle curriculum creates breadth of skills knowledge, while the E-Spiral creates depth of learning. Skills trainers utilize both of these constructs simultaneously. The broadening and deepening of learning creates a foundation in long-term memory that enhances the generalization of skills. Figure 4.1 exemplifies how an individual's knowledge grows in a web shape using these teaching techniques.

As the individual learns, practices, and generalizes information, linkages between skills fortify over time. The increased connectivity of the knowledge base enhances recall and recognition of information. Adaptive responses become more automated, requiring fewer cognitive resources. As the individual builds a foundation of knowledge, cognitive load demands related to skills use decrease. The person becomes able to master complex skill behaviors as a result of the integrated skills knowledge base.

Skills System Session Format

The Skills System session format presents the various tasks within each phase of the E-Spiral. The skills trainer follows these guidelines and designs activities to complete the function of the E-Spiral phase. As the group flows from one discussion point and activity to another, learning happens. Participants do not necessarily need to know this framework, although improving metacognitive understanding about the learning process may increase self-awareness, self-efficacy, and motivation. Table 4.1 presents the curriculum tasks that occur during E-Spiral phases in a skills group.

It is vital that the instructor understand the necessary steps to enhance comprehension and integration while remaining flexible and responsive to what is happening in the group. Under theoretically ideal conditions, approximately equal amounts of time are spent on each of the

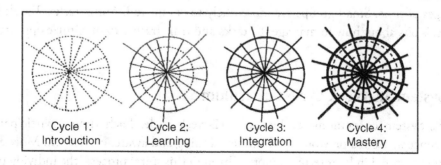

FIGURE 4.1. Learning the Skills System.

TABLE 4.1. Tasks within E-Spiral Phases in a Skills Group

1. Exploring Existing Knowledge Base: *Recalling past learning.*
   - Mindfulness activity to focus attention; describe the experience.
   - Review Skills System terms and Skills Practice Review.
   - Introduce new skills topic.
   - Discussion: Assess existing knowledge; highlight the need for skills.
   - Orient to the relevant context of the new learning.

2. Encoding: *Teaching the new topic.*
   - Direct instruction: Lecture, write on the board, handouts and worked examples.
   - Discussion: Test comprehension of content; prompt clarification.
   - Multimodal tools: Use diagrams, cue pictures, gestures, objects, and video.

3. Elaboration: *Practice new learning and link it to previous learning.*
   - Practice: Practice exercises, worksheets.
   - Discussion: Describing the experience; some self-disclosure; expand awareness.
   - Skills Chains: Link the new skill with other skills in skills chains.

4. Efficacy: *Bridge to real life.*
   - Contextual learning activities: Role play, psychodrama, and *in vivo.*
   - Discussion: Highlighting barriers; personal commitment; troubleshooting for future use of the skill.
   - Plan for home-study activities.
   - Group ending: Mindfulness breathing.

four phases. Realistically, a group rarely moves systematically through all of the phases. There are times when certain discussions and activities require more depth, hence consuming larger percentages of time. Small groups are more likely to complete E-Spiral tasks. The skills trainer makes decisions about how to manage the tasks and time frames to maximize opportunities for learning.

Skills System 12-Week Cycle Curriculum

The Skills System curriculum revolves in a 12-week cycle. Each time a participant revisits familiar concepts from a previous cycle, understanding and awareness deepen. More elaborated information is stored in long-term memory. Through this spiral process, the individual continually integrates new facets of the skills. As the participant learns and practices skills, she gains the ability to utilize skills in increasingly complex situations. The list below presents Skills System topics that are covered during each of the 12 weeks. Chapter 7 presents detailed explanations of how topics may be reviewed, introduced, practiced, and integrated.

- Week 1: Skills List
- Week 2: System Tools
- Week 3: Clear Picture
- Week 4: On-Track Thinking
- Week 5: On-Track Action
- Week 6: Safety Plan
- Week 7: New-Me Activities
- Week 8: Problem Solving
- Week 9: Expressing Myself
- Week 10: Getting It Right
- Week 11: Relationship Care
- Week 12: Skills Review

Progressing through Skills System Content

It is unrealistic to expect group members to learn a skill completely in a 1-hour group session. The 12-week-cycle curriculum forces the group to keep moving through content related to each of the skills. Practitioners may have the urge to spend weeks on one skill to ensure comprehension. Rather than focusing in-depth on one skill for several weeks, the 12-week-cycle curriculum continually tries to broaden skills knowledge. Although in-depth learning of each skill is helpful, the skills trainer integrates the teaching strategies presented in Chapters 5 and 6 within the 12-week curriculum, to expand the breadth and depth of learning for this population over time.

In its entirety, the Skills System is vast. Trainers have to know the complete Skills System, but individuals in the group can progress at different rates through the material, building mastery over time. To reduce cognitive load and facilitate recall, the system itself and the teaching process are broken into more manageable chunks of information. The skills trainer has to rely on his clinical judgment to decide how to introduce and practice these bits of information given the spectrum of factors that impact each diverse group.

Evaluating comprehension can be challenging. A first step may be when the participant uses skills terms without prompting, coaching, or hints. It is a positive sign of generalization when she is able to discuss scenarios from her life in terms of skills language and recounts skills usage in her daily context. More formal means of assessment including skills tests are available online, or the skills trainer can create skills competency evaluations to monitor integration. Ultimately, increases in factors associated with improved quality of life and reductions in behavioral dyscontrol may be ways to gauge comprehension and generalization. As part of the weekly lesson planning process, the skills trainer needs to be mindful of how the group members are progressing.

The skills trainer creates a plan for covering a portion of that week's topic. On the first cycle through the material for a group, the information highlights the different parts of the skill in a general way. With a more seasoned group, the nuances of skills can be explored. The trainer adapts the speed of progression through the skills content to the capacities of each group.

Within each week's lesson plan, unplanned teaching opportunities and challenging events may emerge. It is important to be able to utilize contextual events when possible, although contextual learning can increase cognitive load demands. It is necessary for the trainer to be prepared for the unexpected. It is critical that the trainer know the Skills System inside and out and have an ample bag of teaching tricks to create teachable moments during any and all eventualities.

ALTERNATIVE TEACHING FORMATS

Chapter 5 presents myriad teaching strategies that can be used to create fun and flexible learning experiences. Unfortunately, even when trainers try multiple techniques to engage a group more severe adjustments are necessary. As clear and structured as the E-Spiral and 12-week curriculum are, there are times when it is necessary to take a different approach. Certain clients or group constellations may force the group leader to redesign skills instruction.

Not Using the Handout Notebook

The 12-week curriculum presented in Chapter 7 utilizes the handouts in Appendix A. Although these are a great resource for some, they are a barrier for others. It is possible that individuals who have difficulty engaging in skills training may not like using handouts and the handout notebook. They may perceive it as too simple or babyish. They may feel overcontrolled or that the integrated model strips them of their identity/individuality. The books can be cues that trigger past educational failures and traumatic experiences that happened in special education settings. *Handouts are not necessary*; using a whiteboard is an alternative. The first step with a disengaged individual may be to assess reactions to the use of the notebooks. Individual or group accommodations, such as using certain handouts and worked examples rather than writing on worksheets can be helpful. Completing worksheets verbally and the trainer writing answers on the board can be another option. Shaping integration of the materials can be effective; worksheets may be introduced gradually and used for home study. If a trainer has ample Skills System knowledge, it is possible to develop teaching interventions that do not rely strictly on handouts. Following the E-Spiral concepts of skills review, teaching new material, practicing the skill, and bridging to real life may still be useful guidelines for the adapted curriculum design.

Skills Surfing

The E-Spiral and 12-week curriculum are designed to bring *individuals to the skills*. These techniques rely on a basic level of investment and stability that translates into compliant, motivated learning behaviors. Alternatively, some individuals have difficulty adjusting successfully to this type of learning experience due to developmental, mental health, or environmental factors. When ample creative efforts to bring the individuals to the skills have failed, it may be useful to shift strategies and bring the *skills to the individual*. One technique is called Skills Surfing. E-Spiral and skills concepts are brought to the context of the individuals.

First, Choose Your Board

The trainer decides whether to set an agenda-free group or do a topic-based approach that targets one of the weekly topics of the 12-week curriculum. If there is a predetermined topic (e.g., that for Week 3 is Clear Picture), the trainer can provide a single handout of the Clear Picture Do's or write them on the side of the white board to passively orient group members to the information in a nonthreatening way. Again, it may be useful to shape the group toward tolerating more direct skills training strategies.

If the trainer is dealing with either an advanced group or a willful beginners group, a free-flowing, agenda-free strategy style may be advantageous. This format begins with no predetermined topic and then homes in on skills topics that emerge. The trainer (or a group member) writes concepts on the board that surface from the discussions and activities. It is challenging to plan for a free-flowing group, because the trainer has to design teaching interventions in the moment. This unpredictability can create an energized, creative, and spontaneous learning environment, if managed well. The deeper the trainers understanding of the Skills System, the richer the learning experiences that can be created on the fly.

Wait for or Make Waves

The trainer begins by asking questions to stimulate conversation and then integrates skills concepts during the discussion. The topics can be scenario-based, such as "What is the first day of a new job like?" The group might listen to a song and discuss the relevance of the lyrics or messages. The trainer might bring up a current event or plight of celebrities to cultivate active discussion. The group members could be asked to share a challenge that was faced during the week. It is important to note that working with self-disclosure increases emotional responses and creates cognitive load demands.

As the discussion progresses, topic waves begin to build. The trainer highlights challenges in the scenario that impact people, their ability to manage emotions, and reach personal goals. This wave-making process sets up a relevant context for skills. Indirectly, this works toward Phase 1 of the E-Spiral framework: Exploring Existing Knowledge.

Ride the Wave

The skills trainer assesses points in the discussion to determine when there are opportunities to do Phase 2: Encoding. The trainer waits and jumps on teachable moments, riding minilesson opportunities as they happen. If at all possible, the trainer tries to get the group members to practice what they just learned (Phase 3: Elaboration). With the example of Clear Picture, getting the group to do a breathing exercise might work. The activity does not have to be lengthy, but it does have to be engaging. Alternatively, a discussion about how previous learning fits with the new information would elaborate the learning. After some form of practice, the trainer makes a link to how this skill can be used in the individuals' lives to complete Phase 4: Bridge to Real Life. Perhaps the group members might discuss how they can do breathing at work or in the middle of an argument with someone. Skills surfing may progress through a series of abbreviated E-Spirals rather than by exploring a specific topic in depth.

Using Skills Surfing has advantages and disadvantages. On the one hand, the format is adventuresome, flexible, and fluid. On the other hand, the instruction is less systematic and organized. The advantage of human engagement it offers may be a necessary factor to facilitate any learning for certain individuals and groups. I find that when I am teaching adolescent clients, giving the group members control of group activities can increase engagement (e.g., writing on the board, reading handouts, facilitating discussions, creating rules for activities, or using a time clock). Once they have control, often the group members are more willing to tolerate a structured approach.

The Experiential Approach

The trainer may plan a series of activities that are designed to teach skills concepts in an experiential way and create bridges to the skills materials. Like Skills Surfing, this tactic does not explicitly utilize the E-Spiral framework and 12-week curriculum, but elements of both can guide the progression of this type of learning experience. These types of activities can also be woven into more structured approaches. The next section features a sample group session for teaching Clear Picture through creative, multimodal techniques.

Teaching Clear Picture Experientially

To teach Clear Picture, the trainer may begin with a mindful eating activity to discuss the concept of awareness. A piece of chocolate, a lollipop, or fruit is fun. The trainer can write all of the Clear Picture Do's on the board, highlighting Body Check relative to the exercise. The group members can start seeing how body awareness is linked to noticing other internal experiences (feelings, thoughts, and urges) in the moment.

Next the trainer can show the group a series of pictures of people taken from media. All different people in different situations are useful. Using a set of skills cards of the six Clear Picture Do's (available as a free download at *www.guilford.com/skills-system*), the group member places the cards one by one near the picture and describes what he thinks the person is experiencing using skills language. The group discussion of different interpretations of the picture teaches a dialectical perspective.

In the next portion of the group, group members take a brief walk together, stopping at different locations to get a Clear Picture. Quietly, each person notices changes in the internal and external experience as the walk progresses. The group returns and members share observations, describing experiences of the Clear Picture Do's.

In the final portion of group, the trainer may show a movie clip. For example, there is a YouTube clip (5 minutes) from *The Empire Strikes Back,* in which Yoda uses the Force to lift a spaceship out of the swamp. Luke gets distracted and Yoda coaches him about attentional deployment and helps him reappraise his experiences. It is an entertaining way to discuss Clear Picture; it is a useful link to On-Track Thinking as well.

There are countless creative ways to teach skills. Although it is important to preserve the key skills concepts/principles, there is latitude in how the information is transferred to group members. A trainer may want to explore getting certified through *www.guilford.com/skills-system* to ensure adherence to the Skills System model.

SKILLS KNOWLEDGE INTEGRATION

There may be marked differences in the ways that individuals learn and use the Skills System. While some individuals benefit from progressing systematically through the 12-week curriculum, gradually building skills knowledge, others require a more targeted learning experience. For example, for a person who demonstrates impulsive, destructive behaviors and has more severe learning challenges, focusing on teaching one or two concepts to begin this process may be best. Figure 4.2 shows how the individual in this example may progress from one skills concept (Move Away) to more elaborated responses over time.

Note that this individual does not begin learning Clear Picture, On-Track Thinking, and On-Track Action, because they are too advanced. This person needs to learn concrete steps to interrupt conditioned responses. Beginning with an adaptive response such as Move Away from the risk may help to reduce challenging behaviors. Learning the entire Safety Plan skill would be too complicated and place high cognitive load demands. Next, bringing attention to a person's internal experience will encourage late-stage second-phase processing. Instead of doing the entire Clear Picture, focusing on Notice the Urge is the most relevant to the problematic chain of behavior. To link Notice the Urge and Move Away proactively before engaging in off-track actions would be a positive progression. Next, building in an appraisal skill, Check It, using thumbs up and thumbs down, could expand capacities. As learning continues, skills components are added, such as Noticing the Breathe and doing a New-Me Activity after Move Away. The chain expands according to the individual's needs and abilities over time.

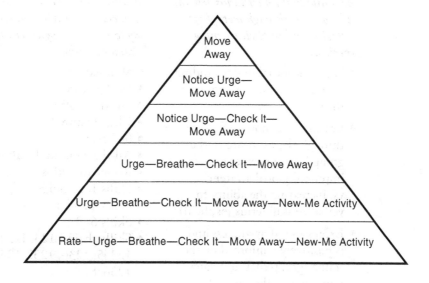

FIGURE 4.2. Example of managing safety.

EVALUATING SKILLS ACQUISITION

All individuals learn the Skills System at different speeds and to varying depths. Bloom's (1956) taxonomy, a framework from the field of education that defines levels of knowledge, can be useful to understand this progression better. This taxonomy was expanded to include both tacit knowledge and explicit knowledge to accommodate the functioning capacities of individuals diagnosed with ID. Although an individual may experience impaired academic skills, he may gain increased awareness and skills through implicit versus strictly explicit means. Table 4.2 describes capacities that are noted at the different levels of understanding and highlights knowledge levels from beginner through Skills System expert.

TRANSITION TO CHAPTER 5

Chapter 5 presents foundational teaching strategies that are used throughout Skills System instruction. The Quick-Step Assessment is a simple framework the skills trainer can use to monitor and adjust for the cognitive load capacity changes an individual experiences. The chapter also reviews basic behavioral strategies that enhance skills learning.

TABLE 4.2. Skills Knowledge Using Bloom's Taxonomy

Levels of understanding	Tacit knowledge concepts (in a progression of learning)	Explicit knowledge concepts (in a progression of learning)
Knowledge	*The individual understands general skills concepts through metaphors, analogies, and implicit learning experiences.* • Has conceptual understanding of skills functions drawn from the skill names. • Learns to be more self-aware through the exposure to the group learning experience (e.g., improved global awareness vs. increasing the ability to verbalize skill terms [explicit]). • Expresses self-awareness and is positively reinforced by the trainer/group that motivates investment, efficacy, and	*The individual uses words and numbers in a formal and systematic way to represent cognitive and behavioral tasks.* • Skill names • Skill pictures • On-track/off-track to goal • Clear Picture Do's • 0–5 scale • All-the-Time and Calm-Only • Recipe for Skills • Skills 1, 2, and 3 • Skills 4 and 5 • Skills 6–9 • Skills chains: 123, 1234, 1235, 12345, 1236, 1237, 1238, 1239, 1236789

	TABLE 4.2 *(continued)*	
Levels of understanding	**Tacit knowledge concepts (in a progression of learning)**	**Explicit knowledge concepts (in a progression of learning)**
Knowledge *(continued)*	increased tacit and explicit knowledge-base development. • Draws from a wider range of strategies to regulate emotions (e.g., general skills concepts vs. creating specific skills chains).	• Has the ability to recall subcomponents of the skills (six Clear Picture Do's, etc.).
Comprehension	*Tacit knowledge is informally acquired rather than learned through explicit instruction; it is therefore difficult for the individual to articulate.*	*The individual has the capacity to explain terms and concepts.* • Answers skills related questions accurately. • Capable of extracting skills concepts from scenarios.
Application	*Evidence of knowledge acquisition translates to improved task performance rather than improved capacities to verbalize terms and concepts.* Social and behavioral functioning improves.	*The individual uses skills to manage real-life situations.* • Can plan and execute skills chains in complex social environments.
Analysis		*The individual can identify, compare, and contrast skills components.* • Can discuss different skills alternatives in relation to varying priorities, needs, and goals. • Is capable of providing skills coaching.
Synthesis		*The individual can combine information from multiple sources to increase knowledge base.* • Is capable of running skills groups and individual skills instruction.
Evaluation		*The individual can design skills training experiences.* • Is capable of training skills coaches. • Understands systemwide applications and implementation issues.

CHAPTER 5

Foundational Teaching Strategies

Chapter 4: Skills Training Treatment Targets and Procedures in the *DBT Skills Training Manual, Second Edition* (Linehan, 2015a) explains about behavioral targets, meeting skills training targets, and managing homework. As with standard DBT, the Skills System mandate is to maximize skills acquisition, strengthening, and generalization. Although individuals with significant learning challenges require enhanced instructional supports to reach these goals, the Skills System builds on elements of DBT teaching, such as clear explanations of instructions, use of handouts, modeling, behavioral rehearsal, behavioral strategies, feedback, coaching, assigning homework, homework/review, behavioral rehearsal/activation, eliciting commitment, and troubleshooting. Awareness of the standard DBT teaching material provides foundational information that helps the Skills System practitioner maintain a DBT perspective as adjustments in skills training are made.

When treating individuals with complex mental health issues, it is necessary to manage the therapeutic relationships strategically within the context of skills groups. The information presented in Chapter 5: Application of Foundational DBT Strategies in Behavioral Skills Training of the *DBT Skills Training Manual, Second Edition* (Linehan, 2015a) can be helpful in managing the teacher–student relationship in ways that foster learning and personal development.

This chapter introduces teaching strategies that are used throughout skills training sessions to manage cognitive load demands and individualize interventions for individual with ID. This information serves as a toolkit for practitioners. Within the category of foundational teaching interventions are several strategies that skills trainers utilize throughout all phases of Skills System instruction. The Quick-Step Assessment is a tool designed to help trainers evaluate (1) the intrinsic cognitive load of an intervention, (2) the individual's cognitive load status in the moment, and (3) how to make necessary adjustment in teaching interventions to reduce cognitive load demands. In addition, behavioral techniques are used during skills training sessions: shaping, positive reinforcement, and contingency management. Understanding these foundational strategies helps the skills trainer be flexible and maximize learning opportunities.

QUICK-STEP ASSESSMENT

The Quick-Step Assessment is a strategy that skills trainers utilize to evaluate, design, and adjust interventions. These strategies are useful in Skills System groups and are helpful for leaders of standard DBT groups when participants struggle to comprehend the material. The assessment is a three-step process.

Step 1: Assess the Cognitive Load of the Intervention

Prior to executing any instructional or therapeutic intervention, it is important that the skills trainer consider the intrinsic cognitive load of the task. Prior to teaching, the trainer needs to assess the size and complexity of the chunk of information that is going to be taught. Instructors quickly evaluate whether the strategies present a high or low cognitive load. High intrinsic (complexity of the material) and/or high extraneous cognitive load (poor design of the intervention) can decrease germane cognitive load (effective processing). Interventions that require the individual to do simultaneous processing of information, manage high volume and interactivity of information, retrieve divergent information, shift rapidly without transition from one topic to another, and/or experience strong emotional responses to the information increase cognitive load demands. It may be possible to reduce cognitive load demands by decreasing the amount of material being taught at that time.

Step 2: Evaluate Cognitive Functioning

In the second step of the Quick-Step Assessment, the skills trainer evaluates whether an individual is cognitively regulated before, during, and after interventions. When an intervention places low cognitive demand on the individual, she is more likely to remain cognitively regulated. Although the learning may tax resources, she is able to engage in the process and learn the material. Conversely, if the cognitive load of an intervention is too high, the individual may become cognitively overloaded. As cognitive demands increase and capacities decrease, states such as confusion and disorganization can happen. During cognitive overload, an individual may experience high-level emotions such as frustration, anger, fear, and shame. Emotional states may further reduce cognitive load capacities. Maladaptive behaviors that function to regulate overwhelming emotions, such as fight–flight responses, can disrupt the individual's and group's learning.

Signs of Cognitive Overload

The following presentations may indicate that the individual is experiencing cognitive dysregulation.

- *Confusion.* The individual may appear unfocused. He may be unable to follow the topic of a discussion, flip though pages indiscriminately, give incorrect answers, or act withdrawn from discussions.
- *Avoidance.* The individual may stare off into space, not answer questions directly, or immediately say, "I don't know," rather than try to answer the question.
- *Impulsivity.* The individual may appear distracted, impulsive, fidgety, and/or disorganized. She may avoid following group rules, offer off-topic comments, fiddle with items, walk around the room, and stare at/engage in side conversations with other people in the group.
- *Discomfort.* The person may display irritability, hostility, crying, panic, refusal, or leave group. He may exhibit flat affect and/or use expressive behaviors if he is uncomfortable.

It is unlikely that the individual will communicate that her cognitive capacities have diminished. In fact, she may try to appear competent, so as not to experience shame related to feeling lost and/or confused. The individual may be interested in participating yet lack the skills to inform the skills trainer about the problem. Skills trainers may misattribute behavior of the individual (which may have been the result of skills trainers' mismanagement of the cognitive load demands) as resistance. In skills groups, generally, the material should be designed for the individual with the lowest cognitive load capacities. This strategy builds the self-efficacy of the other learners; the trainer also can target specific, more advanced questions to individuals with higher capacities to address their learning needs.

Step 3: Choose and Shape Intervention

Skills trainers shape interventions throughout a training session. The lower the cognitive load demand of interventions, the more cognitive resources the individual has available to learn the information. If interventions are well designed, it is more likely that singular concepts and associations between concepts can be learned. The encoding of more associations in long-term memory facilitates recall. The broader and more integrated the knowledge base in long-term memory, the greater the individual's capacity to retrieve and generalize skills in the environment.

When an individual exhibits behavior that indicates he is confused, avoidant, impulsive, or uncomfortable during an intervention, the skills trainer must make adjustments. Skills trainers must learn how to find the delicate balance between reinforcing avoidant behaviors by backing off and flooding the individual by continuing with a high-demand cognitive activity that is overwhelming. The following section highlights strategies the trainer can use to alter the material to improve learning.

ADJUSTING INTERVENTIONS TO REDUCE COGNITIVE LOAD DEMANDS

Several techniques may be utilized to manage cognitive load demands of interventions. A few of these tactics include simplification, task analysis, mnemonics, worked examples, and orienting to new topics and transitions.

Foundational Teaching Strategies

Simplification

An individual with cognitive impairment may have difficulty processing abstract, complex, and interconnected information (American Psychiatric Association, 2013). Simplification of challenging ideas through refinement of language and concepts may reduce cognitive load demands. The simplification process entails finding terms that are easily pronounced, comprehended, applied, and recalled by the individual. For example, the Skills System utilizes the phrase "use sugar" (in Getting It Right) for the concept of reinforcing other people when trying to get one's needs met. An individual with intellectual deficits can pronounce and readily understand the concept of sugar. A participant has existing knowledge that sugar is a sweetener. By saying, "Try using a little more sugar," the participant knows that it means to be nicer or more accommodating. The term "reinforce" (the "R" in the DBT skill DEAR MAN) is long, difficult to pronounce, challenging to comprehend, and less likely to be recalled. Complex terms increase cognitive load demands and reduce the individual's ability to use the skill. Utilizing simple words that rely on knowledge already in long-term memory can improve encoding and, ultimately, recall.

Task Analysis

In task analysis, skills trainers break complex tasks down into component parts. By reducing multicomponent concepts into a progression of single elements, the person is able to complete the entire task one step at a time. For example, if a person wants to ask someone out on a date, there are several tangible and intangible factors to consider when preparing to complete this task successfully. The skills trainer may want to collaborate with the individual to define specific steps that are required to accomplish the goal. The individual needs to learn to perform each step and practice stepping from one step to the next.

Mnemonics

"Mnemonics" are techniques that organize information in ways that reduce the cognitive load of information. Several mnemonic techniques are useful to integrate into intervention design. For example, the use of chunking, metaphors, cue pictures, and acronyms can aid encoding and maximize recall.

"Chunking" information means to organize concepts in ways that improve function of short-term memory by recoding information. For example, the random letters S, N, and F are processed as three units, while B, E, and D are processed as one unit, due to the association the letters have with the object.

"Metaphors" are "bridging strategies" that draw on intuition and existing knowledge of the learner; they provide a "transformation of nonmeaningful information into concrete, meaningful proxies" (Mastropieri, Sweda, & Scruggs, 2000). Metaphors may be words, objects, and/or gestures. These strategies cultivate a semantic knowledge base and teach how things work. For example, a train on a track to a destination is a metaphor for the individual demonstrating goal-oriented behaviors; the Skills System uses the metaphor of being on-track and off-track relative to goals. The trainer can integrate using gestures to make additional points. The instructor can pretend to be standing on the tracks and tip his body far to one side, almost losing balance; this gesture exemplifies how people can begin to head off-track.

Cue pictures, which are used to cue memory, explicitly connect new information with prior knowledge by means of visual stimuli. Thus, cue pictures prompt recall and aid visual encoding. For example, a picture of a TV set represents Clear Picture. Each time the individual sees a TV set in a handout, she knows that using Clear Picture is necessary.

An acronym is created when each letter in a word (e.g., SEALS), represents other secondary concepts (Sugar, Explain, Ask, Listen, and Seal the Deal). It is best if the primary word (SEALS) is associated with the other concepts, to facilitate recall. Acronyms are less helpful for nonreaders. Using the cue picture of a seal or the skills trainer making a noise like a seal can prompt recall of SEALS and Seal the Deal.

Worked Examples

"Worked examples" present completed versions of a concept or problem (Sweller, 1988, 2010). For example, the Emotion Regulation Skills System handouts include worked examples for most worksheets. Worked examples ensure the transfer of accurate information and increase the likelihood that accurate information will be recalled in context from long-term memory Using worked examples reduces cognitive load by eliminating the use of "means–ends analyzing," which occurs when the individual "directs attention to inappropriate aspects of a problem and imposes heavy cognitive load that interferes with schema acquisition and rule automation" (Sweller, 1989, p. 457).

Sweller (1989, p. 457) highlights the importance of "schema acquisition and rule automation" to promote learning. One way of creating adaptive schemata is to use "worked examples" (p. 457) to help the individual integrate accurate information. By reviewing solved problems or demonstrating effective actions, such examples allow the individual to observe how the skill functions. This process facilitates a contextual understanding of the concepts. Studying worked examples promotes increased awareness, knowledge base, and mastery, while minimizing extraneous cognitive load.

Additionally, an individual with ID benefits greatly from repeated demonstrations of effective skills use in various contexts. Reviewing information in different ways helps the individual develop perceptions related to the meaning of the material. This semantic encoding may draw on an individual's strengths rather than relying on perceptual skills that may be more impaired. Semantic knowledge that builds an awareness of how things work enables the person to generalize information from one setting to another. As the individual makes associations about intrapersonal and interpersonal concepts, adaptive coping in diverse settings is possible.

It may be helpful to use both general and personalized worked examples throughout skills training. Utilizing hypothetical situations about fictitious people depersonalizes the scenario, thus reducing the cognitive load demands. As capacities build, transitioning to a review of personal examples enhances relevance, motivation, and contextual learning. Personal examples may stimulate more attention, while also increasing emotionality. Skills trainers use the Quick-Step Assessment to adjust teaching practices to address the needs of each group member.

Orienting to New Topics and Transitions

When changing topics and/or preparing to teach a new concept, orienting is a crucial step. An individual with intellectual challenges may frequently have difficulty managing transitions effectively. Orienting helps the person understand social contexts, which reduces confusion and cognitive load demands: "Great job doing that exercise. Now would it be all right if we take some time to talk about what that activity was like for each of you?" Orienting reduces barriers to learning by decreasing fear of the unknown. As individuals gain skills capacities, they manage transitions more effectively.

Orienting is an essential element within this teaching model; skills trainers continually orient participants to the next steps. For example, instructors provide logistical information that clearly identifies the next activity and where in the skills book the person needs to go. Trainers provide functional validation by clearly explaining the location of the handouts that will be discussed in group. It is helpful to show participants the handout to be sure they are oriented to the current activity.

Additionally, skills trainers ask permission to progress to the next topic as part of the orienting process. For example, asking, "Are we all set to move on?" allows the participants to become ready before moving ahead. Rushing and assuming an individual is prepared to progress can create confusion and disengagement. Importantly, eliciting permission creates a reciprocal relationship or an even playing field in the session within which both parties demonstrate on-track control rather than a hierarchical teacher–student relationship that contains implied power differentials.

When participants have an opportunity to demonstrate self-determination and choice, motivation to learn increases. Carlin, Soraci, Dennis, Chechile, and Loiselle (2001) noted that when an individual with ID is allowed to choose what items to remember, his encoding and free-recall rates improve. As skills trainers offer the opportunity for choice, participants also implicitly learn self-validation and have an opportunity to demonstrate self-determination. Orienting, not only improves encoding and aids transitions, it allows full participation; being fully engaged maximizes emotional learning and personal growth.

DOING THE QUICK-STEP ASSESSMENT

A skills trainer individualizes interventions to fit the a participant's current regulation status. For example, she may ask a group member who is cognitively regulated and actively engaged a more complex question (e.g., "What are the six Clear Picture Do's?"). Questions need to be adjusted for a confused or disengaged participant. Asking a simple question (e.g., "What is the first skill in the Skills System?") may prompt focusing attention and build confidence. If an instructor presents a cognitively overloaded participant with a high-cognitive-load-demand intervention, some form of off-track behavioral expression may occur.

The trainer may want to adjust interventions for an individual who is struggling. Avoiding open-ended questions (e.g., "How do you feel about that?") and asking simple, closed-ended questions (e.g., "Did you think that was helpful?") allow for participation, yet do not increase emotional escalation. When a person is cognitively overloaded, the trainer will want to avoid bringing up hot topics or asking for personal disclosure that may further dysregulate the individual. Giving the individual time to regain composure without interaction may also be helpful.

BEHAVIORAL STRATEGIES

The Introduction to DBT Skills Training offers an overview of relevant contingency management techniques that are used in skills training (Linehan, 2015a, pp. 90-95). Behavioral strategies such as reinforcing contingencies, natural reinforcers, shaping, extinction, punishment, observing limits, exposure, cognitive restructuring, and contingency clarification are all explained.

It is helpful for skills trainers to have an understanding of basic behavioral strategies; my intention in this section is not to educate the trainer about behaviorism but rather to highlight particular ways to integrate elements into Skills System instruction.

Shaping

An individual with learning challenges may need to be taught complex tasks through a gradual process. "Shaping" is a behavioral technique that reinforces steps of successive approximations. The individual is rewarded for reaching objectives that are steps toward a larger goal. It is important to use shaping principles during the Encoding Phase of the E-Spiral to facilitate recall. For example, a learning progression may take steps: A, B, AB, C, and ABC. This type of practice helps the cognitively impaired individual learn to integrate information; schema acquisition is facilitated through this repeated pattern of shaping. Teaching ABCDEFG may introduce more information, yet the person may not have reinforced connections between steps.

There are times in individual or group skills training when it is not possible to teach all the necessary elements of multicomponent concepts. Instructors must individualize and prioritize elements that help most in the immediate situation. Skills trainers address what is relevant in the moment and trust that other opportunities will arise to teach the remainder of the concept at another time. The individual learns the relevant material better in that moment; teaching irrelevant information may waste cognitive resources on impertinent information.

Positive Reinforcement

Skills trainers need to provide positive reinforcement for on-track behaviors that participants demonstrate in the session. Instructors are continually scanning the participants to notice demonstrated effort or improvement by each person and the group as a whole. Clearly labeling a skillful behavior, highlighting the context, and adding positive reinforcement is important—for example: "I saw that put your book away and turned your attention to our activity. Great On-Track Action—Switch Tracks!" Noticing and reinforcing small and large accomplishments are critical.

Contingency Management

Participants may exhibit behaviors that are not harmful to group, yet do not enhance the group process. If a behavior is not helpful to the group process, skills trainers utilize extinction. It is important not to respond to the action, so as not to reinforce the behavior intermittently.

A participant may demonstrate behavioral problems or group-interfering behaviors that negatively impact the group process. If the behaviors are interfering with the skills trainer's ability to teach or the ability of participants to learn, it is necessary to address the problem by orienting the participant to the issue and offering skills coaching to address the situation.

Validate and Orient to the Problem

The skills trainer's first assumption is that the individual does not have the awareness or skills to manage the situation effectively. Therefore, the instructor provides coaching prior to enacting contingencies. Premature contingency management can halt the learning process. Validating and orienting the person to the problem is the first step—for example: "Tim, I know you are excited to jump into this discussion, and your ideas are great. When you interrupt us, it is hard to hear everyone's ideas. It is also hard for us to follow what everyone is saying. Do you know what I mean?" Helping the individual see the problem offers him a chance to self-correct. Humor can also be a lighthearted way of helping someone to adjust behavior. The DBT practice of oscillating between acceptance (validation) and change strategies reduces self-invalidation and promotes synthesis of opposing forces.

Offer Skills Coaching

If the behavior continues, further orientation, corrective feedback, and coaching about effective alternatives may be necessary: "Tim, I think you are doing a little better with the not interrupting, but it is still a problem for the group. Would you like some skills coaching from me or the group to help you stay on-track?" The skills trainer must pay attention to the goal of teaching skills and not offer positive reinforcement for off-track behaviors. Ideally, the co-leader could address these issues so that the leader can continue with the rest of the group.

Coaching during group must be brief and concise. Quickly reviewing Clear Picture and On-Track Thinking with the person can often correct the problem. The following series of questions may be helpful:

- "Would you be willing to Take a Breath?" (Clear Picture)
- "What level of emotion are you feeling?" (Clear Picture)
- "What urges are you having?" (Clear Picture)
- "Is that urge to _____ helpful [thumbs-up] or not [thumbs-down]?" (On-Track Thinking)
- "What skills can you use right now to help you?"
- (If the individual has difficulty self-generating skills options) "Would you like the group to help you think of some options?"
- "What will your On-Track Action be?"

If possible, the skills trainer guides the individual to make a plan to improve the situation. Although these situations can be excellent skills teaching opportunities for the individual and the group, the trainer must determine whether the intervention reinforces the individual's off-track behaviors. When it is clear that the progress of the group is in jeopardy, the individual may need to be asked to take a break for a few moments to gain focus, at which point the the co-leader may engage in individual skills coaching outside of the group room. For individuals who frequently become dysregulated, doing a written Safety Plan and referring to it during group helps the individual practice and decreases the impact on group.

TRANSITION TO CHAPTER 6

Chapter 6 presents detailed descriptions of the teaching strategies used in the 12-week Skills System curriculum. By learning more about the interventions and the progression of strategies, the skills trainer increases the number of instructional tools in his bag of tricks. Having ample resources increases the trainer's efficacy and prepares him to have a flexible style that maximizes teaching opportunities.

CHAPTER 6

E–Spiral Teaching Strategies

This chapter introduces various teaching strategies and activities that are highlighted within the 12-week-cycle curriculum outlined in Chapter 7. These elements are woven together during various phases of the E-Spiral to enhance the learning process. The Quick-Step Assessment and behavioral strategies from Chapter 5 are also integrated into Skills System instruction.

PREPARING FOR A SKILLS TRAINING SESSION

Prior to group, skills trainers make a teaching plan to organize the activities, handouts, exercises, and discussions that will happen during the session. Some trainers copy the curriculum pages and highlight areas of intended focus to use to guide group. A document that lists the E-Spiral activities that will happen in group that day can be easier to read while functioning as a facilitator. Having multiple ideas may help the trainer Switch Tracks as needed. This type of planning can help the trainer be organized and transition effectively if the plan needs to change mid-group. If the trainer becomes flustered or disorganized, it can exacerbate the group members' level of dysregulation. More experienced group leaders may not need written notes and are able to make adjustments as needed to maximize teaching opportunities.

Developmental Differences

Anecdotally, I notice a vast difference in the process of teaching skills to adolescents versus adults. Teaching adolescents requires the instructor to be ready to adjust interventions to ensure that attention, relevance, and learning keep happening. Adolescents' developmental drives for autonomy, identity, and independence need to be managed strategically. There can be an unspoken power differential between the adult leader and the youth that may create collateral conflicts that hinder adolescents' receptivity to skills instruction. Practices such as having the group lead activities, discussions, and exercises can improve investment.

I find that the pace of adult groups is slower. Adult groups tend to move at a more tempered speed, allowing for more reflection and collaboration between the trainer and the group. It is important that trainers understand these developmental differences, so that they may make adjustments in tactics. The skills trainer may use the 12-week curriculum and shift to a Skills Surfing model periodically. Each skills trainer and group is unique.

Progressing through the Material

Using the 12-week curriculum format, during a group's first cycle through the Skills System material, it is important to introduce basic skills information. For example, instructors may plan on reviewing the several handouts in minimal detail to offer a general overview of concepts. Exercises and discussions may be more brief; in-depth exploration of the material will occur in later cycles. As the individual progresses through multiple cycles of the Skills System curriculum, more time is spent on lateral exploration of topics. At that point, the quantity of material introduced is far less important than the quality of the discussions and practice exercises that help an individual integrate concepts.

Teaching plans are adjusted during the group sessions. As the participants share personal information during the various reviews and discussions in the beginning of group, skills trainers formulate how to link the participants' experiences with the new topics. Just as DBT therapists oscillate between acceptance and change strategies (Linehan, 1993a), the Skills System trainer weaves together past and current learning. Practitioners teach through building on existing strengths and motivating the participants by creating relevance. Managing these tasks is a dynamic process; skills trainers are continually making adjustments in the teaching plan to accommodate the changing needs of the group.

The following sections highlight the general structure of a Skills System group. These are suggestions and principles on which to draw when creating a group format. There are many variables (e.g., age, gender, psychiatric profiles, and intellectual functioning) that impact group formation and structure; each trainer has to design skills instruction to fit the group's needs. Just as teaching strategies are adjusted, experimentation with the group format is likely to be necessary. Seeking consultation from myself or other experienced Skills System group leaders can be helpful.

E-SPIRAL PHASE 1: EXPLORING EXISTING KNOWLEDGE BASE

Table 6.1 outlines E-Spiral Phase 1: Exploring Existing Knowledge Base and the teaching strategies in each section.

Welcoming the Group

Greeting people is an important initial element of a skills training session. Instructors engage in lighthearted conversation to initiate a pleasant, egalitarian rapport with participants. During this unstructured time of interaction, skills trainers use the Quick-Step Assessment to evaluate the status of each participant prior to initiating any skills training activities. For example, as the skills trainer engages in chitchat, he is able to evaluate her feeling's rating. Instructors monitor for cognitive overload and immediately begin the process of shaping interventions that reflect the current status of the individual.

TABLE 6.1. E-Spiral Phase 1: Exploring Existing Knowledge Base

Exploring Existing Knowledge Base: Recalling past learning (review)

- Welcome

- Mindfulness activity to focus attention
    Describe questions

- Skills System review

- Homework review
    Disclosure questions
    Clarifying questions

- Orient to new skills topic

- Discussion: Exploring existing knowledge on new topic
    Assessment questions

- Discussion: Orient to the relevant context of the new topic
    Relevant context questions

It is important to be aware that attending a group can elicit strong emotions. If a participant is demonstrating escalated negative behaviors prior to group, it is best to address it before they develop into safety concerns. The individual can be prompted to sit in a quiet area, do a focus New-Me Activity, or take a walk to reduce arousal.

Orienting to Group Process

Once the group members are seated, the trainer goes over the rules for the group and explains any logistics (e.g., time frame of group, schedules, restroom use, cell phone use, breaks, snacks, and transportation). The group discusses any issues that are relevant to be sure all members understand clearly. If the trainer is using the E-Spiral framework to guide the structure of group, he may want to orient the group to the basic format of each session.

Using the formal titles of the four E-Spiral phases that instructors learn is not helpful due to complex language and high cognitive load. Simplifying the terms to give a general orientation can be useful. The first part of group is *review* (Exploring Existing Knowledge Base). The second part of group is *new learning* (Encoding). The third portion is *practice* (Elaboration). The fourth and final section is *real life* (Efficacy). The trainer may want to write these terms on the board and orient the group as shifts in activities occur.

For some groups, this framework may not be necessary and may create extraneous cognitive load. Other groups may benefit from increasing metacognitive awareness about the learning process. This is an example of how the trainer has to have many tools at his disposal, evaluate the needs of the group, and work flexibly to optimize learning experiences.

Mindfulness Activity

Skills training session formally begins with a mindfulness activity to help participants focus attention in the present moment. Specific activities are described in the sample curriculum provided in Chapter 7. The goal of these exercises is to orient the person to the current context, as well as to teach the skill of controlling attention.

The mindfulness exercises in the curriculum utilize tapping a Tibetan singing bowl (my colleagues and I call it "the bell") to begin and end the practice or throughout the exercise to cue attention. It is possible to do the mindfulness exercises without the bell, but everyone generally prefers using it. If a trainer wants to purchase a Tibetan bowl, they are available online for around $50.

Following the mindfulness activity, the participants have a discussion, revealing observations made during the mindfulness exercise. By allowing an opportunity for all participants to describe the experience, individuals practice self-awareness (observing) and self-expression (describing). Mastery of self-awareness behaviors is a crucial primary step that allows for the development of self-acceptance, self-value, and self-trust.

It is crucial that the skills trainer fully explain all activities. Clear, step-by-step directions are necessary to be sure that participants fully understand what the activity is and what they needs to do. It is also helpful to highlight any challenges they may experience and possible solutions for difficulties. For example, when explaining how to do a breathing activity, the trainer may want to discuss how the individual's attention will drift from the breath; the solution is for the participant to notice her attention wandering and bring it back to her breathing.

"Describe" Questions

"Describe" questions are asked to elicit participants' observations related to group activities or experiences. For example, after the mindfulness breathing exercise, the skills trainer may ask describe questions to draw out each group member's experiences of the activity. Instructors query, "What did you notice during that activity?"

Skills System Review

Following sharing about the mindfulness activity, the group reviews the Skills List and the System Tools. The trainer can review the Skills System Review Questions (p. 223) or create fun games that prompt the participants to recall the names and numbers of the skills, as well as, the Feelings Rating Scale, Categories of Skills, and Recipe for Skills. Giving newer members the option of looking at their skills notebooks or the Skills Plan Map (Appendix B, p. 344) during the review offers worked examples that increase participation.

The individual may need hints. Having the cue pictures, inventing gestures, using the initial of the skills, and making sounds can prompt recall and be fun during the review. The goal of the skills review is to store skills knowledge in long-term memory. It is also useful for newer members, who may have joined the group mid-cycle, to review terms of previously covered skills.

The trainer uses the skills review activities as an opportunity to evaluate each participant's skills knowledge. Therefore, it is useful to have every group member participate in this process. Optimally, the individual will move from relying on visual aids to contributing without the materials. The trainer hopes the person will move from knowing a few skills to knowing all of them. The capacity for expanding knowledge of the terms and independent recall increases the likelihood that skills will be utilized in the natural environment.

Different group members demonstrate varying levels of explicit skills knowledge, reflected in their ability to volunteer information. It is important to note that some individuals diagnosed with intellectual disabilities may be developing tacit knowledge versus explicit knowledge. The individual who gains tacit knowledge will be making changes in the way he manages emotions, yet may not readily be able to explain the process. The trainer should be mindful about the different learning styles of each participant and adjust the assessment process accordingly.

Homework Review

Following the Skills System review, the individuals share experiences related to using the skills assigned for practice the previous week. The goal is to cultivate effective skills use in the individual's natural environment. These are important opportunities to discuss internal and external factors that impact skills generalization.

In the context of DBT treatment, the Skills Diary Card (Appendix A, p. 222) is used to record skills practice each day during the week. In addition to encouraging skills practice, the diary card facilitates recall during the homework review period in group. The Skills System Diary Card asks the individual to describe one situation each day, the feelings rating, and skills chain that was used to manage the situation.

During the homework review in group, it may be helpful to use a whiteboard to write down each person's name and the accomplishments; it is important to reinforce adaptive skills use and individual progress positively. Writing down information allows the instructor to link commonalities between individuals' scenarios.

The homework review process serves to prime the individual's memory to retrieve skills information in preparation for new learning. An individual with cognitive impairment learns most effectively when building on existing knowledge schemes. Review helps promote connections and linkage between concepts in long-term memory; continual usage facilitates recognition and recall with less cognitive load demand.

It is important to use the Quick-Step Assessment to evaluate whether scenarios generated in group are useful as teaching examples. If the topic is interesting and applies, it may strike the balance between holding the group's attention and being a good example for skills application. Conversely, if the topic is too provocative and elicits high emotions, cognitive load demands may increase, impeding learning.

Disclosure Questions

The trainer asks for personal examples of skills use during the homework review portion of group meeting—for example: "Our homework was to use On-Track Thinking this week. Who would like to share about using that skill?" The trainer wants the individual to describe times during the week when she used the specific skill and link it to others. The point is less about disclosure of personal information than about skills integration.

Disclosure questions will happen throughout the various E-Spiral phases of group. Personal examples help the group broaden and contextualize learning. For example, questions such as "Has anyone ever had difficulty asking for what they want from people?", "What happened?", and "Did it work out like you wanted?" educate the group about challenges and factors that need to be managed in the natural environment.

It is important to help the individual be efficient with disclosures; instructors have to guide content and time management with the group to ensure that the discussion is focused and allows everyone to participate. While it is often necessary to address human issues that are relevant, detailing highly personal or arousing events may lead to dysregulation of group members. The trainer may ask a participant to discuss a certain topic with the individual therapist or skills trainer after group: "Mary, that sounds like a difficult situation. I am wondering if it would be best for the two of us to discuss that right after group?" If the individual insists on discussing the issue in group, the instructor may have to reorient to the topic and offer skills coaching to the person relating to waiting until the end of group to discuss the issue—for example: "I can hear that you would like to talk about this issue *and* it is difficult to wait sometimes. What skills might help you focus on group until we are able to check in?" Using the word "and" is helpful. It sends a message of validation and acceptance about situations, yet transitions to mobilizing effective behavior.

Clarifying Questions

Clarifying questions may be helpful during homework reviews to promote a deeper and more detailed understanding of a topic. For example, the participant may attempt to describe a situation that happened during the week. The details and time frames may be challenging to follow or vague. Instructors ask clarifying questions, such as "Can you tell us a little more about that so we can clearly understand?" or "Help me understand. On Tuesday you first had an argument with your coworker, and on Wednesday you called your boss?" The participant may need assistance recalling the chain of events due to sequencing deficits.

Additionally, clarifying questions can help the person improve self-awareness—for example, "What body sensations did you notice just before you walked in to meet with your boss?" The skills trainer helps the individual and the group gain clarity and improved understanding; experiencing the process of becoming clearer is an important aspect of learning.

The trainer asks describe, disclosure, and clarifying questions and makes linking statements that highlight commonalities between participants' experiences: "It is interesting that Kevin, James, and Mary, were all dealing with challenging coworkers this week." The instructor consolidates points and moves discussions toward the skills topics that are on the agenda for the group. For example, the leaders may choose to focus on work relationships as a relevant context for learning about the skill for the week. Finding common threads helps create a synthesized body of material that is generated from diverse sources. Additionally, linking provides validation that others are having similar experiences.

Orienting to a New Skills Topic

Once the participants have reviewed skills usage from the previous week (e.g., Week 3—Clear Picture), it is time to introduce the topic for new learning (e.g., Week 4—On-Track Thinking). The instructor gives only a brief overview of the subject. The goal of this introduction is not to teach the material but merely to begin the process of exploring existing knowledge related to the topic.

Discussion: Exploring Existing Knowledge

The trainer cultivates a discussion about the new topic, expanding information that emerged from the homework review. For example, the homework review may have covered the group's experiences using Clear Picture. The discussion that transitions to the new topic (On-Track Thinking) might highlight one or more of those scenarios to prompt more in-depth exploration of what the group members noticed about their thinking and urges in those situations. Focusing on the thoughts and urges in more detail provides the base information for On-Track Thinking—Check It. When the instructor builds from the existing knowledge base and expands the topic to include a small amount of associated new information, cognitive load demands are lower than they are when transitioning to another unrelated topic.

Discussions between group members and the trainers can be useful interventions in Skills System instruction. When participants have an opportunity to self-reflect and express themselves, multiple aspects of growth are served. First, each person is taking skillful action. Additionally, participation in discussions provides an opportunity for the individual to mobilize her Core Self (self-awareness, acceptance, value, and trust) as she joins in the skills exploration. For example, as the person begins to be aware of others and to feel successful, self-awareness is reinforced. Similarly, as the individual listens to others and other people listen to her, self-acceptance is built. Self-value and self-trust develop as the individual interacts and uses skills within training sessions. The person learns implicit lessons about dialectics given that each person has a different perspective and group members can simultaneously coexist and collaborate safely.

Assessment Questions

Assessment questions are designed to assess the individual's existing knowledge of a given topic. For example, if the topic for the session is On-Track Thinking, the skills trainer may ask, "What is the difference between a thought and an urge?" Skills trainers elicit a baseline of information to evaluate each individual's knowledge and abilities.

Participants may offer inaccurate information during discussions. Instructors positively reinforce the participation and communicate that a more accurate answer is still needed—for example: "Good try . . . almost"; "We are getting closer, but we are not quite there . . . let's keep trying." Using the Quick-Step Assessment process, the trainer may adjust his question or give more hints, so that group members understand what he is looking for. To ensure that the group knows which information is accurate, the trainer restates key points, offers positive reinforcement, and writes accurate statements on the whiteboard.

The trainer uses verbal praise to reinforce effective behaviors. If the group members worked together to help each other get the right answer, the group can be praised. If one individual offered the correct answer, perhaps targeting him with praise is best. The trainer reinforces both types of on-track behaviors as soon as they happen in group to encourage more adaptive actions.

The skills trainer can teach a dialectical perspective by carefully constructing her feedback. For example, saying, "Yes, I have noticed that before, too" sends a different message than "You are right." The first option conveys a more dialectical perspective and communicates that there is value or truth in different perspectives. This tactic teaches that there are many sides in a situation versus merely right or wrong alternatives. This dialectical attitude helps teach foundational perspectives that enhance the individual's capacities to engage in reciprocal relationships (being connected with others while maintaining identity). It is more effective to teach dialectics implicitly to individuals diagnosed with intellectual disabilities rather than explicitly. Instructors guide discussions into the gray areas of situations rather than focusing on a black versus white, polarized perspective.

Orienting to Relevant Context

Relevant Context Questions

Motivation and interest are key ingredients for learning; relevant contextual questions are intended to highlight how learning new skills will help participants reach personal goals. For example: "How can off-track urges be a problem at work?" and "If you wanted to get a raise from your boss, how would acting on off-track urges impact that?" If the individual sees that managing emotions, thoughts, and action strategically can improve tangible real-life factors, motivation may be increased.

In addition to stimulating interest, using contextual scenarios in group discussions can help store in long-term memory important information about the individuals, the specific context, and more general social contexts. As the group discusses the myriad internal and external facets that comprise the scenario, this behavior and solution analysis process cobbles together to build a more complete awareness. These bits of information about the situation and skills become integrated into schemata.

Perceptual reasoning is a deficit outlined in criteria for the diagnosis of ID (American Psychiatric Association, 2013). Promoting relevant schema acquisition creates the foundation for improving other deficits area of functioning. For example, expanding mechanisms for awareness and building a skills knowledge base provide the groundwork for improved perceptual reasoning and problems solving. To these ends, linking contextual information shared during the first phases of group with the later discussions in the E-Spiral Encoding, Elaboration, and Efficacy phases has a strong impact on learning and functioning.

During a discussion of relevant context, the trainer leads the group to highlight an important setting (e.g., work). The group members explore their perceptions about effective and ineffective actions in the context (e.g., being focused is on-track, and yelling at coworkers is off-track). The individual may understand that learning skills that help him improve focus at work and decrease coworker conflict may increase the likelihood he will get a raise from the employer.

The E-Spiral—Building Existing Knowledge base phase provides a foundation for building schemata that new learning and elaboration can expand and strengthen.

Some groups, particularly adolescents, have individuals with high levels of emotional dysregulation (e.g., hypervigilance associated with trauma). Exploring real-life contexts may elicit high emotions and cause immediate cognitive overload. It may be necessary to adjust interventions and create relevant, hypothetical scenarios. Unfortunately, generic situations may not mobilize motivation the way real-life ones do. Perhaps finding stories in the media or about celebrities can be impersonal enough to manage cognitive load demands yet stimulate interest that will sustain learning.

E-SPIRAL PHASE 2:
ENCODING ACTIVITIES THAT TEACH THE NEW TOPIC

Table 6.2 outlines E-Spiral Phase 2: Encoding Activities That Teach the New Topic. Once the group members have engaged in Exploring Existing Knowledge Base, they are prepared to learn new information. The goal of the E-Spiral: Encoding Phase is to have the participants learn accurate new skills information. A wide variety of encoding activities are used within the Skills System teaching model.

While direct instruction and teaching points are necessary, multimodal techniques are essential as well. Multimodal teaching strategies provide "dual coding" (Najjar, 1996, p. 14) of verbal and nonverbal stimuli, which may improve recall. Handouts, diagrams, cue pictures, gestures, and objects are many common strategies used to facilitate encoding of information. Skills trainers must be aware of cognitive load demands when integrating materials; the supplemental information must support familiar points versus presenting divergent information. The Skills System instruction blends encoding visual, spatial, acoustic, and semantic information related

---

TABLE 6.2. E-Spiral Phase 2: Encoding

Encoding: Teaching the new topic (new learning)

- Direct instruction that promotes encoding
    Teaching points
    Handouts—summary sheets, introductory handouts, and worked examples
    Diagrams
    Gestures
    Objects

- Discussions that promote encoding
    Content questions

---

to the topic. This multimodal approach helps an impaired learner encode, retain, and retrieve information.

Direct Instruction Activities That Promote Encoding

Teaching Points

Teaching points are excerpts provided within the 12-week-cycle curriculum in Chapter 7. These points are often presented as quotations. The quotes are not intended to prescribe teaching points; rather, they provide a worked example for skills trainers. The teaching points are examples of how to explain the skills concepts. These excerpts are not necessarily meant to be read; rather, they provide the trainer with principles to be translated into her own words. Merely reading the teaching points may be boring and reduce motivation.

Teaching within the Skills System is less oriented around lecture format and more focused on question-and-answer periods. It is important that correct information be generated during the encoding process. Therefore, the trainer asks clear, directed questions to elicit correct answers—for example: "If you are feeling very upset, is your mind usually clear or fuzzy?" Most participants will state that "fuzzy" is the more accurate answer. Guided discovery questions are not a quiz; they are a way to increase participation and motivation by expanding the individual's existing knowledge. In between questions and answers, the trainer presents teaching points about the concept. Beyond encoding and personal growth benefits, this question–answer format allows the trainer to monitor effectively a participant's integration of concepts.

It is useful to assess comprehension following direct instruction. Memory decay may occur for various reasons. Asking a participant to summarize points helps instructors evaluate integration. Summarizing prior to a transition from one topic to another topic helps to reinforce the learning.

Handouts

Handouts may be a key aspect of Skills System instruction and are foundational in the 12-week curriculum provided in Chapter 7. Every group member should have a complete set of handouts. Each type of handout serves different purposes. The summary sheets, introductory handouts, and worked example worksheets are useful during the encoding phase. The summary sheets may have less utility in group but may be helpful for home study or for staff training. The general handouts at the beginning of each section supply important introductory information. The worked example worksheets can be discussed to explain the skills concepts and serve as instructions about filling out the worksheet. Although participants' levels of comprehension of handouts may vary, the sheets can be used to facilitate group learning experiences. An individual diagnosed with moderate-severity ID may not be able to read the handout, but the visual aid components of the sheet can facilitate encoding and recall.

Basic handouts are available in Appendix A, but I encourage skills trainers to create new ones for groups and individual skills training. For example, it may be helpful for skills trainers to individualize handouts. Integrating digital pictures, using fun clip art, and scanning photographs may be beneficial. The practitioners must be careful to keep visual aids simple and clear to help minimize cognitive load demands of the materials.

Reviewing Handouts

Reviewing handouts is generally an interactive process between the skills trainers and participants. The trainer may invite an individual to read the text on the handout or to offer ideas about what the visual aid is communicating. If there are time constraints or there is not a participant who can read the information well enough for the group to clearly understand, the trainer may choose to read. The group and the skills trainer make a plan for how the handout is going to be reviewed prior to going over a page. It is important to engage each participant in the learning process, because it fosters investment and self-efficacy.

Skills trainers must be aware of managing the use of handouts in group. Although handouts provide a framework and visual encoding of information, instructors must be aware that cognitive load increases when an individual engages in multiple activities at the same time (e.g., looking at a handout, listening to the trainer, and answering questions). The trainer uses the Quick-Step Assessment to make adjustments. For example, perhaps the group takes a few minutes to look at the handout first, without talking. The instructor then asks questions, with ample time for the group to reorient to the page if necessary. Transitions increase cognitive load, so shifting rapidly or without orientation from one part of a handout to another can increase demands and reduce learning.

Diagrams

Drawing diagrams on a blackboard, large presentation pad, or whiteboard during discussions can be useful. Diagrams provide visual encoding of information. For example, as the group is discussing how a person can use a Safety Plan, the trainer may draw a diagram of an ascending arc marked with a 0, 1, 2, 3, 4, and 5, and show how a person escalated from a Level 1 emotion up to a Level 5 emotion (harming self, other, or property). Figure 6.1 is an example of a simple drawing that can explain intangible concepts more clearly.

The diagram can show the progression from one level to the next and associated behaviors. Then the group may discuss what skills might have been used to change the outcome. A new arc may be drawn to show what the progression may have looked like if the individual had utilized effective skills earlier in the situation. Visually mapping situations can aid comprehension, because the diagram implicitly teaches relationships between various factors.

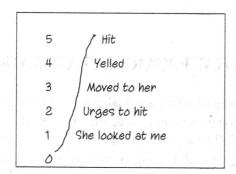 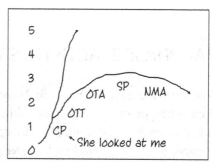

FIGURE 6.1. Examples of diagrams on a whiteboard.

Utilizing different colors makes activities more fun. Use of different colored markers can help the participants understand associations between concepts. For example, using the color orange in every Clear Picture handout creates an association between Clear Picture and orange. Using red to represent On-Track Thinking helps the person see the difference between information in orange and in red. Color coding diagrams can improve organization of information and enhance explicit and implicit learning (Gold, 1972).

Gestures

Gestures are useful techniques during teaching, because they can create tangible representations for abstract concepts. Referencing helpful (on-track to the goal) with a thumbs-up and not helpful (off-track to goal) with a thumbs-down is an example of using gestures. Gestures can draw on common knowledge that requires minimum cognitive load.

Objects

Objects are fun and useful. For example, a Tibetan singing bowl or bell is a basic tool in a Skills System group. Ringing of the bell is a cue to focus during the mindfulness activity; listening to multiple rings may also engage second-phase processing. Other objects, such as pompoms, can be used for Cheerleading thoughts, and red flags can be used to signify risks. Skills trainers can find various objects that represent facets of the Skills System and serve to prompt recall.

Discussions That Promote Encoding

Content Questions

Content questions ask the individual to recall information that has been previously introduced: "What is the first step in the Clear Picture skill?" It is important to expose the group to multiple rehearsals of information, so that material is stored in long-term memory. Asking questions about the separate chunks of information can increase the chances the individual learns a concept and is able to assemble it in skills chains. When the individual gets an answer wrong, the instructor remains positive. Statements such as "Almost!" or "You're close—try again!" instead of "No, that's wrong," are helpful.

SPIRAL PHASE 3: ACTIVITIES THAT PROMOTE ELABORATION

Table 6.3 outlines the E-Spiral Phase 3: Activities that Promote Elaboration. Elaboration is an expanded encoding process that creates "additional memory records that improve the ability of the individual to retrieve the original memory" (Najjar, 1996, p. 14). There are two important aspects of elaboration: (1) expanding knowledge and (2) linking knowledge. In the Elaboration Phase, the participants practice the skills concepts, integrating previous skills knowledge and the new learning.

TABLE 6.3. E-Spiral Phase 3: Elaboration
Elaboration: Practice new learning and link it to previous learning (practice)
• Activities that promote elaboration
Worksheets
Practice exercises
Collaborative feedback
Individual instruction
• Discussion that promote elaboration
Linking questions
Disclosure questions
Expansion questions

Activities That Promote Elaboration

Worksheets

There are many worksheets included in Appendix A of this book. Skills trainers may also design other worksheets for participants. Individualizing worksheets can increase the relevance and impact of the activity. It may be logistically challenging and time-consuming to complete worksheets during group; it may be more advantageous to utilize worksheets as homework assignments.

Individuals in Skills System group often have highly variable levels of academic abilities. Instructors need to personalize the means through which worksheets are completed. One person may be able to complete worksheets independently, while another may require support. The participant may have specific support staff, group members, friends, or family members who help complete paperwork with them. There may be benefits to the person's individual therapist helping to fill out the worksheets. Skills trainers ask participants about their plan to complete the homework assignment prior to leaving group.

Practice Exercises

Practice exercises are a vital aspect of the learning process. For example, when the group is learning about breathing, it is essential to practice breathing. Talking about breathing teaches about the topic, yet the experience of practicing breathing teaches at a broader and deeper level. Contextual learning that does not lead to cognitive overload facilitates retrieval and generalization. Skills trainers should be creative during group and design practice exercises in the moment that integrate the relevant context and content being covered. Trainers should not be reliant solely on the practice exercises provided in this curriculum. For example, if a discussion comes up about voice tone, the trainer can create an impromptu exercise in which each group member says something using a wimpy, then an aggressive, then an assertive tone.

Collaborative Feedback

It is helpful to offer feedback to the individual during and after a practice exercise. Asking the individual if he would like feedback, before offering it, gives him control in the situation and creates a reciprocal interaction between individual and trainer—for example: "Brian, would you like to get feedback about your voice tone?" The trainer can also ask the individual if he would like feedback from the group. Collaborative feedback is intended to explore whether the individual's actions in the exercise would work to reach his desired outcome. An example of a collaborative approach might be "Brian, I noticed that when you were trying to be assertive, you were looking down. Did you notice that?" The trainer may ask Brian more specific questions or ask the group to delve into a topic to cover the point less directly.

Individual Instruction

During discussions or practice activities, it may be necessary to provide individual instruction for certain participants. If the teaching point is relatively brief, doing the individualized teaching in group is beneficial for the individual and the group. Another participant may have the same issue and would gain from the clarification. If the individual has significant difficulties or if review of the material would disrupt group, meeting with the skills trainer following group to create a plan may be a better option.

Discussions That Support Elaboration

Discussions are another important tool in cultivating elaboration. Once the group has worked on practicing the skill, it is helpful to engage in a discussion that links previous and present learning. During this phase, the skills trainer asks questions that link information, promote personal disclosure, and expand awareness of topics.

Linking Questions

Linking questions are designed to foster elaboration of learning through connecting new with past learning. One example might be "You mentioned earlier in group that you hit a housemate when she stared at you. How do you think what we learned about Safety Planning today might have been helpful in that situation?" It is important to be nonjudgmental during discussions; highlighting what behaviors tend to elicit desired results is different than saying a person's choice was good or bad. Skills trainers may comment about experiences, but preaching and being overcontrolling are not effective strategies.

Linking question can also be used to prompt the group to assemble skills chains—for example: "Once Mary does a Safety Plan in that situation, what other skill might be helpful (e.g., New-Me Activities)?" Similarly asking the numbers of the skill chain creates linkages. The trainer wants the group to understand that Safety Plan is a 1234 and adding a New-Me Activity would be a 12345. These types of quantitative activities may be initially challenging, but with practice, quantitative reasoning related to skills can improve.

Expansion Questions

Expansion questions are designed to broaden the scope of the individual's understanding of a concept. For example, the skills trainer may ask, "What other skills would you use in that situation?" Asking the "what–if" questions helps the individual learn about various options and the impact on situations. Participants need to know that different actions work well in diverse circumstances. Expansion questions can help a participant understand unusual situations when traditional approaches may be ineffective. For example, the individual needs to know that yelling at people is an important skill in certain situations; the lessons are about using the right skills at the right time. This is an important aspect of learning how to generalize skills into diverse contexts.

E-SPIRAL PHASE 4: ACTIVITIES THAT ADVANCE EFFICACY

Table 6.4 outlines Activities that Advance Efficacy. Efficacy-oriented exercises are designed to increase the likelihood that the individual will be able to (and want to) perform a skill in her natural environment. There are two important elements of this phase: (1) being able to use the skill in context, and (2) commitment to using the skill. Retrieval of information is improved if the learning and retrieval contexts are similar. Preparing the individual for real life through situational learning promotes generalization and self-efficacy. Unfortunately, contextual learn-

---

TABLE 6.4. E-Spiral Phase 4: Efficacy

Efficacy: Bridge to real life (real life)

- Activities that promote efficacy
    Role play
    Psychodrama
    In vivo

- Discussion promoting efficacy
    Barrier questions
    Wisdom questions
    Commitment questions
    Coaching questions

- Group-Ending Activities
    Homework
    Mindfulness breathing

---

ing and real-life execution of skills creates high cognitive load. It may be necessary to shaping behaviors in activities role play, psychodrama, and *in vivo* practice. Although contextual learning may promote improved integration of skills, these activities may elicit higher levels of emotions. It is important to monitor contextual learning activities carefully to manage cognitive load factors.

Activities That Promote Efficacy

Role Play

Role-play activities are important aspects of Skills System teaching. It is ideal if each participant has an opportunity to participate. Time constraints may impact these activities. Dividing into pairs or small groups may increase opportunities for participation.

The skills trainer and the participants work collaboratively to discuss options and solutions in role-play scenarios. The instructors may request that participants act out various action options to help visualize diverse factors and outcomes. The group can explore how things work and what are natural reactions through role plays. This process provides validation and an experience that advances self-efficacy.

Psychodrama Techniques

Psychodrama enactments often expand on traditional role plays by having additional group members play roles that represent various internal and external components within a situation. For example, if an individual role-plays talking to his house manager, one group member can role-play the participant's On-Track Thinking, and another can articulate Off-Track Thinking. This expanded role-play technique is helpful, because the participant can listen to both types of thinking and make an on-track decision. This technique makes intangible forces (e.g., thoughts) more tangible for participants. Additionally, this exercise helps the individual experience real-life pressures and sensations related to the context within which skills will need to be demonstrated. If the person is struggling, he can ask groupmates to assist as skills coaching voices. Behavioral rehearsal under these contextual conditions helps improve the individual's capacity to perform skills outside of group.

It is important to build the complexity of a psychodrama slowly to manage cognitive load demands. Instructors may want gradually to assemble the players so that the activity does not overstimulate the group. It may be useful to pose the rule that one person speaks at a time. Psychodrama techniques "use active/interactive techniques that stimulate more sensory and affective modes of learning than the verbal modality alone" (Tommasulo, 2005, p. 1). While engaging sensory and emotional aspects might have benefits in this process, when working with individuals who experience significant dysregulation, the skills trainer must proceed cautiously.

In Vivo *Exercises*

In vivo exercises utilize elements of a participant's actual life rather than creating a contrived environment. Support providers and/or family members may be invited to individual skills training sessions for *in vivo* activities. For example, the skills trainer may ask whether the participant wants to practice a skill with her staff, who is in the waiting room. The instructor may function as a skills coach.

Following the exercise, participant and instructor have a rich opportunity to process the experience. The skills trainer gains a firsthand view of both parties and therefore becomes a more effective skills coach for the participant. *In vivo* exercises may be an important vehicle for generalization of skills into daily life and relationships.

Discussions That Promote Efficacy

Discussions can be designed to improve efficacy. For example, participants can discuss common challenges related to using skills and/or communicating each individual's personal commitment to using skills. Through these discussions, participants communicate personal opinions, make a public commitment, and plan for integrating skills into their lives that strengthen the individual's Core Self.

Barrier Questions

Generalization of skills may be difficult due to barriers that are encountered in each unique situation. Emotions, thoughts, action urges, and external forces may interplay to create challenges for the individual. He must learn to become aware of barriers so that contingency planning is possible. Barrier questions are designed to help the individual develop a realistic awareness of challenges he may encounter. For example, the trainer might ask, "How closely will you have to work with that person tomorrow at your job?" or "Will seeing her make it harder to stay on-track?" It is useful to explore specific factors that may happen before, during, and after events that affect the individual's ability to focus on or perform skills.

It is important for the individual to understand that all people are impacted by seemingly small issues; everyone faces challenges and skill barriers throughout each day. The self-invalidation can lower self-efficacy in that the individual perceives herself to be more dysfunctional than other people. Barrier questions are a great way to expand knowledge base about the natural environment, provide validation, and help to create realistic expectations.

Wisdom Questions

Wisdom questions ask the participant to share personal perspectives about a topic: "Which option do you feel would best fit?" or "As you look at all of these choices, which is a fit for you?" Helping the individual to cultivate self-reflection, consider personal perspectives, and find a sense of wisdom are important self-validating behaviors.

Commitment Questions

Commitment questions are a series of queries that guide the individual in deciding whether he is going to engage in a certain behavior. The question first poses whether the person values taking the action. For example, an instructor might ask, "James, when are you going to practice

Getting It Right?" Once the person commits to using the skill, the trainer then tries to get the individual to commit to a plan of action: "James, you mentioned that you wanted to learn to use Getting It Right with your boss. What is your plan to do that?"; "You sound as if you are committed to using skills with your boss. What exactly is your plan?" The trainer can highlight the barriers and double-check whether the individual is willing, ready, and able to start the plan—for example: "We have already talked about all of the things that are going to be difficult about this; are you sure you are ready to give this a try?" It is vital that the individual knows how to seek skills coaching support when challenges are encountered.

Coaching Questions

Coaching questions prompt the participant to consider what skills would be helpful in a situation. Coaching questions are useful during the Efficacy Phase, after the individual makes a public commitment to use skills: "James, what skills are you going to use if your emotions go over a Level 3 when you are talking to your boss?" Coaching questions help create a plan for times when it is challenging to use skills.

Coaching questions may also be helpful when a participant is experiencing stress in skills training. For example, the leader can ask, "What skills could help you handle this exercise?" Depending on the individual's level of skills knowledge, the instructor may offer suggestions to the participant: "Do you think doing a Safety Plan right now would help?" When the individual is over a Level 3 emotion, the instructor may want to ask the individual to go to the waiting area or meet with his support staff individually. If the individual rises above a Level 4 emotion, it may be necessary to move the other participants to another area if there are safety risks.

Group-Ending Activities

Highlighting Home Study Opportunities

At the end of group, the leader assigns homework to be completed between sessions. Home study activities can increase skills knowledge, generalization, and efficacy. As the individual increases knowledge about skills, she is encouraged to participate in ongoing, self-directed, skillful behaviors in daily living. The skills trainer focuses on fostering the individual's internal motivation and commitment to maintain skillful behavior. The following activities are a few home study options that can be assigned by the trainer and/or utilized by the individual for independent study.

Skills Notebooks

Each participant needs to have a skills notebook when he enters skills training (Appendix A, p. 197). The notebook contains all of the skills handouts and homework sheets. The individual can use the notebook to carry any individualized paperwork, such as diary cards or Safety Plans. The participant should control as many decisions about the notebook as possible. He uses the skills notebook to study skills and to teach skills coaches about skills. Skills notebooks and other study materials are available at the Skills System website at *www.guilford.com/skills-system*.

Homework Assignments

The primary homework assignments within the Skills System are to practice skills, in particular the new skill presented during the week. For example, if the skill was Problem Solving, one aspect of the homework would be to use a 1236 skills chain in between groups. Attempting to use the skills chain in context and reporting back about the process, outcomes, and challenges are a valuable part of generalizing skills in the natural environment.

In addition, the trainer may assign worksheets or practice exercises (from this book or created by the trainer) as homework. The individual may complete these sheets independently or with support. The focus of these assignments is not the reading and writing, but the content of the worksheet. It is not critical that the individual fill out the paper. When homework assignments are given, each individual makes a plan about how to accomplish the assignment. The Skills System homework assignments are generally simple, so that a person can be successful. The trainer may give special homework assignments to particular group members for individualized study.

Skills Cards

Skills cards are a fun home study and group activity. Skills flash cards help an individual (or group) learn the components of each skill and the System Tools. Cards give the individual a chance to engage physically to the learn names, numbers, and pictures associated with the skills. An individual or group can put the skills cards in order on a large table or on the floor. The cards can be put together in skills chains to represent skills that were or could be used in a scenario. In group, a trainer can also ask quiz questions and the individual can search the skills cards for the correct answer. Making practice fun enhances skills elaboration and generalization.

The individual can do partnership activities with family members, friends, and/or support providers to enhance skills capacities of both people. The Skills System can create a common skills language, as well as promote a reciprocal relationship between the individual and the other person. As the individual teaches the people around him, he fosters a sense of mastery and self-efficacy.

Skills Games

Skills games are a great way to practice skills. Many games can be adapted as a skills game. Who Wants to Be a Skillionaire or Skills Jeopardy is a fun skills trivia activity. The Trainer or participants develop skills questions and create a game show format. Many other games can be turned into skills activities by setting a rule that in order to take a move or receive a token, for example, the participant must correctly answer a skills question.

Skills Journaling

The person may choose to write in a journal. Focusing on exploring self-awareness, self-expression, and descriptive skills can be advantageous. Ruminating on past issues or current problems may be less helpful than highlighting a problem and writing about possible skills that could be used to manage the difficulty effectively.

Phone Consultation and Skills Coaching

When the Skills System is used in conjunction with DBT, phone skills coaching by the individual therapist is integrated into the treatment model (Linehan, 1993a). This mode of treatment facilitates generalization of skills in the natural environment. It is important to establish and follow mutually agreed upon rules for skills coaching calls.

TRANSITION TO CHAPTER 7

Chapter 7 is a worked example of a 12-week curriculum. The skills trainer should read the entire section through, prior to starting a group. Each week, the trainer focuses on the week's materials, integrating information from Chapters 4–6, to create effective teaching plans for skills groups.

Skills System
12-Week-Cycle Curriculum

Chapter 7 contains a sample 12-week-cycle curriculum. Each week of this framework includes a detailed teaching plan and options for future cycles through the material. Skills trainers will notice that instructions and explanations are presented as quotes. This format is intended to provide a worked example for trainers rather than to prescribe language. All Skills System visual aid materials are contained in Appendix A of this book, beginning on page 197.

It is impossible to predict whether the group will complete a teaching plan. Different settings have varying time frames for group sessions. Additionally, skills trainers must remember that the intellectual abilities of group members are unique. Therefore, the collective capacity of each skills group will be variable. This curriculum is a general guide for instructors. It is unlikely that all of the activities will be completed during the time frames that are available to the group.

It is important that Skills System skills trainers are creative. Skills group leaders are encouraged to develop various skills exercises, games, and practice activities that reflect the capacities, interests, and contexts of the group members. It is important to remember that a creative intervention does not necessarily need to be complex. It is important to keep activities simple and clear so that specific teaching points are made. Overcomplicating interventions may not only increase cognitive load but also muddy the key points you are trying to make. The DBT term "one-mindfully" or "one thing in the moment" (Linehan, 2015a, p. 447) helps the skills trainer remember to have the individual focus on a single element to reap maximum benefit from the experience.

In the event that the group does not complete the outlined material, trainers must determine whether to return to that week's materials during the next group or move on. If the group continues on, the remainder of the previous week's lessons can be addressed when the group returns to those topics in the following cycle through the curriculum. It is challenging to leave material unfinished, yet it may be the best long-term alternative. It is vital that an individual develop a broad understanding of the Skills System, so that she can deepen awareness within the full range of Skills System topics. Focusing on a few elements in depth may increase understanding of those topics, yet hinder development of overall emotion regulation capacities and generalization of Skills System concepts. Although it is difficult, it is recommended that the group leave unfinished topics and progress to the following week's teaching. As the skills trainer gains a fuller understanding of the Skills System and the skills group, it will be easier to create realistic and effective teaching plans.

The 12-week-cycle curriculum presents detailed teaching suggestions. Participants will have a wide variety of responses to the activities and discussion questions. Although the script presented below assumes compliance and participation, the realities may be very different in a skills training session. For example, the trainer may encounter silence, partial answers, irreverent attitudes, belligerence, and/or dissociation all at the same time! It may be necessary for the skills trainer to use his skills during group to remain on-track to the learning goals. The following suggestions may help the skills trainer when the group is not going well.

HELPFUL HINTS FOR THE TRAINER

- Taking a few breaths and getting a Clear Picture of the present moment is helpful.
- The trainer can self-reflect as to whether his mindset, tone, and interventions are on-track. A trainer's attitude can trigger problematic transactions and resistance from the group. Check It, Turn It Up, and Cheerleading may be useful to try. A more careful chain analysis after group may help the trainer make changes in tactics for future groups.
- Utilizing the Quick-Step Assessment to evaluate and adjust interventions is important. Interventions that create high cognitive load can cause group members to experience cognitive overload. Cognitive overload can have myriad presentation that disrupts harmony in group. The trainer makes necessary adjustments to simplify and/or break down topics further—for example, asking questions or framing points in alternative ways to prompt engagement.
- The trainer may consider offering skills coaching to an individual experiencing stress. The trainer may ask questions to elicit Clear Picture and On-Track Thinking as the first steps; if the person is more dysregulated, the trainer may help the individual take an On-Track Action. Reminding the individual about her goal, capacities, and skills can help her get back on-track. To help to normalize the experience, it may be useful to acknowledge that learning new things can be a challenging experience.
- Initiating a brief breathing exercise may help the participants and trainers improve focus. Shifting to a game form can Switch Tracks as well. The trainer needs to be mindful of behavioral principles, in that having off-track group members control the group lesson plan on a long-term basis is not in anyone's best interest.
- If the individual or individuals are emotionally, cognitively, and behaviorally regulated (below a Level 3 emotion), then the trainer may focus on Problem Solving to address elements of the situation that need to be changed or Expressing Myself to communicate about the circumstance. If there is a co-leader or skills coach available, it may be best to utilize that person to do individualized skills coaching, so the leader can remain engaged with the group.
- If a participant is experiencing a Level 3 or higher emotion, Safety Planning is more effective. It may be helpful for the person to focus on a New-Me Activity (e.g., attend to the group, do a Focus New-Me Activity in group), move to a different area in the room, or leave

the group. The individual could do a Focus New-Me Activity in the waiting area (e.g., puzzle or card sorting) and return when she is more on-track.

• If the individual refuses to leave the area, the group may have to evacuate the room. It is essential that the skills trainer notice the early warning signs for an individual who is likely to demonstrate violent behaviors. Taking precautions and intervening efficiently is necessary to protect the well-being of the other group members. Having two exits in a group room is optimal. After a problematic event in group, it may be helpful to debrief the other group members to discuss skills that the participants used to manage the event.

• The trainer may need to be cautious about using significant group time to do skills coaching if it is not pertinent for the topic. It may be necessary to ask a participant who does not regain control to step into the waiting area to do Safety Planning with his support staff. Following the group, the trainer may want to review the event and work with the individual to create an On-Track Action Plan for group.

Facilitating any type of therapeutic group can be challenging. It is impossible to know how each individual is going to react. It may be helpful to have co-leaders or other staff members as resources in case there are difficulties. If the trainer is alone, it may be difficult for him to monitor individuals that leave group in a dysregulated state. If there are risk issues such as these, it is important to have procedures in place to manage dangerous situations.

The following sections present options for leading skills groups. Newer skills trainers will want to review this information prior to group and organize a teaching plan. The trainer may make a copy of that week's curriculum, highlighting key points and handouts to review. A trainer working with a mature group may decide to follow the curriculum in the book, reading teaching points; this could be a more collaborative learning approach. More experienced trainers who know the Skills System concepts well may have more unplanned, organic approaches. Generally speaking, the 12-week curriculum lesson plans in the following sections are merely a guide and should not be followed verbatim if they do not fit for the individual or group.

WEEK 1: THE SKILLS LIST

Preparing for Group

Handouts Needed

✓ Skills System Review Questions (p. 223 of Appendix A)
✓ Skills System Handout 1 (p. 199)
✓ Skills System Handout 2 (p. 200)

E-Spiral Phase 1. Exploring Existing Knowledge Base (Review)

➡ *Welcome group.* "Hello, everyone! How are you all doing today? [Wait for response] OK, it is wonderful to see you all; I am very excited about beginning a skills group with you. Are we ready to get to know each other? We are going to jump in with our first On-Track Action by introducing ourselves. If you are feeling a little shy, notice that feeling and tell us your name anyway! Who is really brave and would like to start?"

Note: Skills trainers may want to consider entering the group and greeting participants in a friendly and positive way. Engaging in chitchat is an opportunity for the skills trainer to better understand who the person is, what is important to her, and how she currently regulates emotions. Trainers can use the information to begin the process of doing a Quick-Step Assessment in group for each member.

When the group is beginning or new members join, participants should introduce themselves to each other. Trainers may begin by having group members share their names. The group leader may also have group members share a piece of fun personal information—for example: "What is your favorite kind of pizza?" or "What is your favorite TV show?" If the group members are already familiar with each other, the leader may request that each person respond to questions such as "What are you hoping to learn from this group?" or "What is one of your goals?" The leader is trying to create a comfortable and safe therapeutic environment. Validating the challenges of starting a new group may be helpful.

After reviewing names, it is important that the group members talk about the goal of the group. The leader asks a few simple questions, such as "What do we study in this group?" or "Why do we do that?" Not all group members may know why they are there. Additionally, they may not be there voluntarily. The trainer may want to validate challenges of joining a group and communicate enthusiasm about helping them reach their personal goals.

➡ *Orient to the mindfulness activity: noticing the breath.* "OK, is everyone ready to learn some skills? Great, let's get started. We are going to begin by noticing our breathing."

Note: After introductions, group leaders want to orient the group to the first group activity. Skills trainers have to be prepared to deal with a client saying "no" to invitations; keep invitations open and move on to interact with an individual who is actively participating. It may be helpful to check in with the nonparticipating person after group to do problem solving, if necessary. Additionally, as mentioned in the previous chapter, this curriculum uses a Tibetan singing bowl (referred to as the "bell") in mindfulness activities. The auditory cue helps the participants to begin and end tasks. Adjust the instructions as needed to accommodate not using a bell or using another mechanism.

Instructions for the mindfulness exercise. "We begin every group by doing a mindfulness practice. Today we will start with a simple breathing exercise. When we focus our attention on our breathing, we are being mindful. We are using our minds to pay attention to our breath. Unfortunately, our minds are not always easy to control. That's why we have to practice being mindful. The cool thing is that when we are mindful, we are very focused on what is happening right now. Noticing our breath is actually a really important skill, and it is so simple. When we notice our breathing, it helps us be aware and focused, even in stressful and emotional situations. Are you ready to hear about what we have to do? Are you ready to give 100% when we do this exercise? OK, first, please sit in a comfortable position with your eyes open. Then I will ring the bell six times [involves tapping the bowl with a small wooden striker]. When you hear the first ring, begin to notice your breathing. Notice how your body feels as the air goes in and out. Notice whether you breathe through your mouth or your nose. Usually our minds try to wander to other things. Sometimes we think of the past or the future. Notice where your mind goes and gently bring your mind back to noticing your breath. You may notice feelings inside of you; notice your emotions and bring your attention back to your breathing. One of our goals is to learn to control and shift our attention; this activity helps us practice that. Do you have any questions?"

Note: Careful and detailed instructions about the tasks and how to reorient are important. After the exercise, the group members review the mindfulness activity and share details describing what they noticed. The trainer may want to write down the observations on the board. It is important to reinforce effort and participation. This exercise is intended to teach awareness of attention and the action of reorienting attention to the breath.

Describe questions. Perhaps choose a few questions to ask: "Were you breathing through you nose or mouth?"; "Where did you feel the breath in your body?"; "Did you notice it in different places: your nose, chest, or belly?"; "Did your breathing change at all?"; "Did you notice the bell sound?"; "Did you notice your attention drifting away?"; "What did you do to bring your attention back?"

➡ ***Orient to Skills System review.*** "Great describing and sharing. After doing our mindfulness practice each week, we will review the Skills List and other important Skills System information. Since it is our first week, we will jump right into new learning. Next week, we will review our skills at this time in group."

Note: In other cycles through Week 1, the skills review can include either answering the Skills System Review Questions (p. 223) or doing a creative skills review activity that prompts recall of the names and numbers of each skill, along with the basics of the Feelings Rating Scale, Categories of Skills, and Recipe for Skills. The trainer uses the review process to evaluate how participants are integrating the information. The weekly assessment helps the trainer to shape and expand each participant's skills knowledge base.

➡ ***Orient to skills practice.*** "Great job! Not only do we have to remember the names and numbers of the skills, but we all have to practice using our skills at home. Each week we will share with each other about a time when we used our skills during the week. So our homework every week is to use our skills and to be willing to talk about it at the next group. The more skills we use the better! Sound OK? Great."

Disclosure questions. "I bet folks are using some skills to handle tough situations. Who would like to tell us about a challenging time this week that they were able to manage? What did you do that was helpful?"

Note: In the first week of Cycle 1, the group discusses existing coping skills that the members used during the week. The leader then can label the skill using the Skills System names. For example, if the individual labels an emotion, the trainer can say, "That's a good Clear Picture." The activity of labeling existing skills can help the individual understand that she already has basic capacities that will be enhanced. Otherwise, in later groups, the trainer will ask more specifically, "Let's talk about how we used Clear Picture this week," depending on the assignment from the week before.

➡️ *Orient to new skills topic.* "I think many of you are already using some of the skills, and you don't know it! Today we are going to talk together about different ways we handle stressful situations. You might feel shy, but it is great to jump in with both feet and share your ideas and opinions. Ready?"

Note: Questions that are provided are samples. The trainer can choose one, none, or all to discuss. Each group marches through the material differently, the trainer capitalizing on available teachable moments.

🗨️ *Discuss existing knowledge about the new topic.*

Assessment questions. "What is stress?"; "What are emotions?"; "What is it like when emotions go high?"

Relevant context questions. "What kinds of situations stress us out?"; "Is it sometimes hard for people to do things that are helpful in these situations?"; "Why do you think that is?"

➡️ *Orient to relevant context of the new topic.* "Great discussion—thank you all. It seems as if all of us have seen or done both helpful and not helpful things when we are in tough situations. Life is very difficult sometimes for all of us. [Cite specific examples given previously in the group.] As we have heard, our thoughts and our feelings can be overwhelming and hard to handle. The Skills System can help us stay on-track even when life gets stressful. We have already learned an important skill today: noticing our breath. It can help in stressful situations. We are already on our way to being Skills Masters."

E-Spiral Phase 2. Encoding: New Learning

➡️ *Orient to new learning: Skills List.* "The Skills System helps us learn how to control our behaviors so that we can reach our goals. These nine skills help us do things that help us feel better and get what we need. Right now we are going to learn the names, numbers, and pictures of the nine skills in the Skills System. How many skills are there in the Skills System?" [Group: "Nine!"; Trainer: "All together, how many?"; Group: "NINE!"] Great, see, you are already getting it! I knew you could do this! Are you ready to learn more about how to handle things well? Great."

Instructions for the encoding activity. "Let's all find Skills System Handout 1. It is on page 199 and it looks like this. [Hold up the page and be sure each participant has the page before continuing.] Would someone like to read, or would you like me to? We are going to read the number and name of each skill. We are also going to discuss each skill picture and what it means. Any questions?"

Note: After reading each skill, the group talks about each skill picture. They discuss the skill and the relevance of the picture to the skill. If a group member reads and the communication is unclear, the skills trainer need to repeat the section so that each group member clearly understands the information. The group needs to move through the teaching material; leaders may have to limit group reading if it hinders progression through the information.

➡ ***Orient to reviewing Skills System Handout 2.*** "Okay, fantastic. Now we have to read Skills System Handout 2: How Our Skills Help Us. It is on page 200 and looks like this. Would anyone like to read?"

Note: This handout is used as an overview to introduce group members to the function of each skill. This handout is not intended to be used as an in-depth teaching tool. A brief explanation about each skill as time allows is useful.

➡ ***Orient to the end of the Encoding Phase.*** "Does anyone have any questions about that handout? Great, now we are going to practice some of what we have learned."

E-Spiral Phase 3. Elaboration: Practice and Linking

➡ ***Orient to the elaboration activity.*** "So, we have gone over the Skills List once, and now we are going to practice it more, so that we can learn and remember the information. The more we go over this, the easier it is to remember the skills when we need them."

Instructions for the elaboration exercise. Note: Sample exercises A–F are listed below; choose one exercise per cycle. Elaboration exercises ask participants to practice recognition and recall of skills material in a noncontextual format. This phase focuses on having participants expand their capacities effectively to demonstrate the tasks with increasingly less support.

The activities listed below can be completed with or without using visual aid materials. The group can begin using handouts as a worked example, then shift away from using the cues as confidence builds. The skills trainer may allow each individual to make a personal decision as to whether she wants to look at the sheet, although prompting the individual to stretch and try to close the book may be helpful at some point.

The exercises below become progressively more difficult; thus, during initial cycles through the curriculum, easier exercises minimize cognitive load demands. Be sure to explain the exercise so that the group members clearly understand the activity. Leaders and groups can invent fun ways to practice the numbers and names of skills that fit the learning needs of the participants.

Options for Basic Review Exercises

A. The skills trainer says a number from 1 to 9 and the group reads the skill name from the handout. The group members try to get quicker and more accurate as the exercise progresses.

B. Using handouts to guide them, the group members put the skills cards representing the numbers, pictures, initials, and skills names in order on a large table or the floor.

C. The leader creates a competition between individuals or teams. She holds up one of the skills cards and ask a question about another element of the skill. For example, if she holds up a card with a "2," the group may have to say the associated skill name, describe the skill picture, or tell the initials. The team that gets it correct gets a point.

D. The group members close their books. A group leader writes 1–9 on the board. The group members try to fill in the blank spaces.

E. With no visual aids, a leader asks the group to say the nine skills in order.

F. With no visual aids, a group leader says a number, and the group members say the skill.

G. A group leader has a client say the first skill, and the next person says the second, and so on.

Describe questions. "How was that exercise for you?"

➡ **Orient to discussion.** "I think you all did a great job with that exercise. Now, we are going to talk together about skills, so that we can begin to understand them a little better."

Note: The goal of an elaboration-oriented discussion is to begin the process of linking, personalizing, and expanding the participants' semantic knowledge related to the new learning; connecting past and present learning increases integration of the material.

Linking question. "Have any of you used skills like these in the past?"

Disclosure question. "Can you tell us about a time in the past when you had problems handling thoughts or emotions?"

Expansion questions. "Has anyone else had a similar experience?"; "Do you think that there are times when knowing skills would help you reach your goals?"

Note: These discussions are not intended to delve into traumatic memory material or detailed accounts of events. The skills trainer listens to the specific point that is being made, then creates a general statement that applies to all participants. For example, "That situation with your coworker sounds difficult. So, are coworker relationships situations in which we need to use our skills? Has anyone else had challenges with coworkers?"

➡ **Orient to the end of the Elaboration Phase.** "I can't believe how much you all know about skills already. We are going to do very well with the Skills System."

E-Spiral Phase 4. Efficacy: Bridge to Real Life

➡ **Orient to efficacy activities.** "It is important to have fun while we are learning, so that we will like doing it. Right now we are going to play a game."

Note: It is important to have group members participate in activities. During the first cycle through the Skills System curriculum, games, worksheets, and role plays are simple and brief. Over time, leaders can design more complex, lengthy activities that foster generalization of skills information.

Instructions for efficacy activities. "I am going to ask the group some questions. Raise your hand if you think you know the answer. If you want to look at your handouts, that's OK. Ready?"

"What is the name of the skill that helps us fix our problems?"

"What skill helps me know what is going on inside and outside of me?"

"What skill is it when I enjoy a cup of tea and have a snack?"

"What skill is it when I do something to get back on-track?"

"What skill is it when I tell someone how I feel?"

"What skill is it when I think about how to handle a situation?"

"What skill is it when I try to get what I want?"

"What skill helps me handle risky situations?"

"What skill is it when I show my friend that I care about them?"

Note: This activity is intended to elicit correct answers. When the individual guesses incorrectly, the skills trainer may say, "Close," "Almost," or "Try one more time," rather than "No, that's wrong." It may be necessary for a leader to give hints so that the group gets the correct answer. These questions are suggestions; trainers may adapt questions to ensure success for the participants.

Review questions. "How do you think that game went?"; "Was it hard to remember the skills?"

➡ *Orient to discussion.* "I thought you all did really well. We are going to take a few minutes to chat together before we leave for the day."

Note: The goal of these efficacy-oriented questions is to help the individual understand realistic challenges related to the topic. The discussion offers an opportunity for self-reflection about the learning. Participants are invited to make a personal commitment and plan for integrating the skill into their lives.

Barrier question. "So far, what is difficult for you about learning the Skills System?"

Wisdom question. "Do you think that it is important for you to learn skills?"

Commitment questions. Asking one or more of these commitment questions can help increase motivation: "Are you willing to face the challenge of trying new things?"; "Are you willing to learn and practice skills in group and in your life?"; "Are you willing to do some homework for group?"

Coaching question. "How can you coach yourself to learn and practice skills?"

➡ *Orient to home study.* "We can see that learning skills is challenging. It also sounds as if we all know that practice will help us get better at skills. We may not love doing homework, so it is a good thing that we have our On-Track Action skill to help us jump into our practicing! This week for homework, we are going to start learning our skills. Perhaps look over your skills handouts. Next week in group, we will review our skills. Also, notice your breath this week as many times as you can. We will talk about when you noticed your breathing and what you noticed about it. Do you have any questions?

"If anyone would like to study skills at home this week, you can do the Skills System Worksheet 1 or 2 (p. 201 or p. 202). You could also review today's handouts. Going over the Skills System Review Questions on page 223 is very helpful. Perhaps you can go over this sheet with staff members. As staff members learn skills, they are able to be skills coaches for us. Talk to me after group if you would like to go over these."

Note: Be sure the group members are clear about the locations of materials. Skills System Worksheets 1, 2, or 3 (pp. 201, 202, or 203, respectively) and the Skills System Review Questions (p. 223) can be completed as self-study or as homework in later cycles through the material. Following group, meet with any individuals to make a plan for completing the worksheets.

➡ *Orient to group ending.* "We ring the bell six times at the end of group. It is a chance to notice our breathing. We take a moment to focus our minds as we go back to our activities. Who would like to ring the bell today?"

Skills System Component Handouts to Review in Future Cycles or for Home Study

✓ Skills System Worksheet 1 (p. 201)
✓ Skills System Worksheet 2 (p. 202)
✓ Skills System Worksheet 3 (p. 203)

WEEK 2: SYSTEM TOOLS

Preparing for Group

Handouts Needed

✓ Skills System Review Questions (p. 223)
✓ Skills System Handout 3 (p. 204)
✓ Feelings Rating Scale Handout 1 (p. 205)
✓ Categories of Skills Handout 1 (p. 211)
✓ Recipe for Skills Handout 1 (p. 216)
✓ Week 2 Practice Activity Worked Example (p. 220)
✓ Week 2 Practice Activity Worksheet (p. 221)

E-Spiral Phase 1. Exploring Existing Knowledge Base (Review)

➡ *Welcome group.* "It is great to see everybody. How are you all doing? Are we ready to learn about skills?"

➡ *Orient to the mindfulness activity: noticing the air going in and out of my nose.* "What do we do first in group? You are right; we ring the bell. Why do we do that? Very good, because we want to focus our minds. OK, today we are going to learn more about breathing. We are going to notice the air going in and out of our noses as we breathe."

Instructions for mindfulness exercise. "Last week we rang the bell and noticed our breathing. Today we are going to ring the bell six times and notice our breathing again. This time we are going to notice the air going in and out of our noses. Our job is to bring 100% of our attention and focus to our noses. Sometimes our minds act like puppies; they jump all around. We have to be the boss of our minds, so that our attention goes where we tell it. So, if your attention drifts to things other than your nose, reel it in [makes a gesture of a fishing reel] and notice the air going in and out of your nose. You may notice other thoughts and feelings, too; notice them, allow them to pass, and bring your attention to your nose. This is important to us, because we have to be able to control our attention; we have to direct our minds to what is helpful to us. We have to get our puppies to listen and mind. Any questions? I will ring the bell, and we will start."

Describe questions. "What did you notice about the air going in and out of your nose?"; "Where else did your attention go?"; "Did you bring your focus back to your breathing?"; "How did you bring your attention back?"

Note: The group shares details about what they noticed. The leader may want to write observations on the board.

➡ **Orient to Skills System review.** "Good job! Now we are going to review the Skills List and the System Tools."

Note: The trainer can choose one of the review exercises A–G in Week 1 (see p. 115).

➡ **Orient to skills practice.** "OK, great job. You guys are really starting to be Skills Masters! Let's shift gears and go over our Skills Practice for this week. Your homework was to practice noticing your breath."

Disclosure questions related to the breath. "Who can tell us about when you noticed your breath this week?"; "What did you notice?"

Disclosure question related to studying skills. "Who had a chance to practice learning their skills?"; "Did any of you look at your notebook?"

Note: Starting with volunteers is helpful, because it gets the discussion started. Low self-efficacy can hinder volunteering. As a client shares, leaders can include a less participatory group member by asking one or more simple, direct questions, which may reduce the barriers for volunteering: "Bill, did you notice your breathing at all during the week?"; "Great, when was that?"; "OK, what did you notice?"

➡ **Orient to new skills topic.** "Great! I am going to ask a few questions that will help us talk about what we already know about handling strong emotions. OK?"

💬 **Discuss existing knowledge about the new topic.**

Assessment questions. "How does stress or strong emotion affect people?"; "How do strong emotions affect our actions?"

Relevant context question. "Do you think that people ever feel so confused that they just react without thinking?"

Clarifying questions. "Have you ever seen that happen?"; "How did it work out for the person?"

➡️ ***Orient to relevant context of the new topic.*** "Today we are going to learn about three important Skills System tools. One is the Feelings Rating Scale. Second is the Categories of Skills. Third is the Recipe for Skills."

E-Spiral Phase 2. Encoding: New Learning

➡️ ***Orient to new learning: System Tools.*** "We use the Feelings Rating Scale, Categories of Skills, and the Recipe for Skills to know which skills to use in every situation. Having these three tools can help us handle even very stressful and confusing situations! Life can be confusing for all of us. Being able to focus our attention and shift our attention helps us be in control of ourselves and our lives. When we know what is going on, we can be on-track. When we are unfocused, often we go off-track. Being focused helps us use our skills well."

Instructions for the encoding activity. "Does that sound OK?"; "Great. We are going to look at four different handouts. Please raise your hand if you have a question or feel lost. How about we turn to Skills System Handout 3 on page 204. What is our plan for reading this handout?"

Note: Skills trainers have many options about how to progress through the handouts, worked examples, and worksheets. This teaching plan reviews four basic handouts that serve as a preliminary introduction to the System Tools. There are worked examples and worksheets listed below that offer expansion of the concepts in these introductory handouts. The supplemental materials can be used in future cycles of the Skills System curriculum. How the leader decides to utilize these materials depends on the status of the group.

There are four handouts to review in this section. The information in the teaching points below is intended as learning tools for trainers, more so than as scripts to be read in group. As the leaders understand the skill concepts, briefer descriptions can be utilized in group that hit main points without being boring.

➡️ ***Orient to reviewing Skills System Handout 3.*** "Now if you are ready, let's turn to page 204, the Skills System Handout 3; it looks like this."

☆ *Section A teaching points.* "The first System Tool is the Feelings Rating Scale. It helps us rate how strong our feelings are. If you were a tiny bit upset, you would rate the emotion a 1. If we were very upset, you would label it as a 4. If you were so upset you were hurting yourself, someone else, or destroying property, the emotion would be rated a 5. We will learn more about the Feelings Rating Scale in the next handout. Any questions?"

☆ *Section B teaching points.* "The second System Tool is the Categories of Skills. Skills 1, 2, 3, 4, and 5 are our All-the-Time skills. We can use them any time, at any level of emotions rated 0–5. Skills 6, 7, 8, and 9 are Calm-Only skills. We use Calm-Only skills *only* when we are calm. This means we cannot use skills 6, 7, 8, and 9 when we are over emotion Level 3. We have to learn when we can use each skill and when we need to wait to use a skill until we are a little calmer. We will learn more about this on the Categories of Skills Handout 1 (p. 211). Any questions?"

☆ *Section C teaching points.* "It is important that we link skills together in skills chains, one after another, especially when we have strong emotions. The Recipe for Skills helps us remember to link together more skills when we are more emotional. Skills Masters use even more skills than the Recipe for Skills tells us to! The more skills we use, the more on-track to our goals we are. Any questions?"

➡ **Orient to Feelings Rating Scale Handout 1.** "Good job! Now we are going to take a few minutes to learn more about the Feelings Rating Scale. Please turn to page 205. This is the Feelings Rating Scale Handout 1."

☆ *Feelings Rating Scale Handout 1 teaching points.*

   ☆ "When we are at a Level 0 emotion, we are not having that emotion. For example, Level 0 sadness means that the person is not sad at that time."

   ☆ "A Level 1 emotion is a tiny emotion. We have a Level 1 emotion when we have a tiny reaction to something. For example, if have Level 1 sadness, I might feel an empty sensation in my chest or feel like looking at the ground."

   ☆ "A Level 2 emotion is a small emotion. We may notice different body sensations that a Level 2 emotion causes. At Level 2 sadness, I might notice my face changing, and my smile disappears; my shoulders may drop, because I feel a heaviness. My heart may begin to pound more, and my breathing may be affected. A Level 2 emotion may be a little uncomfortable, if it is a painful emotion."

   ☆ "A Level 3 emotion is a medium emotion. A Level 3 emotion will cause body sensations. For example, I might have a stomachache, feel the urge to pace, and feel muscle tension at Level 3 sadness. I am able to talk and listen and be on-track. It is more difficult to be focused when at a Level 3 emotion, and I may have more off-track urges, but I am able to let them pass and stay focused on doing what works to reach my goal. We can still use All-the-Time and Calm-Only skills at a Level 3 emotion, but it is important to be careful in case the level increases. If the emotion is even a tiny bit over a Level 3, then we use only All-the-Time skills, *not* Calm-Only ones.

   ☆ A Level 4 emotion is a strong emotion. If it is a painful emotion, we will be very uncomfortable. For example, I would cry at Level 4 sadness. I also might want to get angry about what is making me sad. I might have urges to scream, swear, and storm around. At this level, it is difficult to focus, and action urges will be strong. At a Level 4 emotion, we do not use Calm-Only skills, even though we may have the urge to do so. We wait until we are below a Level 3 emotion."

   ☆ "A Level 5 emotion is an overwhelming emotion. At Level 5, we harm ourselves, others, or property. At Level 5 we have to use All-the-Time skills to get back in control. Any questions?"

Content questions. "What might make you have a Level 1 emotion?"; "What would the emotion be?"; "How would your body feel?"; "What might make you have a Level 2 emotion?";

"What would the emotion be?"; "How would your body feel?"; "What might make you have a Level 3 emotion?"; "What would the emotion be?"; "How would your body feel?"; "What might make you have a Level 4 emotion?"; "What would the emotion be?"; "How would your body feel?"; "What might make you have a Level 5 emotion?"; "What would the emotion be?"; "How would your body feel?"

➡ **Orient to Categories of Skills Handout 1**. "The Feelings Rating Scale might seem harder than it really is; you will get it! Now we are going to learn more about Categories of Skills from the Categories of Skills Handout 1 on page 211. It looks like this. All set?"

➡ **Review Categories of Skills Handout 1**.

☆ *Teaching points*. "There are two Categories of Skills. Skills 1, 2, 3, 4, and 5 are called All-the-Time skills. [Perhaps ask the group what skills 1–5 are.] These skills can be used at any level of emotion: 0, 1, 2, 3, 4, and even 5. The other Category of Skills, Calm-Only, can *only* be used when we are having emotions between Levels 0 and 3. If we are even a tiny bit over Level 3, we do not use Calm-Only skills! Any questions?"

Assessment questions. "What is it like when we use Expressing Myself at a Level 4?", "What kinds of behaviors do we have at a Level 4 when we try to solve our problems?"

➡ **Orient to Recipe for Skills Handout 1**. "The last handout reviewed here is on page 216 of Appendix A. The Recipe for Skills Handout 1 looks like this. Everyone ready?"

☆ *Teaching points*. "The Recipe for Skills tells us how many skills at least we need to use in a situation. We add at least one skill to our skills chain for every level of emotion, including Level 0. At Level 0 we are using Clear Picture to know what is going on. At a Level 1 emotion, we have to link at least two skills. At Level 1, we will use Clear Picture and On-Track Thinking. This is a 12-skills chain. At a Level 2 emotion, we have to use at least three skills. Again, we use Clear Picture, On-Track Thinking, then take some kind of On-Track Action. This is a 123 skills chain. At a Level 3 emotion, we link at least four skills. Once again, we use Clear Picture, On-Track Thinking, On-Track Action, and at least one more skill that we think will help us reach our goals. If we are at a Level 4 emotion, we use at least five skills. These five skills have to be skills 1–5, because we cannot use any Calm-Only skills at a Level 4 emotion. At a Level 5 emotion, we have to use at least six skills. Once again, at Level 5, we cannot use Calm-Only skills, so all six skills have to be All-the-Time skills. Often we double up on On-Track Actions or New-Me Activities to help us focus and feel better. Any questions?"

Content questions. "At a Level 1, how many skills do we need?", "At a Level 2?", "At a Level 3?", "At a Level 4?' and "At a Level 5?"

➡ **Orient to the end of the Encoding Phase**. "We have learned a lot today. We learned how to put our skills together. It takes time to understand how to use these tools. Practicing is very important."

E-Spiral Phase 3. Elaboration: Practice and Linking

➡ *Orient to the elaboration activity.* "If it is OK, let's turn to page 220, which says Week 2 Practice Activity Worked Example on the top and looks like this. All set? We will read through this together. [The group reads through the worked example together.] Next we are going to complete the Week 2 Practice Activity Worksheet (p. 221) together. Who is willing to share a stressful situation that happened this week that we can use as an example?"

Note: The trainer decides on a topic. The topic needs to be interesting enough to hold the group's attention, yet not so intense that it cognitively overloads anyone in group.

Describe questions. "How was that exercise for you?"

➡ *Orient to discussion.* "I thought that was fun. Working together like that is what skill? Right—Relationship Care! Now we are going to have a discussion before we finish for the day."

Linking questions. "Is using the Skills System different from how you have handled emotions in the past?"

Disclosure questions. "Have there been times in the past when you were confused about what to do in a stressful situation?"; "What did you do?"; "How did it work?"

Expansion question. "How can the Feelings Rating Scale, Categories of Skills, and Recipe for Skills help you when you are upset or confused?"

➡ *Orient to the end of the Elaboration Phase.* "Great discussion. I think we are ready to move on to another activity. OK?"

E-Spiral Phase 4. Efficacy: Bridge to Real Life

➡ *Orient to the efficacy activity.* "Now we will play a game to practice using the Feelings Rating Scale, Categories of Skills, and the Recipe for Skills.

"I will say an emotion and the level. For example, Mad Level 3. We will then figure out together which skills we can use. At Mad Level 3, we can use both our All-the-Time and Calm-Only skills, right? Then we are going to figure out how may skills we have to use, at least, in that situation using the Recipe for Skills. So at a Level 3 feeling, we have to use four skills, right? OK, Sad Level 2?"

Note: The trainer continues to generate different feelings and rating levels, so that the group members can practice deciding whether all of the skills are available or only the All-the-Time skills, and how many skills are possible. The group members can also generate questions for other participants to answer. Depending on the cognitive abilities of the group, the trainer may want to write the Categories of Skills on the board or prompt more vulnerable learners to look at their handouts.

Review question. "How was that exercise for you?"

➡ **Orient to discussion.** "Wonderful job—that isn't easy! We are going to talk now about some of the challenges we face when we use skills like these. OK?"

Barrier question. "So far, what is hard about using the Feelings Rating Scale, the Categories of Skills, and the Recipe for Skills?"

Wisdom question. "Do you want to be able to use these tools?"

Commitment questions. "Are you willing to learn and practice using these tools?"; "When are you going to use these tools in your life?"

Coaching question. "How can you coach yourself to practice using these tools?"

➡ **Orient to home study.** "That was a good discussion—thank you. That helps me understand what is challenging for you. Our homework this week will be to practice using the Feelings Rating Scale, the Categories of Skills, and the Recipe for Skills. Whenever you think of it, label and rate what you are feeling. Think about whether you are over or under a Level 3 emotion. Ask yourself if you are able to talk and listen, and to be on-track. Try to remember which category of skills you can use and how many skills would be helpful. Any questions?

"Also, if anyone is interested in doing home study this week, you can look at the handouts that we have gone over. You could look over the worked examples in that section of your skills book. You could also do the worksheets. Check in with me after group if you need to make a plan for home study."

➡ **Orient to group ending.** "I thought you all did well. We ring the bell six times at the end of group. It is a chance to notice our breathing. We take a moment to focus our minds as we go back to our activities. Who would like to ring the bell today?"

System Tools Handouts to Review in Future Cycles or for Home Study

✓ Feelings Rating Scale Handout 2 (p. 206)

☆ *Teaching points.* This handout is a home-study tool for participants and staff to review the Feelings Rating Scale. Understanding the Feelings Rating Scale helps the individual become more organized and more able to integrate skills at lower levels of emotional arousal. It is critical that the individual learn the difference between Emotion Levels 4 and 5. At Level 4, the person may feel horrible, yet she is not acting in an out-of-control way. At Level 5, she is taking actions that harm herself, others, or property. A participant may say that she is at a 4.5 level to express being nearly out of control. If the person is in the group and states that she is currently at Level 5, the leaders can ask, "Are you hurting yourself, others, or property right now?" The person can then adjust the rating to a Level 4, if she is extremely uncomfortable, yet she is not taking abusive actions.

✓ Feelings Rating Scale Worked Example 1 (p. 207)

☆ *Teaching points.* The group reviews this worked example, which shows how the events prompted different levels of emotion. This sheet is presented using a scenario that links all of the answers to help the individual learn how emotions and situations can interact in escalating patterns.

✓ Feelings Rating Scale Worksheet 1 (p. 208)

☆ *Teaching points.* This worksheet is intended to have the individual practice associating events with levels of emotion. Feelings Rating Scale Worksheet 1 does not have to describe a specific situation, as did the previous worked example. The participant can list events that would lead to levels of emotion that are not associated with each other. For example, losing keys might be a Level 2 frustration, and losing a child would be Level 5 sadness.

✓ Feelings Rating Scale Worked Example 2 (p. 209)

☆ *Teaching points.* This worked example focuses on how a singular emotion can escalate. This is useful to help the individual understand the merits of early skills intervention.

✓ Feelings Rating Scale Worksheet 2 (p. 210)

☆ *Teaching points.* This worksheet asks individuals to be aware of how a specific emotion affects them as their emotions escalate.

✓ Categories of Skills Worksheet 1 (p. 212)

☆ *Teaching points.* This worksheet asks the individual to fill in the names and categories of the skills.

✓ Categories of Skills Worked Example 1 (p. 213)

☆ *Teaching points.* This worked example shows the Categories of Skills that may be used at different levels of emotion.

✓ Categories of Skills Worksheet 2 (p. 214)

☆ *Teaching points.* This worksheet asks the individual to circle the Categories of Skills that may be used at different levels of emotion.

✓ Categories of Skills Worksheet 3 (p. 215)

☆ *Teaching points.* This worksheet asks the participant to write in an emotion and a rating level. The person then circles which Categories of Skills may be used in that situation.

✓ Recipe for Skills Worked Example 1 (p. 217)

☆ *Teaching points.* This worked example sheet shows how many skills are needed at different levels of emotions.

✓ Recipe for Skills Worksheet 1 (p. 218)

☆ *Teaching points.* This worksheet lists emotions and ratings; the individual circles the number of skills that are necessary.

✓ Recipe for Skills Worksheet 2 (p. 219)

☆ *Teaching points.* This worksheet requests that the participant write down emotions and ratings. The individual then circles how many skills are necessary at that level of emotional escalation.

WEEK 3: CLEAR PICTURE

Preparing for Group

Handouts Needed

✓ Skills System Review Questions (p. 223)
✓ Clear Picture Handout 1 (p. 225)
✓ Clear Picture Worked Example 1 (p. 227)

E-Spiral Phase 1. Exploring Existing Knowledge Base (Review)

➡ *Welcome group.* "Hi, everybody; how is it going today? Are we ready to learn about skills? Does anyone remember what we do to start group? [Wait for answer.] You are right; we ring the bell. Why do we do that? [Wait for answer.] Very good—because we want to focus our minds. We are going to learn even more about breathing today!"

➡ *Orient to the mindfulness activity: notice air filling my belly.* "Last week we rang the bell and noticed our breathing. We learned how to turn our attention to the air going in and out of our noses."

Instructions for the mindfulness exercise. "Today we are going to pay attention to our breathing again when the bell rings. We will breathe in though our noses again, and this time, we are going to try to feel the air going deep into our bellies. When we do belly breathing, we feel our tummies get bigger. Putting your hand on your belly might help you focus attention there. You might notice your pants or your belt getting tighter as your belly fills with air. How about we try it a few times before we ring the bell? [Observes each participant.] That looks good. So, I will ring the bell six times. We all will shift our attention to our belly breathing. If your attention drifts away from your belly breathing, try to bring your focus back to the belly breaths. If you notice emotions, gently bring your attention back to your breathing. If you notice other thoughts, gently bring your focus back to . . . ? [Wait for response.] Right, your belly breathing! Let's try to keep our puppies in control. We want to practice being the boss of our minds. All set? Any questions?"

Note: Leaders observe the participants and provide individual instruction to those who have difficulty performing the breathing task. Additionally, it may be helpful for the leader to use the gesture of two hands turning a car steering wheel when he refers to turning attention. The metaphor can be expanded to include acting as though the steering wheel is hard to turn (rusty or lacking power steering), exemplifying how there are times when our attention is difficult to shift.

Describe questions. "What did you notice about the air filling your belly?"; "Where else did your attention go?"; "Did you bring your focus back to your belly breathing?"; "How did you bring your attention back?"

Note: The group members share details about what they noticed. The leader may choose to write observations on the board.

➡ *Orient to Skills System review.* "Every week, we will review the Skills List, the Feelings Rating Scale, the Categories of Skills, and the Recipe for Skills. It is important that we learn these things inside and out, backward and forward."

Note: Group leaders can utilize the Skills System Review Questions (p. 223 in Appendix A) or create another way to review this material. The goal is to practice recalling the information, so that the terms and concepts become learned and automatic. A basic review of exercises (A–G) in Chapter 1 (beginning on p. 115) addresses the names and numbers of the nine skills. The list below is a more inclusive list of options that incorporate the skills names and the System Tools. The trainer and/or the group can choose which review activities best suit the needs of the group.

Examples of Advanced Review Activities

- The trainer asks the group the questions on the Skills System Review Questions (p. 223).
- The trainer asks the group to list the names, numbers, initials, categories, and functions of each skill.
- The trainer names an emotion and a rating level. The group says which Categories of Skills can be used and the minimum number of skills needed according to the Recipe.
- The group sorts the laminated skills cards to put them in order using the Categories of Skills cards and subsets of skills (i.e., placing the six Clear Picture Do's cards under Clear Picture card).
- The trainer has the group look at the Skills Plan Map (Appendix B) and asks different skills questions related to making skills chains.

➡ *Orient to skills practice.* "I think we are doing well; it does take time. The more we practice, the easier it will be to remember these things. This week's homework was to practice using the Feelings Rating Scale, the Categories of Skills, and the Recipe for Skills. Right?"

Disclosure questions. "Who can talk to us about what it was like to use the Feelings Rating Scale?"; "Who can tell us about practicing using the Categories of Skills?"; "Who can tell us about using the Recipe for Skills?"

➡ *Orient to new skills topic.* "Great! Let's see what we already know about getting a Clear Picture."

🗨 *Discuss existing knowledge about the new topic.*

Assessment question. "When we are focused, are our minds clear or fuzzy?"

Relevant context questions. "How do people handle things when they are in Clear Mind?";

"How do people handle things when they are in Fuzzy Mind?"; "What happens to our emotions when we are in Fuzzy Mind?"

Clarifying questions. "How does Clear Mind help people get to their goals?"; "How does Fuzzy Mind keep people from reaching their goals?"; "What does it mean to be in Emotional Mind?"; "What is our thinking like in Emotional Mind?"; "How do you think noticing your breathing can help you handle emotions?"; "How can noticing our breathing help us manage Off-Track Thoughts?"

➡ *Orient to relevant context of the new topic.* "From our discussion, it sounds like we agree that emotions and thoughts can become overwhelming. Sometimes we block or avoid emotions. Unfortunately, that makes things worse. Noticing emotions and thoughts helps us know what is really happening inside and outside of us. When we are clear, we can see where we are going; when we are fuzzy, we cannot. Clear information about ourselves and our situation helps us make decisions that lead us to our goals. Our Clear Picture skills will help us get a clear mind, so that we can take actions that help us reach our goals. Any questions?"

E-Spiral Phase 2. Encoding: New Learning

➡ *Orient to new learning: Clear Picture.* "Today we are going to learn about the first skill in the Skills System. Skill 1 is Clear Picture. You can tell by the name of the skill that we will be learning how to have a clear mind."

Instructions for encoding activity. "If you are ready, let's turn to page 225. This is the Clear Picture Handout 1. [Holds up the page.] This is what it looks like. OK, what is our plan for reviewing this? Would anyone like to read?"

Note: When group members read, it is important that the leader restate terms so that the group is very clear about the information.

➡ *Review Clear Picture Handout 1*

☆ *Teaching points for Clear Picture Handout 1.* "When we get a Clear Picture, we focus 100% on what is happening inside and outside of us right now. We pay attention to what is happening so that we understand the facts of the situation. When we are clear about the facts, we can make skills plans to reach our goals. When we are fuzzy or try to change the facts, we end up off-track.

"We get a Clear Picture by going through the Clear Picture Do's. These are things we do to become aware of what is happening inside and outside of us in the moment. We take a Breath, Notice our Surroundings, do a Body Check, and Label and Rate Emotions using the 0- to 5-point scale, Notice Thoughts, and Notice Urges. When we go through the Do's, it is like taking a picture of what is happening right now. It is like taking a snapshot. [Snaps fingers to show how quickly and easily this can be done.]

"It is important to have a clear picture of situations, so we can figure out how to do what works. It helps us make strong Skills Plans. If we have a fuzzy picture, we usually do what does not work. We need a Clear Picture of ourselves, others, and the situation to make on-track choices that help us reach our goals."

➡ *Orient to Clear Picture Worked Example 1.* "Does anyone have any questions about that handout? OK, now we are going to learn more about getting a Clear Picture. Let's turn to page 227. This is the Clear Picture Worked Example 1. It looks like this." (Holds the page up.) "Would anyone like to read?"

➡ *Review Clear Picture Worked Example 1.* The group reviews the worked example. If this worked example is not relevant to the population being treated, skills trainers can create a worked example on a copy of the Clear Picture Worksheet 2 (p. 228). The group leader tries to explain each concept, so the participants understand each step of the Clear Picture. It is not necessary that the participant be able to recall each concept initially; that knowledge base will build as the person is exposed to Clear Picture repeatedly.

➡ *Orient to ending Encoding Phase.* "Does anyone have questions about Clear Picture so far? OK, are we ready to practice some of the things we have learned?"

E-Spiral Phase 3. Elaboration: Practice and Linking

➡ *Orient to the elaboration activity.* "Great, let's practice getting a Clear Picture!"

Instructions for the practice exercise. "I am going to say one of the Clear Picture Do's and then I will ring the bell. When I ring the bell, I would like you to do the Do. For example, when I say, 'Notice the Breath,' we will all listen to the bell and pay attention to our breathing. Then I will ring the bell and say, 'Notice Surroundings.' As the bell ring fades, we will all notice what is happening around us. We will do this for Body Check, Label and Rate Emotions, Notice Thoughts, and Notice Urges. Together we will listen to six rings, and we will do all six Clear Picture Do's. If you get lost, notice what getting lost is like and try to follow along at the next bell ring. Any questions? [Wait for response.] Great, here we go."

Describe questions. "What did you notice about your breath?"; "What did you notice when you noticed surroundings?"; "What did you notice during the Body Check?"; "What emotion did you notice, and how strong was it?"; "What thoughts did you notice?"; "What urges did you notice?"

➡ *Orient to discussion.* "Good job. Now we are going to take a few minutes to talk a little more about what it is like to get a Clear Picture."

Linking questions. "Have you ever had a Clear Picture in the past?"; "What actions did you take?"; "Have you been in Emotional Mind?"; "What actions did you take?"

Disclosure questions. "What is it like to be more aware of things inside and outside of you?";

"Can it be difficult to see how things really are?"; "What do you do when it is hard to face what is really happening?"

Expansion questions. "What other skills do we use with Clear Picture?"; "How can having a Clear Picture help you reach your goals?"; "Does a fuzzy or clear picture help you reach your goals?"; "Why?"

➡ ***Orient to the end of the Elaboration Phase.*** "That was a good discussion. I was thinking that it would be helpful to read a story that teaches us more about how we use Clear Picture in our lives."

E-Spiral Phase 4. Efficacy: Bridge to Real Life

➡ ***Orient to efficacy activities: reading a story.*** "I will read this story, and we will answer some questions when we are done. Is everyone all set?"

Instructions for the efficacy activity. Story: "There is a man named Robert, and he is 22 years old. Robert works in a grocery store, stocking shelves. One day at work, Robert was kneeling and putting cans on a bottom shelf. Suddenly an older lady pushed her cart into him when he was working. He did not see the woman coming toward him; he only felt the cart hitting him. Robert did a Body Check and noticed a sharp pain in his back. Right away, he knew he had to get a Clear Picture, because he was feeling confused at a Level 4. He noticed an urge to scream, 'Look out! What are you doing? Didn't you see me working here?' As he stood up to see what had happened, he took a few breaths. He checked around him and saw the old woman looking the other way at some spaghetti sauce. He noticed the thought, *I don't think she knows that she ran into me.* Robert did another Body Check, and the pain in his back was nearly gone."

Review questions.

"Do you think Robert had a Clear Picture of the situation?"

"Can you point out the six Clear Picture Do's?" (Write them in the order in which they happened on the board.)

"When did he think to take a breath?"

"How long did it take for Robert to do the Clear Picture Do's?"

"Do you think Robert ended up screaming at the woman?"

"What do you think he did next?"

"What would have happened if he had yelled at that old woman?"

"Do you think Clear Picture helped Robert reach his goals?"

➡ ***Orient to discussion.*** "It sounds like Robert is learning to be a Skills Master. Before we finish for the day, we are going to have a brief discussion. OK?"

Barrier questions. "What is hard about taking a few seconds to get a Clear Picture?"; "We have to use Clear Picture all day. What is difficult about that for you?"

Wisdom questions. "Would the Clear Picture Do's help you?"; "Do you think you want to use Clear Picture?"

Commitment question. "When will you use Clear Picture?"

Coaching question. "How can you coach yourself to use Clear Picture every day, all day?"

➡ *Orient to home study.* "This week our homework will be to jump in with both feet to practice Clear Picture. As many times as you can, take a few seconds to notice your breathing, surroundings, body, feelings, thoughts, and urges. You might find that the more you practice, the more quickly you can do the Do's. We can learn to do it in a snap! [Snaps fingers.] At first it might be hard to remember all six Clear Picture Do's. Try to take a few seconds to be aware of what is happening inside and outside of you before you take action. Good luck; we will talk about it next week. Also, if you want to study skills at home, review all the handouts we have gone over so far. You can also do Clear Picture Worksheet 1 (p. 226), in which you write the name of the clear Picture Do, and Clear Picture Worksheet 2 (p. 228), in which you list what you notice in the moment. Ask someone to help you write if you need to."

➡ *Orient to group ending.* "As you know, we ring the bell six times at the end of group. We do one ring for each of the Clear Picture Do's. It is a chance to notice what is happening inside and outside of us right now. We take a moment to get a Clear Picture as we go back to our activities. Who would like to ring to bell today?"

Clear Picture Handouts to Review in Future Cycles or for Home Study

Note: Skills trainers use these handouts, worked examples, and worksheets to develop teaching plans in future cycles through the Skills System curriculum. Orienting, questions, exercise, and skills practice are created to teach expanded material through subsequent cycles.

✓ Clear Picture Summary Sheet (p. 224). The summary sheet can be used during the encoding phase to explain concepts as teaching points. It may be too boring to read in group, but having different group members read different sections can break it up. Summary sheets are helpful for home study and for teaching skills to skills coaches.

✓ Clear Picture Worksheet 1 (p. 226)

☆ *Teaching points.* This worksheet helps participants practice recalling the six Clear Picture Do's.

✓ Clear Picture Worksheet 2 (p. 228)

☆ *Teaching points.* This worksheet is helpful for participants to use in the moment at home. The pictures prompt the individual to Take a Breath, Notice Surroundings, do a Body

Check, Label and Rate Emotions, Notice Thoughts, and Notice Urges. This is a useful activity for the person to do when he or she needs to get a Clear Picture.

✓ Review Clear Picture: Breathing Handout 1 (p. 229)

☆ *Teaching points.* The Clear Picture Breathing Handout 1 guides the participant to focus attention on breathing to tolerate distress. The handout shifts the person's focus from the stressful situation to awareness of breathing. The awareness of breathing shifts from being aware of current breathing to doing diaphragmatic or belly breaths. Belly breathing can help the individual remain regulated so that she can think things through. The last step is to practice patterned breathing by counting to 4 on the inhalation and to 4 on the exhalation.

✓ Review Clear Picture: Notice Surroundings Handout 1 (p. 230)

☆ *Teaching points.* This worksheet helps the participant understand how we observe our surroundings. Practice exercises can include sensory awareness activities.

✓ Review Clear Picture: Notice Surroundings Worked Example 1 (p. 231)

☆ *Teaching points.* Clear Picture: Body Check Worked Example 1 (p. 233) helps participants understand how to get a Clear Picture of their body parts.

✓ Review Clear Picture: Notice Surroundings Worksheet 1 (p. 232)

☆ *Teaching points.* This worksheet helps the participant understand how to get a Clear Picture of their surroundings.

✓ Review Clear Picture: Body Check Worked Example 1 (p. 233)

☆ *Teaching points.* This worked example describes different sensations that an individual may feel in different parts of the body.

✓ Review Clear Picture: Body Check Worksheet 1 (p. 234)

☆ *Teaching points.* This handout is used by the individual to describe what is observed in different parts of her body in different situations.

✓ Review Clear Picture: Body Check Worked Example 2 (p. 235)

☆ *Teaching points.* This worked example reviews possible body sensations at different levels of anger.

✓ Review Clear Picture: Body Check Worksheet 2 (p. 236)

☆ *Teaching points.* This worksheet helps the participant associate body sensations and an emotion. Increasing awareness can help assist the individual in Labeling and Rating Emotions.

✓ Review Clear Picture: Body Check Exercise (p. 237)

☆ *Teaching points.* This is a progressive relaxation exercise to help the individual tighten and then loosen different parts of his body.

✓ Review Clear Picture: Label and Rate Feelings Handout 1 (p. 238)

☆ *Teaching points*. Clear Picture: Label and Rate Feelings Handout 1 introduces 11 different emotions. These labels serve as a starting point to describe many other emotions that people experience; it is fun to have the group brainstorm a list of all different emotions.

✓ Review Clear Picture: Label and Rate Feelings Handout 2 (p. 239)

☆ *Teaching points*. This handout teaches the participant how emotions function. The participant comes to understand that events prompt emotions. The person learns that chemical changes happen in the body when emotions happen. People communicate what is happening inside of them through their facial expressions and body language. Awareness of these factors can help individuals understand themselves and other people better. It is important for the participant to understand that emotions create action urges. This would be an opportunity to educate the group about "fight–flight" responses. By being aware of these forces, the participant is better able to observe them, describe them, and make decisions versus reacting quickly without thought.

✓ Review Clear Picture: Label and Rate Feelings Worked Example 1 (p. 240)

☆ *Teaching points*. This worked example lists events that may elicit various emotional responses.

✓ Review Clear Picture: Label and Rate Feelings Worksheet 1 (p. 241)

☆ *Teaching points*. This worksheet asks participants to list situations that elicit specific emotions. This activity helps individuals understand links between prompting events and their emotional responses.

✓ Review Clear Picture: Notice Thoughts Handout 1 (p. 242)

☆ *Teaching points*. The Clear Picture: Notice Thoughts Handout 1 teaches participants that thoughts are continually produced by the brain. It is important that the individual understand that some thoughts are helpful and others are not. The goal is for the person to observe thoughts and allow unhelpful thoughts, or off-track thoughts, to pass without taking action. The metaphor of thoughts being like city buses can be helpful, because the individual only gets on a bus that is heading to the desired destination. Getting on the wrong bus, or responding to off-track thoughts, will hinder the individual from reaching goals.

✓ Review Clear Picture: Notice Thoughts Worked Example 1 (p. 243)

☆ *Teaching points*. This worked example sheet highlights thoughts that can elicit certain emotions. It is important that the individual understands how thinking patterns can affect emotional status.

✓ Review Clear Picture: Notice Thoughts Worksheet 1 (p. 244)

☆ *Teaching points*. This worksheet gives the individual an opportunity to list thoughts that may elicit specific emotions.

✓ Review Clear Picture: Notice Urges Worked Example 1 (p. 245)

☆ *Teaching points.* This worked example highlights how situations create thoughts and emotions that lead to action urges.

✓ Review Clear Picture: Notice Urges Worksheet 1 (p. 246)

☆ *Teaching points.* The individual writes down a situation, a thought, a feeling, and possible action urge that might result.

✓ Review Clear Picture: Notice Urges Worked Example 2 (p. 247)

☆ *Teaching points.* This worked example outlines examples of urges that a person may experience when having specific emotions.

✓ Review Clear Picture: Notice Urges Worksheet 2 (p. 248)

☆ *Teaching points.* This worksheet asks the individual to list urges that the participant notices when experiencing certain emotions. Increasing awareness of emotions and action urges facilitates management of action urges.

✓ Review Clear Picture: Notice Urges Worked Example 3 (p. 249)

☆ *Teaching points.* This worked example sheet demonstrates how action urges intensify as an emotion strengthens.

✓ Review Clear Picture: Notice Urges Worksheet 3 (p. 250)

☆ *Teaching points.* This worksheet asks the individual to observe action urges that occur at increasing levels of emotion. This activity helps the participant improve awareness of affective experiences; enhanced awareness during preliminary escalation can result in proactive skill use.

WEEK 4: ON-TRACK THINKING

Preparing for Group

Handouts Needed

✓ On-Track Thinking Handout 1 (p. 252)
✓ On-Track Thinking Worked Example 1 (p. 253)
✓ On-Track Thinking Worksheet 2 (p. 255)
✓ On-Track Thinking Worked Example 2 (p. 256)
✓ On-Track Thinking Worksheet 3 (p. 257)
✓ On-Track Thinking Practice Activity (p. 258)

E-Spiral Phase 1. Exploring Existing Knowledge Base (Review)

➡ *Welcome group.* "Hello, everybody! It is wonderful to see you all! How are you doing today?"

➡ *Orient to the mindfulness activity: breathing at the same time as the bell rings.* "Are we ready to get started with our mindful breathing?"

Instructions for the mindfulness exercise. "Today we are going to practice being the bosses of our minds and bodies. We are going to practice being aware of and controlling our breathing. During this exercise, I will ring the bell, and we will all take a belly breath in and out while the tone of the bell is happening. I am going to wait until the sound of the bell has disappeared completely before I ring the bell again. Once the sound is gone, I will ring the bell again, and all of us will take a second belly breath. I think you will notice that the sound lasts for several seconds, so we have to slow our in and out breaths down to fit how long the ring is. Try to make adjustments in the speed of your breathing so you don't have to hold your breath too long for the next rings. We will do this six times. If you notice your mind drifting to other things, try to bring your mind back gently to the ringing of the bell and your belly breathing. If you struggle with the timing of the breathing, you might judge yourself or have feelings. If you feel emotions, notice them and bring your attention back to the bell and the breath. Our goal is to work together 100% with the bell; other things can wait until the exercise is over. Any questions? Let's practice this a few times so we are all clear about how to make our in and out breath last as long as the bell's sound."

Describe questions. "What was that like?"; "Were you able to breathe with the bell?"; "What was challenging about that?"; "Were you able to bring your attention back to your breath and the bell if it wandered?"

➡ *Orient to Skills System review.* "You guys are really doing well. Learning about breathing is an important skill. The cool thing is that we always have our breath with us. If we need to focus, all we have to do is bring our attention to our breathing. It is time for our skills review."

Note: The skills trainer can choose a Basic Review Activity from Week 1 (p. 115) or an Advanced Review Activity from Week 3 on page 127 or create a new one.

➡ *Orient to skills practice.* "Very good—I think we are doing well. OK, let's talk about how we did practicing Clear Picture this week."

Disclosure questions. Choosing one or more of these questions can help participants review the use of Clear Picture: "Who used Clear Picture?"; "Could you tell us how it went?"; "Which of the Clear Picture Do's did you do?"; "Which of the Clear Picture Do's didn't you do?"; "Did you find that Clear Picture was helpful?"

➡ *Orient to new skills topic.* "It sounds as if using our skills helps us focus more and feel better. It also sounds as if we can feel pretty out of control and uncomfortable when we don't use our skills. Unfortunately, it is really hard to reach goals when we are off-track. I am going to ask a few questions that will help us to share what we already know about thinking things through."

🗩 *Discuss existing knowledge about the new topic.*

Assessment questions. "What is it like to be confused?"; "What kinds of situations make people confused?" (Brainstorm this list on the board.)

Relevant context questions. "What kinds of plans do we make when we are confused?"; "What kinds of actions do we take when we are in Fuzzy Mind?"; "What kinds of plans do we make when we are in Clear Mind?"; "What kinds of actions do we take when we are focused?"

Clarifying questions. "When we take actions when we are fuzzy or unfocused, how does it usually turn out?"; "When we take actions when we are focused and clear, how does it usually turn out?"

➡ **Orient to relevant context of the new topic.** "It is important to use On-Track Thinking because, as we know, life can be confusing. We experience stress and strong emotions every day. It is difficult to reach goals when we are upside down or out of our minds. So, to reach our goals, we have to be in our minds and make good plans. Getting organized helps us handle stressful situations. On-Track Thinking helps us think clearly so that we can handle what is happening inside and outside of us to reach our goals. Any questions?"

E-Spiral Phase 2. Encoding: New Learning

➡ **Orient to new learning: On-Track Thinking.** "OK, today we are going to learn about Skill 2, On-Track Thinking. We use On-Track Thinking after we get a Clear Picture. On-Track Thinking helps us check our urges, create on-track thoughts, and use skills plans to handle every situation.

Instructions for the encoding activity. "Now we are going to learn about the different parts of On-Track Thinking. Please turn to page 252. This is the On-Track Thinking Handout 1."

Note: The skills trainer reads through the handout.

➡ **Review On-Track Thinking Handout 1.**

☆ *Teaching points for On-Track Thinking Handout 1.* "When we do Clear Picture, we are finding out what is happening inside and outside of us in a situation. We do On-Track Thinking before we take any actions; we have to be sure to have an on-track skills plan before we move ahead. When we notice an urge to take action, first we stop and Check It. We take a few seconds and Check It to see whether the urge is helpful or not helpful to us. We ask ourselves, "If I do this, will it help me reach my goals?" We give helpful thoughts a thumbs-up and unhelpful thoughts a thumbs-down. When we notice that an urge is not helpful, we create a Turn It Up thought. Turn It Up thoughts are ones that coach us not to take the off-track action. I may Turn It Up by thinking about all the negative things that will happen in my life if I do the off-track action. Turn It Up could also be when I coach myself to be new-me. We do not want to get on the off-track city bus, because it is not going where we want to go! We Check It, Turn It Up to thumbs-up thinking, and Cheerlead. It is hard to stay on track sometimes, and off-track thoughts sneak back into our minds. So we use lots of Cheerleading to help us keep working toward our goals.

"Making lemonade out of lemons is an important type of On-Track Thinking. This means that when life gives us something difficult (sour lemons), we add sugar and look on the bright side. We have a Clear Picture that the situation is difficult, and we try to see it in a positive way. Making lemonade can help us deal with tough situations in ways that make us feel better.

"Once we have Checked It and Turned It to on-track thinking, we make a Skills Plan. This is when we think about what skills will help us in this situation. First, we check to see whether we can use Calm-Only skills at this time using the Category of Skills. If we are over a Level 3 emotion, we use All-the-Time skills. [Asks the group to list verbally the All-the-Time skills and the Calm-Only skills.] Then, using the Recipe for Skills, we figure out how many skills to use. We have to be sure to use enough skills. Then, we decide what other skills will help us reach our goals. We think about whether we need to use a Safety Plan. Safety Plans help us handle risky situations. Maybe doing a New-Me Activity would be helpful. It may help us keep busy and focused. If we are under a Level 3 emotion, we might want to use Problem Solving to fix problems, Expressing Myself to communicate, Getting It right to get what we want, and Relationship Care to balance relationships. We keep Cheerleading ourselves to be sure we stay on-track! Any questions?"

Content questions. "What are the different steps in On-Track Thinking?"

➡️ *Orient to On-Track Thinking Worked Example 1.* "There is a lot to learn about On-Track Thinking. Let's go through On-Track Thinking Worked Example 1 on page 253 together. It looks like this."

Note: The On-Track Thinking Worked Example 1 is self-explanatory. Skills trainers read through the worksheet with the group.

➡️ *Orient to On-Track Thinking Worked Example 2.* "Let's look a little closer at how we use Check It, Turn It Up, and Cheerleading thinking to help us reach our goals. Please turn to the On-Track Thinking Worked Example 2 on page 256 together. It looks like this."

Note: The group members discuss how taking action on the urge works against the goal. They may also talk about how the Turn It Up thought helps them move toward the goal, and how Cheerleading helps them stay on track.

➡️ *Orient to the end of the Encoding Phase.* "Excellent job! Any questions about On-Track Thinking so far?"

E-Spiral Phase 3. Elaboration: Practice and Linking

➡️ *Orient to On-Track Thinking Worksheet 2.* "Great, are we ready to practice On-Track Thinking? Now we are going to fill out On-Track Thinking Worksheet 2 together. Turn to page 255. This is what it looks like."

Instructions for filling out the worksheet. "This worksheet helps you to practice checking urges. I will read a list of eight urges. You will think about each one and decide whether the urge would be helpful or unhelpful for you in this moment. If it is helpful, circle the thumb that goes up. If the urge is not helpful, circle the thumb that goes down. If you have a hard time reading, you can get the person next to you to help, or you can just show the group a thumbs-up or thumbs-down for your answer. Any questions?"

☆ *Teaching points for On-Track Thinking Worksheet 2.* "Each of us has to decide what is on-track and off-track for ourselves. No one can tell you what is right for you; we have to search within ourselves to find those answers. This worksheet is a chance to practice looking inside to see if an urge is helpful or unhelpful. Our goals change, so we have to be sure to check within our hearts to find out whether something is helpful or unhelpful in this moment. Every situation is different. So it is best to check urges each time you use On-Track Thinking. Any questions?"

Note: If time allows, it would be helpful to review On-Track Thinking Worked Example 2, (p. 256) complete On-Track Thinking Worksheet 3 (p. 257) as a group activity.

Disclosure questions. "What were these exercises like for you?"; "How did you decide whether the urge was helpful or unhelpful?" and "How long did it take for you to Check the Urge?"; "Have you used Turn It Up and Cheerleading before?"; "Can it be difficult?"

➡ **Orient to discussion.** "You all did really well with that. We are going to talk together for a few moments about using On-Track Thinking."

Linking question. "How is On-Track Thinking different from how you have thought in the past?"

Disclosure questions. "Have you ever just reacted quickly without thinking things through?"; "How did that work?"

Expansion questions. "What other skills do you use with On-Track Thinking?"; "When can On-Track Thinking help you in your life?"

➡ **Orient to the end of Elaboration Phase.** "Now that we know a little more about On-Track Thinking, are we ready to read a story together?"

E-Spiral Phase 4. Efficacy: Bridge to Real Life

➡ **Orient to the Group Practice Activity.** "We are going to go through a scenario for a practice activity to see how Clear Picture and On-Track Thinking go together. Let's turn to the On-Track Thinking Group Practice Activity (p. 258)."

Instructions for the efficacy activity. "We will read through this story about Jill; she is late for work. We will work together to fill in the blanks."

Describe question. "Did you feel like that story helped you see how we put all the steps together?"

➡ **Orient to discussion.** "I thought you guys did an awesome job. We have worked with lots of handouts today, and you all really did a good job hanging in there. It isn't easy to use skills, but you will find it gets easier and easier with practice. On-Track Thinking is one of the toughest skills! Let's talk for a few minutes about some of the challenges of using skills before we finish for today."

Barrier question. "What is difficult about using On-Track Thinking for you?"

Wisdom question. "Do you think it is important for you to use On-Track Thinking?"

Commitment question. "Are you going to use On-Track Thinking?"

Coaching question. "How can you get yourself to use On-Track Thinking?"

➡ *Orient to home study.* "It sounds as if we know it is hard, and we still have to use skills. When we understand this, we really are on our way to being Skills Masters. Skills Masters practice skills outside of group. So this week we will work on using On-Track Thinking. Practice whenever you have a chance do Clear Picture and On-Track Thinking. Good luck!

"Also, if you want to study skills at home, review all the handouts we have gone over so far. You can also do On-Track Thinking Worksheet 1 (p. 254). Choose a situation, and fill out the worksheet. You can do it by yourself or ask a staff member to help. Any questions?"

➡ *Orient to group ending.* "As you know, we ring the bell six times at the end of group. We do one ring for each of the Clear Picture Do's. It is a chance to notice what is happening inside and outside of us right now. We take a moment to get a Clear Picture as we go back to our activities. Who would like to ring the bell today?"

On-Track Thinking Handouts to Review in Future Cycles or for Home Study

✓ On-Track Thinking Summary Sheet (p. 251). The summary sheet can be used during the encoding phase to explain concepts as teaching points It may be too boring to read in group, but having different group members read different sections can break it up. Summary sheets are helpful for home study and for teaching skills coaches the skills.

✓ On-Track Thinking Worksheet 1 (p. 254). The individual chooses a situation to review and completes each of the questions.

WEEK 5: ON-TRACK ACTIONS

Preparing for Group

Handouts Needed

✓ On-Track Action Handout 1 (p. 261)
✓ On-Track Action Handout 2 (p. 262)
✓ On-Track Action Handout 3 (p. 263)
✓ On-Track Action Handout 4 (p. 264)
✓ On-Track Action Handout 5 (p. 265)

✓ On-Track Action Handout 6 (p. 268)
✓ On-Track Action Worked Example 2 (p. 270)
✓ On-Track Action Worksheet 2 (p. 271)

E-Spiral Phase 1. Exploring Existing Knowledge Base (Review)

➡ *Welcome group.* "How is everyone doing today? OK, ready to learn some skills? Great! What activity do we do to start group? [Pause for response.] Exactly—we ring the bell. All set?"

➡ *Orient to the mindfulness activity: Body Check.* "Today we are going to notice the breath and then do a Body Check. Practicing a Body Check can help us be more self-aware. The more we notice what is happening inside us, the clearer we are. It helps us label and rate our emotions when we notice how our body is reacting to a situation."

Instructions for the mindfulness exercise. "OK, I will ring the bell, and we will begin by noticing the breath. On the second ring, we will move our attention to noticing other body sensations, such as the texture of chair that you are sitting on or the hardness of the floor under your feet. You may notice aches, pains, or muscle tightness. You may notice muscle relaxation and calmness in your body. Notice whatever is happening in your body. If your mind drifts away from doing the Body Check, gently bring your mind back to your body. I will ring the bell six times, then we will share what we noticed. Any questions?"

Describe question. "What did you notice during your Body Check?"
Note: It may be helpful to write the different observations on the board.

➡ *Orient to Skills System review.* "Fantastic! How about we go through our Skills System review?"
Note: The skills trainer can choose a Basic Review Activity from Week 1 (p. 115) or an Advanced Review Activity from Week 3 on p. 127 or create a new one.

➡ *Orient to skills practice.* "Great! It is getting a little easier, isn't it? Okay, let's go over our homework. This week we were going to practice using Clear Picture and On-Track Thinking."

Disclosure questions. "Who would like to share about how they use Clear Picture and On-Track Thinking this week?"; "How did it work?"; "Do you wish you had done anything differently?"

➡ *Orient to new skills topic.* "That is a good start. Shall we talk about taking On-Track Actions?"

🗨 *Discuss existing knowledge about the new topic.*

Assessment questions. "Are there times when people have urges to go off-track?"; "What kinds of things make us want to go off-track?"; "Do people feel out of control sometimes?"; "Why do you think that happens?"; "What is wisdom?"

Relevant context questions. "What is it like to be off-track?"; "Do you ever feel as if you are stuck off-track, and you can't get back on-track?"; "Do you ever want to get back on-track but don't do anything to make that happen?"

Clarifying questions. "Do off-track actions help us reach our goals?"; "Where do off-track actions take us?"; "Do On-Track Actions help us reach our goals? How?"

Note: It is helpful to orient participants to the possible short-term benefits of off-track actions to validate the urge. Then, highlighting the long-term results can help participants make an informed decision.

➡ *Orient to relevant context of the new topic.* "From our discussion, it is clear that we all have Off-Track Urges. It sounds like it is hard to stay on-track. We have to use Clear Picture and On-Track Thinking to stay on-track. Thinking about being on-track must be followed by action. Taking action means that we do something on-track."

E-Spiral Phase 2. Encoding: New Learning

➡ *Orient to new learning: On-Track Action.* "Great discussion. Today we are going to learn about On-Track Actions. We will learn about how we get a Clear Picture, use On-Track Thinking, and take an On-Track Action reaching toward our goal. This is a 123 skills chain. When we use skills 123, it helps us act in Wise Mind. Let's turn to page 261. We are going to work on the On-Track Action Handout 1. It looks like this. All set?"

Instructions for encoding activity. "Great, we are going to go through the handout together. I will talk a little about each main point; then we will have a discussion, OK?"

☆ *Teaching points for On-Track Action Handout 1.* "Clear Picture and On-Track Thinking help us do On-Track Actions. First, we use Skill 1, Clear Picture, to know what is happening inside and outside of us. We check our emotions, thoughts, and urges and Turn It Up to Skill 2, On-Track Thinking. Then we make a skill plan and figure out what our On-Track Actions, Skill 3, will be to reach our goal. When we start with Skills 1, 2, and 3, we can usually stay on-track to our goals. [Points to the line that leads to the star.] Using skills 123 together helps us be in Wise Mind. In Wise Mind we are balancing having emotions *and* thinking clearly to be on-track. Sometimes we are in Emotional Mind and have a Fuzzy Picture. Often when we are out-of-balance with our emotions, we have off-track thinking that leads to off-track actions. [Points to the line that leads to the crash site.] The good news is that once we are off-track, we can get back on-track by doing 1, 2, 3 Wise Mind! What are skills 1, 2, 3? Right: Clear Picture, On-Track Thinking, and On-Track Action! Staying on-track is as easy as . . . [Says '1, 2, 3' with everyone at once.] Right: 1, 2, 3! Any questions?"

➡ *Orienting to On-Track Action Handout 2.* "OK, let's learn more about On-Track Actions. Turn to page 262. On-Track Action Handout 2 looks like this. Ready?"

☆ *Teaching points for On-Track Action Handout 2.*

1. "There are lots of different kinds of On-Track Actions. An On-Track Action is the first step toward our goals. For example, if we want to learn skills, practicing at home is an On-Track

Action. Practicing will help us be a Skills Master. Throwing our skills book in the garbage would probably be an off-track action in that situation." (Optional: Refer to On-Track Action Handout 3 on p. 263.)

2. "Sometimes we need to do the On-Track Action of Switch Tracks when we are heading off-track. It might be helpful to do an On-Track Action that is opposite of our Off-Track Urges to Switch Tracks. When we do the opposite of our urge, we are doing Opposite Action."

Assessment question. "What does the word 'opposite' mean?"

For example, if we want new friends, and we are standing in the corner at a party, we may need to take actions to be very friendly and introduce ourselves to people rather than hiding in the corner. Our urge may be to hide, yet we take an Opposite Action and jump into the social situation with both feet. Doing the opposite may be a great idea to help us reach our goal." (Optional: Refer to On-Track Action Handout 4 on p. 264.)

3. "It is often helpful to make an On-Track Action Plan. Doing on-track things every day that make us healthy and happy can help us feel good and make on-track choices. For example, if we eat well, exercise, and sleep in balanced ways, we are less grumpy and moody. When we feel good, we are more able to be on-track." (Optional: Refer to On-Track Action Handout 5 on p. 265.)

4. "There are times when we need to Accept the Situation. Sometimes we have done everything we can in a situation, and we just have to accept what is happening. We may not like it, but we have to realize that it must be accepted. The great thing is that we have skills to deal with waiting for things to get better! Skills Masters learn to make the best of a bad situation or make lemonade when life gives us lemons." (Optional: Refer to On-Track Action Handout 6 on p. 268.)

5. "There are times when we need to Turn the Page. For example, if we broke a favorite mug, we can be sad for a while, but at some point, we are dwelling on problems. When we dwell on problems for too long, it can make us more emotional. We have to learn when enough is enough for ourselves. We may have the urge to get stuck on certain things, but getting stuck can keep us from our goals. Any questions?" (Optional: Refer to On-Track Action Handout 7 on p. 269.)

Note: If time allows, try to review the On-Track Action Handouts (3–6).

☆ *Teaching points for On-Track Action Handout 3 (p. 263).* This handout explores the first type of On-Track Action—Take a Step to My Goal. The group reviews the handout to see that the individual in the picture does Clear Picture, On-Track Thinking, and Takes an On-Track Action of doing a Safety Plan—Move Away to reach his goal. After that his On-Track Action is to do a New-Me Activity (playing solitaire), which helps him focus. The boxes above show what skills he can choose as On-Track Actions at 0–5 and 0–3 feelings.

☆ *Teaching points for On-Track Action Handout 4 (p. 264).* The group reviews this handout that explains On-Track Action—Switch Tracks. The example is self-explanatory. Giving examples for jumping in with both feet and doing the opposite will be helpful.

☆ *Teaching Points for On-Track Action Handout 5 (p. 265).* This handout outlines different components of an individual's On-Track Action Plan. It is important to focus on the concept of balance versus absolute rules. The individual needs to be able to make adjustments as her life changes.

☆ *Teaching Points for On-Track Action Handout 6 (p. 268).* This handout describes when we may consider practicing acceptance. The group members go through each instance and discuss examples.

☆ *Teaching Points for On-Track Action Handout 7 (p. 269).* The group members review this handout and discuss the process and challenges associated with Turning the Page.

➡ *Orient to the end of the Encoding Phase.* "On-Track Actions are our friends! They keep us on-track! Are we ready to practice On-Track Actions?"

E-Spiral Phase 3. Elaboration: Practice and Linking

➡ *Orient to the elaboration activity: On-Track Action Worked Example 2 and Worksheet 2.* "OK, we are going to fill out a worksheet together (p. 267), but first let's look at a completed one (p. 266) to get an idea about how to do it."

Note: The group can read the answers on the worked example and discuss how each is an On-Track Action. There are different options for how to complete the On-Track Action Worksheet 2. The leader can write each answer on the board or participants can do their own and share. As a fun alternative, the trainer can put the concepts (the five types of On-Track Actions and the other six skills listed on the sheet) on slips of paper and put them in a basket. A group member picks a slip of paper and the group has to brainstorm an On-Track Action to fit the prompt. This format for an exercise can be used in many ways to vary from reviewing handouts.

Disclosure question. "How did that exercise go for you?"

➡ *Orient to discussion.* "OK, let's talk a little more about On-Track Actions."

Linking questions. "This is a 123 skills chain: What does this mean?"; "How is this different from what you have done in the past?"

Disclosure questions. "When was a time when it was difficult to do an On-Track Action?"; "What was going on that made it difficult?"

Expansion questions. "What are other skills we use with On-Track Action?"; "Could On-Track Action help you in your life?"; "At home?"; "At work?"; "In your relationships?"; "When you deal with family members?"

➡ *Orient to the end of the Elaboration Phase.* "Great discussion. It is important for us to understand how to use our skills in difficult situations. In tough situations, it is easy to go off-track and hard to reach goals."

E-Spiral Phase 4. Efficacy: Bridge to Real Life

➡ *Orient to efficacy activities: role-play a scenario.* "So, now we are going to do a role play. We are going to have a little, tiny argument! I am actually going to irritate you on purpose, so that you can practice Clear Picture, On-Track Thinking, and On-Track Action. Who would like to start?"

Instructions for the efficacy activity. "I am going to walk up to you and accuse you of stealing my CD. As I am talking, I would like you to quickly get a Clear Picture and do On-Track Thinking. I am not going to keep talking too much, because I want you to have time to figure out what to do. Once you make a Skills Plan, take an On-Track Action. You can ask the group for help whenever you need to. Now, group members, if you have suggestions, raise your hand. Our volunteer may point to you, and you can give the advice. He can ask for volunteers or try to handle it on his own. We are going to do this slowly to practice putting these skills together. Any questions?"

Note: It is helpful for the skills trainer to stop and prompt the group members to help the participant through the Clear Picture Do's, On-Track Thinking, and figuring out an On-Track Action that fits for the participant. If a psychodrama format was used, different group members could offer coaching on specific skills (e.g., Clear Picture and On-Track Thinking). Depending on the group's level of skills knowledge, the trainer gauges how much depth to go into, as well as how much support to offer.

Disclosure questions. "Did you get a Clear Picture?" [review each of the Clear Picture Do's]; "Did you use Check It?"; "Turn It Up?"; "Cheerleading?"; "What was your skills plan?"; "Did you take an On-Track Action?"; "Were you in Wise Mind?"

➡ ***Orient to discussion.*** "Great job on the role play. Before we finish, would it be OK if we have a brief discussion about some of the challenges involved in taking On-Track Actions?"

Barrier question. "What is difficult about using On-Track Action?"

Wisdom question. "Do you feel it is important for you to use On-Track Action in your life?"

Commitment question. "When will you use On-Track Action?"

Coaching question. "How can you coach yourself to use On-Track Action when you feel stuck?"

➡ ***Orient to home study.*** "Good discussion about On-Track Actions. Homework time! This week we are going to practice using On-Track Actions. Let's try to take actions that are Taking a Step to my Goal. Also, please practice Switching Tracks when you have off-track urges. If you want to study skills at home, you can review all the handouts we have gone over so far. You can look at On-Track Action Worked Example 1 (p. 266) and complete On-Track Action Worksheet 1 (p. 267). Perhaps find someone to help you, if you need it. Any questions?"

➡ ***Orient to group ending.*** "As you know, we ring the bell six times at the end of group. We do one ring for each of the Clear Picture Do's. It is a chance to notice what is happening inside and outside of us right now. We take a moment to get a Clear Picture as we go back to our activities. Who would like to ring the bell today?"

On-Track Action Handouts to Review in Future Cycles or for Home Study

✓ On-Track Action Summary Sheet (p. 260). The summary sheet can be used during the encoding phase to explain concepts as teaching points. It may be too boring to read in group, but having different group members read different sections can break it up. Summary sheets are helpful for home study and for teaching skills to skills coaches.

✓ On-Track Action Handouts 3–7 (pp. 263–265, 268–269). If the group was not able to review On-Track Action Handouts 3–7, the individual can complete these in future cycles, during individual therapy, or while at home.

✓ On-Track Action Worked Example 1 and On-Track Action Worksheet 1 (pp. 266–267). The individual reviews the worked example to understand better the concept of an On-Track Action Plan. She then fills in the worksheet, developing her own On-Track Action Plan.

✓ On-Track Action Worksheet 3 (p. 272). This worksheet is a practice linking different On-Track Actions in skills chains.

WEEK 6: SAFETY PLANS

Preparing for Group

Handouts Needed

✓ Safety Plan Handout 1 (p. 274)
✓ Safety Plan Worked Example 1 (p. 275)
✓ Safety Plan Handout 2 (p. 277)
✓ Safety Plan Worked Example 2 (p. 278)
✓ Safety Plan Handout 3 (p. 280)
✓ Safety Plan Handout 4 (p. 281)
✓ Safety Plan Worked Example 3 (p. 283)
✓ Safety Plan Worksheet 4 (p. 284)

E-Spiral Phase 1. Exploring Existing Knowledge Base (Review)

➡ *Welcome group.* "Welcome back! How is everyone doing today? Well, how about we get started?"

➡ *Orient to the mindfulness activity: Noticing surroundings.* "Are you ready to do our mindfulness exercise? [Wait for response.] Great!"

Instructions for the mindfulness exercise. "OK, I will ring the bell and we will begin by noticing the breath. I will ring it a second time and we will shift our attention from the breath to noticing our surroundings. Noticing Surroundings is one of the Clear Picture Do's. We use our five senses to notice what we see, hear, smell, taste, and touch. If your mind drifts to something other than your breath and surroundings, gently bring your mind back. Having a Clear Picture about what is happening around us helps us make on-track choices. Having a Fuzzy Picture about what is happening around us can help us go off-track."

Describe questions. "What did you notice during this exercise?"; "Did your mind drift?"; "Were you able to bring your mind back?"

➡ *Orient to Skills System review.* "Good observations. Now, how about we do our Skills System review?

Note: The skills trainer can choose a Basic Review Activity from Week 1 (p. 115) or an Advanced Review Activity from Week 3 on page 127 or create a new one.

➡ *Orient to skills practice.* "Great job—we are getting there! Now, we are going to review our skills practice. We were practicing doing On-Track Actions this week. Let's not forget how we also use Clear Picture and On-Track Thinking to do what works."

Disclosure questions. "Who would like to share about how they used On-Track Actions this week?"; "What were some of the positive things people did as an On-Track Action?"; "Did anyone Switch Tracks?"; "What did we do that was opposite of Off-Track Urges?"; "Who used 123 Wise Mind?"; "What things did you have to accept this week?"; "Did anyone Turn the Page on something this week?"

➡ *Orient to new skills topic.* "Excellent! Before we get started on our now skill for this week, can we talk about what we already know about keeping ourselves safe?"

💬 *Discuss existing knowledge about the new topic.*

Assessment questions. "What does the word 'risk' mean?"; "What is a risky situation?"

Relevant context questions. "What are some examples of risky situations that you have noticed?"; "How do we know when a situation is not safe?"; "What are some situations that may be helpful to avoid?"

Clarifying questions. "What can happen if we move toward risky situations?"; "What happens if we move away from risky situations?"

➡ *Orient to relevant context of new topic.* "Sometimes there are difficult situations in life. Much of the time, it is best that we face challenging situations so that we learn how to deal with them. Sometimes, avoiding can make things worse. Other times, situations should be avoided, because there is risk that can cause us problems. In these situations, we use our Safety Plan. We use our Clear Picture and On-Track Thinking to make these important decisions."

E-Spiral Phase 2. Encoding: New Learning

➡ *Orient to new learning: Safety Plan.* "The Safety Plan is the fourth skill in the Skills System. Safety Plans help us handle risky situations. We are going to go over several handouts today; it seems like a lot! I do not expect us to learn all about Safety Plans today, but we will review the three types of Safety Plans, the three Levels of Risk, and the three things we can do when we notice risk."

Instructions for the encoding activity. "Let's get started by turning to page 274. Safety Plan Handout 1 looks like this. All set?"

Note: The skills trainer reads the handout.

☆ *Teaching Points for Safety Plan Handout 1.* "Safety Plans help us handle risks that come from both inside and outside of us. Inside risks are ones that happen inside our bodies. When we have TUFFs [Off-Track <u>T</u>houghts, <u>U</u>rges, <u>F</u>eelings, and <u>F</u>antasies], we need to use Safety Plans. TUFFs make it more difficult for us to stay on-track.

"Things, such as people, places, or things, can be outside risks. Certain people, places, or things can cause us problems. These Outside risks can make us have off-track Thoughts, Urges, Feelings, and Fantasies that make the situation dangerous for us or other people. Any questions?"

➡️ *Orient to Safety Plan Worked Example 1.* "Let's turn to the Safety Plan Worked Example 1 on page 275. It looks like this."

☆ *Teaching point for Safety Plan Worked Example 1.* "Let's read through this worksheet together to learn more about inside and outside risks."

➡️ *Orient to Safety Plan Handout 2.* "OK, good start. Now let's learn about the three levels of risk. Please turn to page 277. Safety Plan Handout 2 looks like this."

Note: The leader reads through the handout with the group.

☆ *Teaching Point for Safety Plan Handout 2.* "There are three Levels of Risk: low, medium, and high. To identify risk, we ask ourselves (1) how much damage can the risk cause and (2) how close is it to us? In a high-risk situation, there is a chance for serious damage or the thing is very close to us. In a medium-risk situation, the risk can cause us problems or is in our area. In low-risk situations, the risk may cause us some stress or it is far away from us.

"So, the more damage something can cause, the higher the risk. The closer the risk is to us, the higher the risk. For example, if a rattlesnake is next to us, it is high risk. If the snake is 100 feet away, the risk is lower. Any questions?"

➡️ *Orient to Safety Plan Worked Example 2.* "OK, let's look at the example on page 278; it looks like this."

➡️ *Orient to Safety Plan Handout 3.* "Great! I know there is a lot to learn about Safety Plans. It will take some time learn it; we take one step at a time. OK, let's turn to page 280 to see the three types of Safety Plans."

☆ *Teaching Point for Safety Plan Handout 3.* "Let's read this together to learn about the three types of Safety Plans. We have to do more Safety Planning as the situation becomes more risky. For example, in a low-risk situation, it might be all right to just do a Thinking Safety Plan. In a medium-risk situation, it is usually best to do a Thinking and Talking Safety Plans. In a high-risk situation, it is helpful to do Thinking, Talking, and Written Safety Plans to be sure the danger is managed well."

Note: The leader or group reads through the handout with the group.

➡ *Orient to Safety Plan Handout 4.* "So far we have learned about low, medium, and high risks. We have also learned about written, talking, and thinking Safety Plans. Next we are going to learn about what we do in these situations to handle risk. Please turn to page 281. The Safety Plan Handout 4 looks like this."

Note: The leader or group reads through the handout with the group.

☆ *Teaching point for Safety Plan Handout 4.* "When there is a low risk, it may be possible to focus on the New-Me Activity that we are doing at the time. For example, if I notice a small issue far away, I can just focus on my activity. I am not ignoring the problem; I am choosing to focus on something helpful. Next, if there is a risk that is closer or will cause me problems, I move away to get distance between me and the risk. For example, I may move my seat in a room if someone is bothering me, then continue focusing on my New-Me Activity. If there is a high-risk situation, I will want to leave the area completely. I want to be sure I cannot hear, see, talk to, or touch the risk. For example, I would go to my room and close the door."

Content questions. "Why is it dangerous to be able to see, hear, talk to, or touch the risk?"; "How do we know where to go when we have to move or leave an area?"; "Why is it good to do a New-Me Activity?"; "What New-Me Activities are helpful to focus on?"; "How far away do we need to go when we move away?"; "How do we focus our attention on our activity when there is a low risk?"; "How do we know when we should do a Safety Plan to avoid a situation and when it is best to try to face a difficult situation?"

➡ *Orient to end of the Encoding Phase.* "There are many parts of the Safety Plan skill: Levels of Risk, types of Safety Plans, and actions that we take to handle risky situations. How about we move on to practice Safety Planning?"

E-Spiral Phase 3. Elaboration: Practice and Linking

➡ *Orient to elaboration activity: Safety Plan Worked Example 3.* "OK, we are going to put all of these new things together into a written Safety Plan. Please turn to page 283. The Safety Plan Worked Example 3 looks like this."

Instruction for practice exercise. "We are going to read through this Safety Plan together and talk about it."

Disclosure question. "What are your thoughts about Safety Plans?"

➡ *Orient to discussion.* "OK, I know you have done Safety Plans in the past; let's talk about that a little bit."

Linking questions. "What does it mean that this is a 1234 skills chain?"; "What is it like to do a Safety Plan in Wise Mind?"; "How is Safety Plan different from what you have done in the past?"

Disclosure questions. "Were there times when you did not use a Safety Plan and wish you had?"; "What happened?"

Expansion questions. "What are other skills we use with Safety Plans?"; "Are there times in your life that you could use a Safety Plan?"; "At work?"; "At home?"; "With family?"; "With friends?"

➡ ***Orient to the end of the Elaboration Phase.*** "It sounds like there are times when we need to use Safety Plans. I'm glad we are learning this today!"

E-Spiral Phase 4. Efficacy: Bridge to Real Life

➡ ***Orient to efficacy activities: Safety Planning Worksheet 3.*** "OK, I think we are ready to do a Safety Plan together. Let's turn to page 282. The Safety Plan Worksheet 3 looks like this. Who would like to share a risky situation that happened this week that we could go through and do a Safety Plan for? [Wait for response.] Very brave, thank you!"

Note: It is important to pick a scenario that is interesting, yet not highly arousing for the volunteer or the group. A medium- or low-risk situation is best to review.

Instructions for the efficacy activity. The trainer leads the person through the Safety Plan. The trainer focuses on moving through the Safety Plan rather than stopping to do Expressing Myself or Problem Solving about the situation. The group is encouraged to participate. The trainer and group ask questions to foster thinking about different options and check the fit of each. Together the trainer, the volunteer, and the group make the Safety Plan.

Disclosure questions. "How do you think this Safety Planning went?"; "Do you think the Safety Plan would have helped?"; "Do you have any questions about Safety Plans?"

➡ ***Orient to discussion.*** "That was very good; everyone was helpful. Before we finish up today, I would like us to talk together about some of the challenges of doing Safety Plans."

Barrier questions. "What is difficult about using a Safety Plan?"; "What is it like to have to walk away from situations, especially ones that we enjoy but know are risky?"; "What is it like to have to stop doing something we like because of someone else?"

Wisdom question. "Do you think Safety Plans are important for you to use?"

Commitment question. "When can you use Safety Plans in your life?"

Coaching question. "How can you coach yourself to use Safety Plans?"

➡ ***Orient to home study.*** "Great job today! There is a lot to learn about Safety Plans. Practice can really help. So, this week, please practice noticing risky situations. Think about whether the risk is low, medium, or high. Think about whether you should do a Thinking, Talking, and/ or Writing Safety Plan. Also, decide whether it is best to refocus, move away, or leave the area completely. Are there any questions? [Wait for response.] Good luck!

"Also, if you want to study skills at home, review all the handouts we have gone over so far. You can also do Safety Plan Worksheets 1, 2, 3, and 4."

➡ *Orient to group ending.* "As you know, we ring the bell six times at the end of group. We do one ring for each of the Clear Picture Do's. It is a chance to notice what is happening inside and outside of us right now. We take a moment to get a Clear Picture as we go back to our activities. Who would like to ring the bell today?"

Safety Plan Handouts to Review in Future Cycles or for Home Study

✓ Safety Plan Summary Sheet (p. 273). The summary sheet can be used during the encoding phase to explain concepts as teaching points It may be too boring to read in group, but having different group members read different sections can break it up. Summary sheets are helpful for home study and for teaching skills coaches the skills.

✓ Safety Plan Worksheet 1 (p. 276)

☆ *Teaching Points.* The individual lists specific inside and outside risks that he experiences.

✓ Safety Plan Worksheet 2 (p. 279)

☆ *Teaching points.* The individual lists specific low, medium, and high risks on Safety Plan Worksheet 2.

✓ Safety Plan Worksheet 3 (p. 282)

☆ *Teaching points.* The individual thinks of a different situation that happened to her and circles the type of risk, level of risk, type of Safety Plan, and how she would handle the risk.

✓ Safety Plan Worksheet 4 (p. 284)

☆ *Teaching points.* The individual writes down (or has assistance in writing) information about a risky situation. She then determines the level of risk and on-track ways to manage the situation.

WEEK 7: NEW-ME ACTIVITIES

Preparing for Group

Handouts Needed

✓ New-Me Activities Handout 1 (p. 286)
✓ New-Me Activities Handout 2 (p. 287)
✓ New-Me Activities Handout 3 (p. 289)
✓ New-Me Activities Handout 4 (p. 291)
✓ New-Me Activity Handout 5 (p. 293)

E-Spiral Phase 1. Exploring Existing Knowledge Base (Review)

➡️ *Welcome group.* "Hi, everybody. How are we doing today? Ready for some mindfulness?"

➡️ *Orient to the mindfulness activity: noticing emotions.* "Today we are going to notice our emotions as we listen to the bell."

Instructions for the mindfulness exercise. "I will ring the bell one time and we will bring our attention to the breath. On the second ring, we will turn our attention to noticing any emotions we are having. Notice the sensations and then label what emotion it is. If your mind starts to wander to other things, gently bring your mind back to the emotion. Notice the emotions come and let them go without needing to act on them or make them stronger by focusing on the issues. Learning to turn our minds to and from emotions helps us manage them. OK, here goes; let's focus on emotions. Any questions?"

Describe questions. "How was that for you?"; "What emotions did you notice?"; "Did your mind drift?"; "Did you notice urges to take actions?"; "Were you able to bring your mind back to your emotions?"

➡️ *Orient to Skills System review.* "Great job with Clear Picture. OK, how about we review our skills, System Tools, and the Clear Picture Do's."

Note: The skills trainer can choose a Basic Review Activity from Week 1 (p. 115) or an Advanced Review Activity from Week 3 on page 127 or create a new one.

➡️ *Orient to skills practice.* "Great, on to homework! How did we do this week practicing Safety Plans?"

Disclosure questions. "Who would like to tell us about a thinking Safety Plan they did this week?"; "Who can tell us about doing a Talking Safety Plan this week?"; "Who can tell us about doing a Written Safety Plan this week?"; "Did anyone wish he or she had used a Safety Plan this week?"

➡️ *Orient to new skills topic.* "Good start. Safety Plans take time to learn; you all will get it. Now, let's talk about what we know about doing New-Me Activities."

🗨️ *Discuss existing knowledge about the new topic.*

Assessment questions. "After people walk away from a risky situation, what do they do then?"; "What do you think 'new-me' means?"; "What do you thin 'old-me' means?"; "What are some activities that help you stay on-track?"

Relevant context questions. "What is the difference between an on-track activity and an off-track activity?"; "How do we decide if an activity is helpful or not helpful?"

Clarifying questions. "Why do people choose New-Me Activities?"; "Why do people choose off-track activities?"

➡️ *Orient to relevant context of the new topic.* "New-Me Activities help us in many ways. We are going to learn about how to choose the right activities at the right time to help us reach our goals."

E-Spiral Phase 2. Encoding: New Learning

➡️ *Orient to new learning: New-Me Activity.* "We are going to learn about New-Me Activities today! We are going to read through five New-Me Activity Handouts. Let's turn to page 286. The New-Me Activities Handout 1 looks like this."

Instructions for the encoding activity. The group reads through the New-Me Activities handouts and discusses different activities. "Would anyone like to read or should I?"

☆ *Teaching points for New-Me Activities Handout 1.* "This handout introduces the four different types of New-Me Activities. Different activities help us do different things. Some help us focus, feel better, distract us, and are fun. We have to learn to do many different New-Me Activities and to choose the one that helps most in the moment. Handouts 2–5 go into detail about each kind."

➡️ *Orient to New-Me Activities Handout 2 (Focus).* "Now let's learn more about Focus New-Me Activities. Please turn to page 287. The New-Me Activities Handout 2 looks like this."

☆ *Teaching points for New-Me Activities Handout 2.* "Focus New-Me Activities help us focus our attention. We have to concentrate and pay attention carefully when we do these activities. Let's brainstorm a list on the board of each kind of activity on the handout."

Note: It is particularly important that each individual has accessible activities that fit his means and logistical situation.

Content questions. "What are different things we can organize and sort?"; "What kind of things can you clean?"; "When is it helpful to use Focus New-Me Activities?"

➡️ *Orienting to New-Me Activities Handout 3 (Feel Good).* "Now we are going to look at page 289. It is the New-Me Activities Handout 3 that shows us Feel Good New-Me Activities. It looks like this."

➡️ *Review New-Me Activities Handout 3.*

☆ *Teaching points for New-Me Activities Handout 3.* "Feel Good New-Me Activities use our senses to make us feel more comfortable and happy. When we are feeling stressed or upset, it can help to do an activity that soothes and makes us feel better. Let's read these and brainstorm on the board a list of activities that utilize each of our senses that help us feel good."

Content questions. "What do you enjoy looking at?"; "What are things that you enjoy listening to?"; "What do you enjoy touching?"; "What do you enjoy smelling?"; "What do you enjoy tasting?"; "When is it helpful to use Feel Good New-Me Activities?"

➡️ *Orient to New-Me Activities Handout 4 (Distraction).* "On to Distraction New-Me Activities Handout 4. It is on page 291, and it looks like this."

☆ *Teaching points for New-Me Activities Handout 4.* "Sometimes, we are overwhelmed and need to chill out and take a break. If we have done everything we can to fix a situation, there are times when it is best to Distract My Mind and/or Distract My Body. When we distract, we are switching our focus from one situation to another. We are focused on the new activity and Turning the Page from the one that is bothering us.

"It is important that we use Distract New-Me Activities when we have used all necessary skills in a situation and we need to wait, relax, or get our mind off of the situation. We don't want to distract, if we need to deal with the situation. Distracting ourselves when we need to focus may lead us off-track. Knowing when and how to Distract My Mind and Distract My Body is important. We have to use Clear Picture and On-Track Thinking to figure out whether a Distraction New-Me Activity is an On-Track Action. Let's brainstorm a list on the board of activities that are useful to distract us."

Content questions. "What are things that help you get your mind off of your problems?"; "When is it helpful to distract ourselves?"; "When is it not helpful to distract ourselves?"

➡️ *Orient to New-Me Activities Handout 5 (Fun).* "Fun New-Me Activities are next! Please turn to page 293. The New-Me Activities Handout 5 looks like this."

☆ *Teaching points for New-Me Activities Handout 5.* "It is important to do activities that are fun. Doing activities that we enjoy helps us have a higher quality of life. If we do not do things that give us joy, we tend to get depressed. Let's brainstorm on the board a list of activities that people find fun."

Content questions. "What sports do you like to watch?"; "What hobbies do you enjoy?"; "What kind of crafts do you like to make?"

Note: It is important that the group discusses realistic options, so that the participants can readily integrate the activities into their lives.

➡️ *Orient to the end of the Encoding Phase.* "We have come up with many great new ideas today. It's time to practice!"

E-Spiral Phase 3. Elaboration: Practice and Linking.

➡️ *Orient to the elaboration activity.* "We are going to do a New-Me Activity right now!" Today we are going to do some drawing. Here are some markers and paper. We are going to draw for a few minutes."

Instructions for the practice exercise. "We are going to draw something, anything you wish. It can be a house, a person, a car, a tree, a boat, mountains—anything. It does not have to be fancy. The activity is to use your skills to jump into this activity with both feet! I know that not everyone is going to love this New-Me Activity. So for those of you who think you can't draw or are embarrassed, we are going to do an On-Track Action and give 100% effort to drawing. As we are drawing, we may notice our minds starting to insult our drawings or ourselves; we have to allow those off-track thoughts to pass and gently bring our attention back to our picture. Does this sound similar to how we control our attention when we ring the bell? It does to me! We want to stay focused on our picture, not on off-track thoughts or feelings. If we say nice things to other people about their drawings, what skill is that? [Wait for response.] Right— Relationship Care! If we say nice things to others, they might say our drawing is good. That might make us feel better! You can draw anything you want for 5 minutes. If you want to share the picture and even a story about what it is, great. Sharing our pictures might be stressful, so we may have to do another On-Track Action to make ourselves give 100% to this activity. Does everyone have something to draw on and to draw with? Any questions?"

Note: The trainer may want to offer verbal praise evenly across the group for effort, skill use, and drawings.

Disclosure questions. "Did you use Clear Picture and On-Track Thinking while you were drawing?"; "How was that activity for people?"; "What was helpful about it?"; "What was difficult about it?"; "Did you have to do an On-Track Action?"; "Were you able to jump in with both feet?"

➡ *Orient to discussion.* "Great, we are going to talk for a few minutes about doing New-Me Activities."

Linking questions. "New-Me Activities are a 1235 skills chain; what does this mean?"; "What is it like when we do a New-Me Activity in Wise Mind?"; "What is a 12345 skills chain?"; "In the past, have you ever been bored because you did not do enough New-Me Activities?"; "What was that like?"

Disclosure questions. "Did you use skills 1235 during this activity?"; "Who can describe a time when using a New-Me Activity really helped you feel better?"; "Who can describe a time when you had to do an On-Track Action because you didn't feel like doing anything?"; "Who can describe a time when you chose the wrong New-Me Activity to do?"; "What happened?"; "How can you tell when your New-Me Activities are in balance?"

Expansion questions. "What other skills do we use with New-Me Activities?"; "How can New-Me Activities help you reach your goals?"

➡ *Orient to the end of the Elaboration Phase.* "That was a great discussion. Guess what? We are going to practice a New-Me Activity again!"

E-Spiral Phase 4. Efficacy: Bridge to Real Life

➡ *Orient to efficacy activities: Group game.* "That was a great discussion. Guess what? We are going to practice a New-Me Activity again! Game time!"

Note: The skills trainer presents a game that will be fun for the group. This is an opportunity for the group leader to be creative. The trainer can make up an activity or bring in some kind of game that fits the ability level of the group members. The game should be simple, short, and fun. The goal is for all members to participate and to experience joy. It can be a skills game, such as Skills Man (similar to hangman, but each correct answer adds a body part to a person standing rather than a person hanging). In Skills Man someone draws a number of blank spaces that represent skills terms, and the group guesses the letters and ultimately the term. Team skills Jeopardy can be fun; the trainer or group members generate questions.

Instructions for the efficacy activity. The skills trainer gives clear, step-by-step directions. Be sure all participants are ready prior to beginning.

Disclosure questions. "Was this activity a Focus, Feel Good, Distraction, and/or Fun New-Me Activity?"; "Did you use 1235?"; "How was that activity for you?"; "Did you have fun?"; "Was there anything challenging about it?"

➡ *Orient to discussion.* "Let's talk a little more about some of the challenges we face when we do New-Me Activities."

Barrier questions. "What is difficult about doing New-Me Activities?"; "Is it difficult to ask people to join you?"; "How can we deal with that?"

Wisdom questions. "Are New-Me Activities important for you to do?"; "Do you need to do more New-Me Activities?"

Commitment question. "What new New-Me Activities will you try?"

Coaching question. "How can you coach yourself to do a different New-Me Activities?"

➡ *Orienting to home study.* "Great group today. Now it is homework time! This week we are going to practice doing all four kinds of New-Me Activities. We will do at least one Focus New-Me Activity, one Feel Good New-Me Activity, one Distraction New-Me Activity, and one Fun New-Me Activity. Skill Masters will try new New-Me Activities! Also, please go over the Problem Solving Summary Sheet on page 295 for next week. Any questions?

"Also, if you want to study skills at home, review all the handouts we have gone over so far. You can also do New-Me Activities Worksheets 1, 2, 3, and 4."

➡ *Orient to group ending.* "As you know, we ring the bell six times at the end of group. We do one ring for each of the Clear Picture Do's. It is a chance to notice what is happening inside and outside of us right now. We take a moment to get a Clear Picture as we go back to our activities. Who would like to ring the bell today?"

New-Me Activity Handouts to Review in Future Cycles or For Home Study

✓ New-Me Activity Summary Sheet (p. 285). The summary sheet can be used during the encoding phase to explain concepts as teaching points It may be too boring to read in group, but having different group members read different sections can break it up. Summary sheets are helpful for home study and for teaching skills coaches the skills.

✓ New-Me Activities Worksheet 1 (p. 288)

☆ *Teaching points.* The client lists New-Me Activities that help her focus attention.

✓ New-Me Activities Worksheet 2 (p. 290)

☆ *Teaching points.* The participant writes down New-Me Activities that help the body to feel good.

✓ New-Me Activities Worksheet 3 (p. 292)

☆ *Teaching points.* The client lists New-Me Activities that help provide distraction.

✓ New-Me Activities Worksheet 4 (p. 294)

☆ *Teaching points.* The individual writes down Fun New-Me Activities that he or she likes to do.

WEEK 8: PROBLEM SOLVING

Preparing for Group

Handouts Needed

✓ Problem Solving Summary Sheet (p. 295)
✓ Problem Solving Worked Example 1 (p. 296)
✓ Problem Solving Worksheet 1 (p. 297)
✓ Problem Solving Handout 1 (p. 298)
✓ Problem Solving Worked Example 2A (p. 299)
✓ Problem Solving Worked Example 2B (p. 301)
✓ Problem Solving Worked Example 2C (p. 303)

E-Spiral Phase 1. Exploring Existing Knowledge Base (Review)

➡ *Welcome group.* "Welcome back! How is everybody today? Ready to go?"

➡ *Orient to the mindfulness activity: Breathing and Rating Emotions.* "Last week, we noticed emotions when we rang the bell. This week we are going to notice emotions again, and this time we are going to rate the emotions."

Instructions for the mindfulness exercise. "I will ring the bell one time and we will notice the breath. On the second ring we will shift our attention to notice an emotion. We notice the sensation and label it, like happy, sad, or anxious. We then will rate how strong the emotion is using the Feelings Rating Scale. If you have time during the six rings to label and rate another emotion, try to. We label and rate emotions and let them pass. If your mind drifts to things in the past or future, bring your mind back to the emotions you have right now. It is important to be able to focus your attention on a task. It is also important to be able to notice, label, rate, and allow emotions to pass like clouds in the sky. Any questions?"

Describe questions. "How was that exercise?"; "What did you notice about rating your emotions?"; "Where did your attention go during this exercise?"

➡️ *Orient to Skills System review.* "It is time for us to review our skills, System Tools and the Clear Picture Do's."

Note: The skills trainer can choose a Basic Review Activity from Week 1 (p. 115) or an Advanced Review Activity from Week 3 on page 127 or create a new one.

➡️ *Orient to skills practice.* "Great, let's talk about how our practice of New-Me Activities went this week?"

Disclosure questions. "Who can tell us about the Focus New-Me Activities they did?"; "Who can tell us about the Feel Good New-Me Activities they did?"; "Who can tell us about the Distraction New-Me Activities they did?"; "Who can tell us about the Fun New-Me Activities they did?"

➡️ *Orient to new skills topic.* "Sounds as if we did a lot of interesting things this week. Would it be OK if you talked a little about what we already know about Problem Solving?"

💬 *Discuss existing knowledge about the new topic.*

Assessment questions. "How do we know when we have a problem?"; "What is it like to solve problems when we are in Emotional Mind? Fuzzy Mind? Wise Mind?"

Relevant context questions. "What are some examples of on-track Problem Solving?"; "What are some examples of off-track Problem Solving?"

Clarifying questions. "What happens when people try to do Problem Solving when they are upset?"; "How does that usually work out?"; "What happens if we do Problem Solving when we are clear and calm?"; "How does that usually work out?"

➡️ *Orient to relevant context of the new topic.* "Knowing how and when to fix problems is important. Life gives us challenges all the time. If we try to fix problems at the wrong time, we can make things worse. If we don't know how to solve problems, we can also make things worse. The goal of our skills is to make our lives better and to reach our goals."

E-Spiral Phase 2. Encoding: New Learning

➡️ *Orient to new learning.* "We are going to learn about Problem Solving today. Problem Solving, Skill 6, is a Calm-Only skill. This means that we, and anyone we are talking to, have to be below a Level 3 emotion when we are solving problems. Problem Solving helps us fix problems, so we can reach our goals. Knowing when and how to fix problems is important. I hope you had a chance to review the Problem Solving Summary Sheet (p. 295) during the week."

➡️ *Orient to Problem Solving Worked Example 1.* "Let's start by going over the Quick Fix worked example on page 296. This is what it looks like. We can do a Quick Fix when the situation is simple and clear. When situations are confusing, it is better to do all the steps in Problem Solving. We will go over those steps after we see how to do a Quick Fix."

Note: The trainer goes through the Quick Fix example and the group discusses the concepts and the scenario. The group can refer to the Problem Solving Summary Sheet (p. 295) for explanations of specific concepts as needed.

E-Spiral Phase 3. Elaboration: Practice and Linking

➡️ *Orient to elaboration activity: Problem Solving Handout 1.* "Now we are going to learn about how to do Problem Solving when we have medium and large problems. Let's turn to page 298 to Problem Solving Handout 1. It looks like this."

☆ *Teaching points for Problem Solving Handout 1.* "There are three basic steps to Problem Solving. First we get a Clear Picture of the Problem. Second, we fast-forward and Check All Options that we have for fixing the problem. Third, we make Plans A, B, and C for solving the problem. Ready to learn more?"

➡️ *Orient to Problem Solving Worked Example 2A.* "Let's turn to page 299, so we can learn more about getting a Clear Picture of the problems by turning to Problem Solving Worked Example 1. It looks like this. Everyone all set?"

☆ *Teaching points for Problem Solving Worked Example 2A.* "There are four steps to do when we get a clear picture of the problem. First, we think about what we want to happen. Second, we think about what is in our way. Third, we focus on the one part of the situation that we want to fix. Fourth, it is helpful to think about how big the problem is. Some problems are more serious than others. Small problems are often not too serious and cause low-level feelings. Medium problems cause higher-level feelings (Levels 3 and 4) and take more steps and time to fix. Large or overwhelming problems are very serious and often cause us to have Level 4 or 5 feelings, may take weeks/months/years to fix, and change our lives in serious ways.

"In this situation, the person wants to buy sneakers and there isn't enough money. Is this a small, medium, or large problem? If we react like the sneakers are a large problem, what might happen to our actions?"

➡️ *Orient to Problem Solving Worked Example 2B.* "Great, we know what we want and what the problem is. Now we move on to Check All Options. Turn to page 301, to Problem Solving Worked Example 2B. It looks like this."

Note: The trainer or group reads through the worked example explore options, fast forwarding to determine the pros and cons of each option.

☆ *Teaching points for Problem Solving Worksheet 2B.* "Turn to page 302. When we Check

All Options, we think of many different ways to solve a problem. For each option, we fast forward to see what the pros and cons are. The pros of an option are helpful results. [Makes the thumbs-up gesture.] The cons of an option are the unhelpful results. [Makes the thumbs-down gesture.] Once we look at several options, we check the fit to choose the best option for us.

"Problem Solving takes a lot of thinking and focus. It takes time and energy to fast-forward each idea to see what might happen if we make that choice. This is why it is a Calm-Only skill. When we are calm, we can think of options, pros, and cons. When we are upset, we rush to solutions that make us feel better in the moment. We don't take time to think clearly. In Fuzzy Mind, we have a hard time focusing on what is good in the long term."

Note: Some group members may understand pros and cons quickly. Other participants will comprehend the concepts when the worked example is reviewed.

Content questions. "Can you think of any other options?"; "What would be the pros of your ideas?"; "What would be the cons of your ideas?"; "Which option do you think is the best?"; "What does it mean for something to fit in the short term but not the long term?"

➡ *Orient to Problem Solving Worked Example 2C.* "It will help us to go through an example of this. Please turn to page 303, to the Problem Solving Worked Example 2C. It looks like this. We have gotten a clear picture of the problem, checked all the options, and found the best option. Now we are ready to make Plans A, B, and C."

☆ *Teaching points for Problem Solving Worked Example 2C.* "Once we figure out our best option, we have to make plans. We use Clear Picture, On-Track Thinking, and On-Track Actions to help us do Problem Solving. We call our favorite idea Plan A. Usually we have to take several steps to fix problems well. We determine who we need to talk to. We plan what we are going to say and how we are going to say it. We focus on doing what works to fix our problem.

"Sometimes we start Plan A and find out that our favorite plan will not work. It can be upsetting. So we come up with a Plan B, so that we are prepared when things go wrong with Plan A. Plan B is a backup plan; it may help us get part of what we want. It may make sense even to make a fallback plan, Plan C, in case Plans A and B do not work. Plan C will help us stay on-track. Any questions?"

➡ *Orient to discussion.* "If it is OK with you, I would like to ask a few questions that will help us understand Problem Solving even better."

Linking questions. "Problem Solving is skills chain 1236; what does that mean?"; "What is it like to solve problems in Wise Mind?"

Disclosure questions. "Who can describe a time when you have done on-track Problem Solving in the past?"; "Who can describe a time when they did off-track Problem Solving in the past?"

Expansion question. "What do we do if we notice we are doing off-track Problem Solving?"

➡ *Orient to the end of the Elaboration Phase.* "Very interesting discussion. Problem solving can be pretty complicated. That is why we must be below a Level 3 emotion. We need to take time to carefully solve problems. We also may need to talk to our friends, coaches, and therapist to help us think things through. OK, let's step it up another notch. How about solving one of our own problems?"

E-Spiral Phase 4. Efficacy: Bridge to Real Life

➡ *Orient to efficacy activities: Problem Solving Worksheet 1.* "We are going to practice doing a Quick Fix of a group member's problem now. Please turn to page 297, it looks like this. Who would like to tell us a simple problem that the group can use to practice doing a Quick Fix?"

Note: The trainer leads the group through the Quick Fix using an example provided by a group member. It is important that the group understand when a Quick Fix will work (e.g., when the solution is fairly clear) and when the expanded version of Problem Solving is needed.

Describe question. "What did you learn about Problem Solving in that exercise?"

➡ *Orient to discussion.* "We are just about done for today, but first, how about chatting for a few minutes about the challenges of Problem Solving?"

Barrier questions. "What is difficult about doing a Quick Fix?"; "What is difficult about going through all the steps of Problem Solving?"; "Is it hard to tell the difference between when we do a Quick Fix and full Problem Solving?"

Wisdom question. "Is it important for you to know how to solve problems?"

Commitment question. "Are you going to use Problem Solving?"

Coaching question. "How can you coach yourself to use Problem Solving?"

➡ *Orient to home study.* "Great group; homework time! This week we are going to practice doing Problem Solving. Please read or have someone read to you the Expressing Myself Summary Sheet on page 306. Any questions?

"Also, if you want to study skills at home, review all the handouts we have gone over so far. You can also do worksheet 1, 2, 3, and 4 if you like."

➡ *Orient to group ending.* "As you know, we ring the bell six times at the end of group. We do one ring for each of the Clear Picture Do's. It is a chance to notice what is happening inside and outside of us right now. We take a moment to get a Clear Picture as we go back to our activities. Who would like to ring the bell today?"

Problem Solving Handouts to Review in Future Cycles or for Home Study

✓ Problem Solving Summary Sheet (p. 295). The summary sheet can be used during the encoding phase to explain concepts as teaching points. It may be too boring to read in group, but having different group members read different sections can break it up. Summary sheets are helpful for home study and for teaching skills coaches the skills.

✓ Problem Solving Worksheet 1 (p. 297)
✓ Problem Solving Worksheet 2A (p. 300)
✓ Problem Solving Worksheet 2B (p. 302)
✓ Problem Solving Worksheet 2C (p. 304)
✓ Problem Solving Worksheet 3 (p. 305)

WEEK 9: EXPRESSING MYSELF

Preparing for Group

Handouts Needed

✓ Expressing Myself Summary Sheet (p. 306)
✓ Expressing Myself Handout 1 (p. 307)
✓ Expressing Myself Worked Example 1 (p. 308)
✓ Expressing Myself Handout 2 (p. 310)
✓ Expressing Myself Handout 3 (p. 311)
✓ Expressing Myself Handout 4 (p. 312)
✓ Expressing Myself Worked Example 2 (p. 313)
✓ Expressing Myself Worksheet 2 (p. 314)

E-Spiral Phase 1. Exploring Existing Knowledge Base (Review)

➡ *Welcome group.* "Hi, everyone! How are we doing today? Are we ready to get started? [Wait for response.] Great, it is time to ring the bell."

➡ *Orient to the mindfulness activity: Noticing Thoughts.* "Last week we did a mindfulness activity of noticing and rating our feelings. Today we are going to practice the next Clear Picture Do, Noticing Thoughts. Are we ready?"

Instructions for the mindfulness exercise. "OK, I will ring the bell and we will bring our attention to our breath. On the second ring we will shift our attention to notice thoughts going through our minds. Notice a thought in your mind and let it go. When you notice a thought, watch it pass like a city bus driving by. We are only going to watch thoughts and not get on any of the buses! We will allow thoughts to pass without thinking more about that thought or taking action. We will let the bus pass by and look for another bus. If our attention drifts from Noticing Thoughts, we will gently bring our minds back to our thoughts. Practice of Noticing Thoughts is helpful. There are many times when we need to watch thoughts and not take actions. Any questions?"

Describe questions. "What was it like to watch thoughts?"; "Did your mind drift at all?"; "Were you able to bring your attention back to Noticing Thoughts and allow them to pass?"

➡ *Orient to Skills System review.* "Great job. It is time to review our skills."

Note: The skills trainer can choose a Basic Review Activity from Week 1 (p. 115) or an Advanced Review Activity from Week 3 on page 127 or create a new one.

➡ *Orient to skills practice.* "We are really getting good at this! How about we review how we used Problem Solving this week?"

Disclosure questions. "Who would like to share how the Problem Solving went this week?"; "Did anyone do a Quick Fix?"; "Did anyone do Problem Solving?"

➡ *Orient to new skills topic.* "The skill we are going to learn about today often helps us with Problem Solving, Getting It Right, and Relationship Care. Let's spend a few minutes talking about what we know about Expressing Myself."

🗨 *Discuss existing knowledge about the new topic.*

Assessment questions. "What does it mean when someone is expressing herself?"; "Why do we express ourselves?"; "How do we express ourselves?"; "When do we express ourselves?"; "How does it go when we express ourselves when we are in Emotional Mind?"

Relevant context questions. "Did you have to express yourself to anyone when you were trying to solve problems this week?"; "Are there on-track ways to express ourselves?"; "Are there off-track ways to express ourselves?"

Clarifying questions. "What happens to our relationships when we do on-track expressing?"; "Do we reach our goals?"; "What happens when we use off-track expressing?"; "Do we reach our goals?"

➡ *Orient to relevant context of the new topic.* "Expressing Myself helps us communicate well with other people. Having clear communication helps us feel better about ourselves, our lives, and relationships. It helps us solve problems, get what we want, and keep our relationships in balance."

E-Spiral Phase 2. Encoding: New Learning

➡ *Orient to new learning.* "We are going to learn what 'Expressing Myself' is, why it is helpful, how we can do it well, and when is best to use it. It is important to remember that Expressing Myself is a Calm-Only skill and can be used *only* when we are at a Level 0–3 emotion. Are we ready to get started?"

➡ *Instructions for the encoding activity.* "Let's begin by turning to page 307. Expressing Myself Handout 1 looks like this."

☆ *Teaching points for Expressing Myself Handout 1.* "This handout will help us begin to understand more about what 'Expressing Myself' is. Let's read through it and discuss the points; perhaps we can add some things to it, as well."

➡ ***Orient to Expressing Myself Worked Example 1.*** "We are now going to turn to Expressing Myself Worked Example 1 on page 308. It looks like this. Let's read through it and discuss it together."

➡ ***Orient to Expressing Myself Handout 2.*** "Good start. Let's check out Expressing Myself Handout 2 on page 310. It teaches us why we use Expressing Myself. It looks like this. All set?"

➡ ***Orient to Expressing Myself Handout 3.*** "OK, so now we are going to learn more about how we use Expressing Myself by reading through this handout and discussing the points. Let's turn to Expressing Myself Handout 3 on page 311."

➡ ***Orient to Expressing Myself Handout 4.*** "Next, we are going to learn about when we use Expressing Myself. Let's turn to page 312. We will read through and discuss the points."

➡ ***Orient to Expressing Myself Worked Example 2.*** "As we can see, there are many parts to Expressing Myself. Sometimes it can be helpful to plan what we are going to say to someone to be sure the messages come out like we want. So, let's turn to page 313, to the Expressing Myself Plan worked example. We will read through this together and chat about it."

➡ ***Orient to the end of the Encoding Phase.*** "Great discussion about all these parts of Expressing Myself planning. Are we ready to practice putting all the parts together to practice Expressing Myself?"

E-Spiral Phase 3. Elaboration: Practice and Linking

➡ ***Orient to the elaboration activity.*** "Today we are going to use a worksheet to help us practice expressing what is in our minds and in our hearts. Let's turn to Expressing Myself Worksheet 1 on page 309. Each of us will practice how we would share a thought, a concern, a need, a feeling, a like, a dislike, a hope, and a dream. Please tell the group who in your life you would say this to and demonstrate how you would say it."

Note: Writing is optimal in this exercise. The trainer can either fill in this worksheet as a group activity listing each person's responses on the board (if the individuals in the group are unable to write) or each group member can take a few minutes to write down responses, then verbally express them to the group.

Disclosure questions. "What was it like to use Expressing Myself?"; "Were any responses more difficult to express?"

➡ *Orient to discussion.* "Great, I feel like I know you all a little better! Would it be all right if I asked you a few more questions that will help us understand Expressing Myself better?"

Linking questions. "Expressing Myself is skills chain 1237; what does that mean?"; "Who can describe a time in the past when he did on-track Expressing Myself?"; "What is Expressing Myself like in Wise Mind?"; "Who can describe a time when she did off-track Expressing Myself?"

Disclosure questions. "What happened when you used on-track Expressing Myself?"; "How did it make you feel about yourself and your life?"; "What happened when you did off-track Expressing Myself?"; "How did it make you feel about yourself and your life?"

Expansion questions. "What other skills do we use with Expressing Myself?"; "What do you do if you notice you are doing off-track Expressing Myself?"; "What can you do instead?"; "In what parts of your life can Expressing Myself help you?"; "At work?"; "At home?"; "With family?"; "With friends?"

➡ *Orient to the end of the Elaboration Phase.* "Good discussion. It sounds as if Expressing Myself is an important skill."

E-Spiral Phase 4. Efficacy: Bridge to Real Life

➡ *Orient to efficacy activities: Worksheet.* "Great, I think we are ready to use Expressing Myself in our lives. We are going to make plans to use the Expressing Myself skill this week. Let's turn to the Expressing Myself Worked Example 2 on page 313."

Instructions for the efficacy activity. "We are going to read through the worked example that shows us how to make an Expressing Myself Plan. Making a plan can help us prepare for communicating with people, so that it goes well. Once we read through this worked example, we are each going to make a plan."

Note: The group members can do this activity verbally or by writing on the sheet. Going through each step of the plan with each group member is ideal, but time may not allow it. Having a few people complete it verbally may be helpful. The group may have previously practiced what is important to say to someone in the elaboration exercise, so perhaps choosing which of those are most important to share could be a way to save time. This worksheet can be assigned for homework.

Disclosure questions. "How was it to make an Expressing Myself Plan?"; "Do you think it will help you express yourself?"

➡ *Orient to discussion.* "Before we finish up for today, we are going to talk about some of the challenges we face when we use Expressing Myself. OK?"

Barrier question. "What is difficult about using Expressing Myself?"

Wisdom question. "Do you want to learn how to use Expressing Myself?"

Commitment question. "When are you going to use Expressing Myself?"

Coaching question. "How can you coach yourself to use Expressing Myself when you need it?"

➡ *Orient to home study.* "Good discussion! Time for homework! This week we are going to practice use of Expressing Myself. We are going to practice communicating what we think and feel. Remember, Expressing Myself is a Calm-Only skill, so when can we use it? [Wait for response.] Right—when *both* people are below a Level 3 emotion! Good luck! Also, if you want to study skills at home, review all the handouts we have gone over so far."

➡ *Orient to group ending.* "As you know, we ring the bell six times at the end of group. We do one ring for each of the Clear Picture Do's. It is a chance to notice what is happening inside and outside of us right now. We take a moment to get a Clear Picture as we go back to our activities. Who would like to ring the bell today?"

Expressing Myself Handouts to Review in Future Cycles or for Home Study

✓ Expressing Myself Summary Sheet (p. 306)
✓ Expressing Myself Worksheet 2 (p. 314)

WEEK 10: GETTING IT RIGHT

Preparing for Group

Handouts Needed

✓ Skills System Review Sheet (p. 315)
✓ Getting It Right Handout 1 (p. 316)
✓ Getting It Right Handout 2 (p. 317)
✓ Getting It Right Handout 3 (p. 318)
✓ Getting It Right Handout 4 (p. 319)
✓ Getting It Right Handout 5 (p. 320)

E-Spiral Phase 1. Exploring Existing Knowledge Base (Review)

➡ *Welcome group.* "Hi, everyone. How are we doing today? Ready to build some skills? [Wait for response.] Excellent! How about we start with mindfulness?"

➡ *Orient to mindfulness activity: Noticing Urges.* "Last week we worked on noticing our thoughts. Today we are going to practice the Clear Picture Do, Noticing my Urges. OK?"

Instructions for the mindfulness exercise. "Great. I will ring the bell once and we will focus our attention on our breath. On the second ring we will bring our attention to noticing any urges we are having. An urge is a feeling inside of us that makes us want to do something or to take an action. We will notice the urge and allow it to pass, without taking action. If your mind drifts to something other than Noticing Urges, gently bring your mind back to the bell and the urges. We have to be able to experience an urge and not take action until we Check It. Any questions?"

Describe questions. "What urges did you notice?"; "How did you handle the urge?"; "Did your mind drift?"; "Were you able to bring your attention back to Noticing Urges?"

➡️ *Orient to Skills System review.* "Handling urges is very important; all of us have urges that make us want to go off-track. Noticing the off-track urges and allowing them to pass is difficult *and* important! Let's review our skills so the are fresh in our minds."

Note: The skills trainer can choose a Basic Review Activity from Week 1 (p. 115) or an Advanced Review Activity from Week 3 on page 127 or create a new one.

➡️ *Orient to skills practice.* "OK, how about we talk about our skills practice for the week? Who would like to share about using Expressing Myself this week?"

Disclosure questions. "What different ways did you use Expressing Myself?"; "When did you use it?"; "How did it work out for you?"

➡️ *Orient to new skills topic.* "Great job. Today we are going to talk about getting things that we need from people. Let's talk for a little bit about what we already know about getting people to give us what we need and want."

💬 *Discuss existing knowledge about the new topic.*

Assessment questions. "Has anyone ever asked you for something in an on-track way?"; "What happened?"; "Has anyone ever asked you for something in an off-track way?"; "What happened?"

Relevant context questions. "How does it work when people want to help us?"; "Do people want to help us when we are on-track or off-track?"; "Why is that?"

Clarifying questions. "How do we feel when people help us?"; "How do we feel when people refuse to help us?"

➡️ *Orient to relevant context of the new topic.* "It sounds like Problem Solving, Expressing Myself, and Getting It Right are important skills to help us make our lives happier. Knowing what to say and how to say it really helps us reach our goals. Getting It Right can give us more joy; Getting it Wrong can lead us off-track!"

E-Spiral Phase 2. Encoding: New Learning

➡ *Orient to new learning.* "We are going to learn about Getting It Right today; it is Skill 8 in the Skills System. Ready to get started? Let's turn to page 316. Getting It Right Handout 1 looks like this. Got it?"

Instructions for the encoding activity. The skills trainer reads through the handout. This handout functions as an introduction.

➡ *Orient to Getting It Right Handout 1.* "Getting It Right is how we get what we want from other people. We will go through five handouts to learn how to Get It Right."

☆ *Teaching points for Getting It Right Handout 1.* "Getting It Right is a Calm-Only skill. This means that we have to be below a Level 3 emotion if we are going to use it. We have to remember that the person we are talking to has to be below a Level 3 emotion, too. So, if we notice that the person is starting to get upset or overly excited, we should step back and get a Clear Picture of the situation. We will want to do On-Track Thinking to decide what to do. We have to be careful, because when we want things, we can become nervous and impatient. These feelings can make us want to rush. Rushing Getting It Right usually makes it turn out wrong."

➡ *Orient to Getting It Right Handout 2.* "Let's start with being in the Right Mind. Please turn to page 317. Getting It Right Handout 2 looks like this. Has everyone found the page?"

Note: The group discusses each of the points about Right Mind. The individual must understand that being in the Right Mind is critical to reaching goals.

➡ *Orient to Getting It Right Handout 3.* "OK, let's keep going. Please turn to page 318. The Getting It Right Handout 3 looks like this. We are going to learn about talking to the Right Person now. All set?"

Note: The group members or the trainer read through this handout. A discussion about who people go to for particular issues is helpful. Support teams can be complex systems; an individual with significant cognitive disabilities may not have a clear understanding of who to talk to about certain issues.

➡ *Orient to Getting It Right Handout 4.* "Great! Not only do we have to be in the Right Mind and talk to the Right Person, we have to choose the Right Time and Place. Let's turn to page 319. Getting It Right Handout 4 looks like this. Ready?"

Note: The group and/or skills trainer reads through this handout. The group discusses the reasoning for each of the points.

➡ *Orient to Getting It Right Handout 5.* "Awesome! Now let's learn about using the Right Tone. Please turn to page 320. Getting It Right Handout 5 looks like this. Did you find it?"

Note: The group and/or trainer reads through this handout. The group discusses the reasoning for the each of the points.

➡️ *Orient to Getting It Right Handout 6.* "Almost there—one more handout to review. We are going to learn about the Right Words: SEALS. SEALS stands for Sugar, Explain, Ask, Listen, and Seal the Deal. Let's turn to page 321. Getting It Right Handout 6 looks like this. All set?"

Note: The group and/or trainer reads through this handout. The group members discuss the reasoning for each of the points.

➡️ *Orient to ending Encoding Phase.* "OK, let's learn more about how to Get It Right."

E-Spiral Phase 3. Elaboration: Practicing and Linking

➡️ *Orient to the elaboration activity.* "OK, we are going to practice Getting It Right. Let's turn to the Getting It Right Worked Example 1 on page 322 first. Let's read through this example, then work as a group to complete a Getting It Right Plan together."

Note: Once the group members review the worked example, they choose a scenario to use that is relevant to making a Getting It Right Plan. After this plan is complete, this scenario may be used in a role play instead of the scenario in the worked example. Ideas: Asking a coworker, housemate, friend, or family member for something or to stop doing something. Choosing highly emotional topics will increase cognitive load demands, decreasing integration of the concepts. The key is to pick something interesting/fun but not dysregulating.

Instructions for the worksheet. "First you have to figure out what you want before you can make a plan. So, perhaps you can think about things you need from people in your life. We will make a Getting It Right Plan and role-play after that. Who needs something from someone that we can use as an example? Any questions?"

Note: The trainer and group choose the broadest topic that is salient for the group and suitable for a role-play exercise. The group members work together with the individual to address each aspect on the Getting It Right Plan.

➡️ *Orient to discussion.* "Let's talk a little more about getting what we want from people."

Linking questions. "The skills chain for Getting It Right is 1238; what does that mean?"; "Have you ever gotten something from someone in the past?"; "What worked?"; "What is Getting It Right like in Wise Mind?"; "Have you ever used Getting It Wrong and not gotten what you wanted?"; "What happened?"

Disclosure questions. "What parts of Getting It Right are you good at?"; "What parts of Getting It Right do you need to work on?"

Expansion questions. "What other skills do we use with Getting It Right?"; "How can Getting It Right help you in your life?"; "What is something that you need or want in the future?"; "How are you planning to get it?"

➡ *Orient to the end of the Elaboration Phase.* "It is great when we know how to get what we want; let's practice Getting It Right some more!"

E-Spiral Phase 4. Efficacy: Bridge to Real Life

➡ *Orient to efficacy activities: role play.* "Ready for a role play? We can choose the topic of the role play. We can use the scenario in the worded example of the person asking for more hours, or we can use the scenario for which we just made a plan. Any thoughts about which we should do? A volunteer to begin?"

Note: Once the group decides on the topic, the trainer sets up the role play. The following instructions apply when the group chooses the worked example option.

Instructions for the efficacy activity. "You are going to talk to your boss about adding another day to your work schedule. I will play the boss to start with and may have someone else jump into that role once we get going. The situation is that you work 2 days a week now, and you would like to work 3 days a week in the future. Are you in the Right Mind? Are you over a Level 3 emotion? Am I the Right Person? Is this the Right Time and Place? Did you call me ahead of time to set up a meeting? Are you just showing up at my office? Where is this role play taking place so that you get more hours from me? Think about the tone and words you want to use. Remember SEALS: Sugar, Explain, Ask, Listen, and Seal a Deal. You can do this."

Note: Skills trainers will adjust the boss's responses for each participant. Hitting the "pause" button can give the group a chance to chat about what is happening and to offer feedback and coaching. Helping the individual shape behaviors to be effective is the goal.

Disclosure questions. "How was that role play for you?"; "What did you learn about Getting It Right?"

➡ *Orient to discussion.* "Before we head home, let's talk about some of the challenges of using Getting It Right."

Barrier questions. "What is difficult about Getting It Right?"; "What do you do if you think you have all the steps right and the person still says no?"

Wisdom question. "Do you think that Getting It Right is important for you?"

Commitment question. "When are you going to try to use Getting It Right?"

Coaching question. "How are you going to coach yourself to use Getting It Right?"

➡ *Orient to home study.* "Homework time already! This week we are going to practice Getting It Right. What are the parts of Getting It Right? [Allows the group to answer.] That is correct: Right Mind, Right Person, Right Place, Right Time, Right Tone, and Right Words. You remembered that after only one day. Very good!

"Also, if you want to study skills at home, review all the handouts we have gone over so far. You can also do Getting It Right Worksheet 1 on page 323.

"This is a great worksheet to use if you want to make a good plan to Get It Right."

➡️ *Orient to group ending.* "As you know, we ring the bell six times at the end of group. We do one ring for each of the Clear Picture Do's. It is a chance to notice what is happening inside and outside of us right now. We take a moment to get a Clear Picture as we go back to our activities. Who would like to ring the bell today?"

Getting It Right Handouts to Review in Future Cycles or for Home Study

✓ Getting It Right Summary Sheet (p. 315). The summary sheet can be used during the encoding phase to explain concepts as teaching points. It may be too boring to read in group, but having different group members read different sections can break it up. Summary sheets are helpful for home study and for teaching skills coaches the skills.
✓ Getting It Right Worksheet 1 (p. 323)

☆ *Teaching points.* This worksheet helps the individual plan ahead to do Getting It Right successfully. The client can complete this sheet independently or with support.

WEEK 11: RELATIONSHIP CARE

Preparing for Group

Handouts Needed

✓ Relationship Care Handout 1 (p. 326)
✓ Relationship Care Handout 2 (p. 327)
✓ Relationship Care Handout 3 (p. 329)
✓ Relationship Care Handout 4 (p. 330)
✓ Relationship Care Handout 5 (p. 331)
✓ Relationship Care Handout 6 (p. 333)
✓ Relationship Care Handout 7 (p. 334)

E-Spiral Phase 1. Exploring Existing Knowledge Base (Review)

➡️ *Welcome group.* "Welcome, everyone! How are we doing today?"

➡️ *Orient to the mindfulness activity: six rings, one for each of the Clear Picture Do's.* "We are going to learn about Skill 9, Relationship Care, today! Are we ready to get started with mindfulness?"

Instructions for the mindfulness exercise. "Today we are going to go through all six of the Clear Picture Do's as we listen to the bell. I will say, 'Notice the Breath,' and ring the bell. We will all take a belly breath. Then I will say, 'Body Check,' and ring the bell. As the bell rings, we will all do a Body Check. Then I will say, 'Notice Surroundings,' and ring the bell. We will all notice our surroundings. Next I will say, 'Label and Rate Emotions.' I will ring the bell, and we will notice and rate our emotions using the 0- to 5-point scale. Then I will say, 'Notice

Thoughts,' and I will ring the bell. We will all Notice Thoughts that are in our minds. Last, I will say, 'Notice Urges.' I will ring the bell, and we will all Notice Urges. If you feel your mind drifting off, gently bring your mind back to following the directions. This exercise helps us pay attention, shift our focus, and practice Clear Picture. Any questions?"

Describe questions. "How was that exercise for you?"; "Were you able to follow the instructions?"

➡️ **Orient to Skills System review.** "Ready to review our skills?"

Note: The skills trainer can choose a Basic Review Activity from Week 1 (p. 115) or an Advanced Review Activity from Week 3 on page 127 or create a new one.

➡️ **Orient to skills practice.** "OK, time to review our skills practice for the week. We were working on Getting It Right."

Disclosure questions. "Who can tell us about using Getting It Right?"; "Did anyone Get It Wrong?"

➡️ **Orient to new skills topic.** "As we have learned, relationships are an important part of our lives. Let's take a few minutes to talk about what we know about Relationship Care."

💬 *Discuss existing knowledge about the new topic.*

Assessment questions. "What does the word 'relationship' mean?"; "What does the word 'care' mean?"; "What does it mean to balance a relationship?"

Relevant context questions. "What do people do to keep relationships in balance, or on-track?"; "What are things that make relationships go off-track?"

Clarifying questions. "How does it feel when our relationships are on-track?"; "What is it like when our relationships are off-track?"; "What happens to our relationships when we are in Wise Mind?"

➡️ **Orient to relevant context of the new topic.** "Relationships can be wonderful when they are on-track and stressful when they are off-track. Relationship care can help us manage our relationships so they add to the quality of our lives."

Note: Relationship Care is a complex skill that integrates several other skills. The trainer has to decide what elements are most important to address for a group. The teaching notes for all eight handouts are below; some are lengthy due to the complexity of relationships. The E-Spiral Elaboration and Efficacy phase activities depend on which Relationship Care handouts are covered. The tactic presented here reviews the first six handouts, with brief discussions on points during the Encoding phase and focus on the Finding Middle Ground during the Elaboration and Efficacy phases.

E-Spiral Phase 2. Encoding: New Learning

➡ *Orient to new learning: Relationship Care Handout 1.* "Ready to get started learning about Relationship Care? Let's turn to page 326. Relationship Care Handout 1 looks like this."

Instructions for the encoding activity. Note: The skills trainer can decide how best to read through the material in all of the Relationship Care handouts. This handout is an overview of the different parts of Relationship Care.

☆ *Teaching points for Relationship Care Handout 1.* "There are three types of Relationship Care that we are going to learn. First, we will learn about building On-Track Relationships with ourselves and other people. Second, we will learn how to Balance On-Track Relationships by having One-Way- and Two-Way-Street Relationships. Third, we will learn how to Change Off-Track Relationships using Finding Middle Ground and Steps of Responsibility."

➡ *Orient to Relationship Care Handout 2.* "Let's turn to page 327, the Relationship Care Handout 2. It looks like this."

☆ *Teaching points for Relationship Care Handout 2.* "We build On-Track Relationships with ourselves as we learn skills that help us become more self-aware. We are able to understand what is happening inside and outside of us. When we start being self-aware, we also learn to accept ourselves. The more we find out about ourselves, other people, and life, the clearer it becomes that life is hard for us all sometimes. We realize that we are as perfect as the next person; we are all perfectly human. We learn to accept that we are doing the best we can. As we become self-aware and self-accepting, we begin to value things about ourselves. We realize we have strengths. We start believing in our abilities and our skills. We try new things and meet new people. As we keep practicing skills every day, all day, we begin to trust that we can handle most anything that comes our way. We know how to get a Clear Picture, and we stop and think things through. We learn that deep in our hearts that we will be OK—no matter what. So, as we practice skills and Relationship Care with ourselves, we learn to be self-aware, self-accepting, self-valuing, and self-trusting.

"We also learn how to be aware of, accept, value, and trust other people. We use Clear Picture and On-Track Thinking to decide when a relationship is on-track or off-track. We use Safety Plans to be sure we keep relationships safe. We use On-Track Actions to help us handle off-track urges that can harm relationships. New-Me Activities help people in relationships share experiences. Problem Solving helps people work together to fix problems between them and in the world around them. Expressing Myself helps people know how other people think and feel. All these skills are important parts of having On-Track Relationships. Relationship Care makes us aware of all the things we do to keep our relationships on-track. Any questions?"

➡ *Orient to Relationship Care Handout 3.* "There are many different types of relationships. Let's turn to page 329, Relationship Care Handout 3, to see about some of the different kinds. It looks like this."

Note: The group discusses these options and adds more to a brainstormed list on the board.

The goal is to teach participants about how different relationships are and the need to be flexible and adapting in each different situation.

➡ ***Orient to Relationship Care Handout 4.*** "Great, how about we move on to Relationship Care Handout 4? This helps us learn different things we can do to make relationships closer and more distant as we need to. It is on page 330 and it looks like this."

Note: The skills trainer can lead a discussion about the points, emphasizing the need to make decisions in the moment that reflect the person's wisdom. Other options can be added on the board.

➡ ***Orient to Relationship Care Handout 5.*** "Let's turn to Relationship Care Handout 5, which introduces Two-Way-Street and One-Way-Street Relationships. It is on page 331. It looks like this."

☆ *Teaching points for Relationship Care Handout 5.* "Sometimes we have Two-Way-Street Relationships with people, which occurs when both people talk and listen to each other, taking turns. There is a balanced give-and-take between people. Each person cares about what the other person is thinking, feeling, and saying. A Two-Way-Street Relationship can help people work together well. It takes two people to maintain a Two-Way-Street Relationship. Even when we work very hard to keep a Two-Way-Street Relationship working, there are times when it gets out of balance. We may have to repair the relationship to fix the problem. Feeling cared for in a relationship and being able to give caring back adds to the quality of our lives.

"There are times when we try to have a Two-Way-Street Relationship with someone, but it doesn't work out. Then it might be a One-Way-Street Relationship. We may feel we are giving, but we do not feel heard or that the other person is giving back. If the other person is bothering us, we may decide that we do not want to have a Two-Way-Street Relationship, and we stop having an equal give-and-take. It is important to notice when relationships are two-way or one-way streets. We use Clear Picture, On-Track Thinking, and On-Track Actions to make on-track relationship decisions in the moment."

➡ ***Orient to Relationship Care Handout 6.*** "Good points. OK, there are times when we need to change off-track relationships. Since we have relationships with ourselves and other people, let's begin with learning how we get the relationship with ourselves back on-track when it is off-track. If you are ready, turn to Relationship Care Handout 6 to learn more about how to do this. It is on page 333, and it looks like this."

Note: The trainer goes through the points and has a brief discussion about the relevance of each. Additionally, the group talks about challenges related to making the changes from off-track to on-track.

➡ ***Orient to Relationship Care Handout 7.*** "There are times even in great relationships that things go off-track. It is important to know how to repair relationships with other people. Finding Middle Ground and Steps of Responsibility help us get relationships back on-track. Let's go to Relationship Care Handout 7 to learn more about Finding Middle Ground on page 334.

☆ *Teaching points for Relationship Care Handout 7.* "There are times when relationships go off-track and we feel something isn't right between us and another person. Use of Finding Middle Ground can help us talk to some one to work out differences. We use all of our Calm-Only skills in Finding Middle Ground, so we have to be sure we are below a Level 3 emotion when we are doing it.

"When we notice a relationship problem, it is helpful to start with Problem Solving. We think about the issues and get a clear sense of the problem. If we check our options and decide Plan A is to try to work it out together, we decide how we are going to use Expressing Myself. Talking in person, on the phone, in letters, in e-mail, and texting all work differently. We think about whether we are in the Right Mind, when is the Right Time and Place, and what is the Right Tone and the Right Words.

"We plan out whether we want to use Sugar and how we are going to Explain our concerns and side of the relationship story. In Finding Middle Ground, we want to know both sides of the story, so we ask questions to understand the other person's side of the story. If there is something I want from the person, maybe for him to act differently, I Ask for it.

"Sometimes one or both people get upset. Emotion levels can go up when people are blaming each other. Using 'I statements' such as 'I was hurt by how you said that' can be more helpful than insulting someone by saying something like 'You are rude.' Continuing to talk and listen so both sides understand each other better can lead to win–win solutions. When two people work together to get a relationship back on track, they are Finding Middle Ground. Every situation is different, and that is why we may have to use many skills to repair relationships. We may have to use a 1236789 skills chain!"

➡ *Orient to Relationship Care Handout 8.* "OK, let's turn now to Relationship Care Handout 8 on page 337."

☆ *Teaching Points for Relationship Care Handout 8.* "When we have made a mistake that hurts another person, it is helpful to do the Steps of Responsibility. Doing these steps can help us keep self-respect and the respect of other people. First, I admit the problem; I tell the person what I did. I try to explain what I did and how I may have harmed the person. This is really difficult, because I may feel ashamed.

"Next, I apologize for what I did that I feel was a problem. I have to think about what exactly I wish I had done differently and what I wish I had not done. Then, I Commit to Changing my behavior in the future. I let the person know that I am going to try not to do it again. I finish doing the Steps of Responsibility, then do an On-Track Action that shows the person I mean what I am saying. Doing the Steps of Responsibility helps me regain self-trust and trust with the other people I have harmed. Completing Relationship Care Worksheet 4 (p. 339) can help teach the Steps of Responsibility.

"There are times when relationship ends. Sometimes we end a relationship, and other times, the other person ends the relationship. Relationships naturally change and end. People move in different directions and to different locations, or people die. We have to use all of our skills to manage the situation when people leave us before we are ready. It is important to get skills coaching in situations when we feel overwhelmed with sadness and hurt.

"Sometimes, we choose to end relationships. If a relationship is off-track and we can't fix it, we may want to end it. We might tell the person we are moving on, or we may just stop paying attention to the relationship, so that it just drifts apart. We have to use Clear Picture to know how we feel about our relationships and On-Track Thinking to make sure we do what fits for us. Problem Solving can help us figure out how to fix relationship problems. We are taking good care of ourselves when we keep our relationships in balance and change Off-Track Relationships."

➡️ *Orient to the end of the Encoding Phase.* "Relationships are complicated! We have to use all of our skills to be able to do Relationship Care. We are going to talk more about different relationships so that we can learn how to handle all the different, changing relationships in our lives."

E-Spiral Phase 3. Elaboration: Practice and Linking

➡️ *Orient to the elaboration activity.* "Please turn to the Relationship Care Worked Example 1 (p. 335) and Relationship Care Worksheet 3, the Finding Middle Ground Plan (p. 336). We will first go through the worked example; it looks like this. Let's read through this example to see how we might try to fix a relationship problem."

Instructions for the practice exercise. "Great, now we are going to make a Finding Middle Ground Plan using a relationship problem of someone in the group. We are also going to do a role play after we make the plan. Would anyone like to share a relationship problem that he or she would like to fix?"

Note: The trainer and group discuss the options and pick one that will work well. The answers are written on the board as the group members discuss each part of the plan. If no one volunteers, the trainer can invent a relevant scenario.

Disclosure question. "What did you learn from this exercise?"

➡️ *Orient to discussion.* "Let's talk a little more about how we have used Relationship Care in the past, OK?"

Linking questions. "What is it like to use Relationship Care in Wise Mind?"; "This is a 1236789 skills chain; what does that mean?"

Disclosure question. "Have you ever tried to fix a relationship problem in the past?"

Expansion question. "Do you think you could try Finding Middle Ground with anyone in your life?"

➡️ *Orient to the end of the Elaboration Phase.* "Are we ready to do a Finding Middle Ground role play?"

E-Spiral Phase 4. Efficacy: Bridge to Real Life

➡ *Orient to efficacy activities: "OK, this role play will help us practice changing an off-track relationship."*

Note: The individual who volunteered the scenario plays herself. The trainer asks for another participant to be the person with whom she has a conflict. The trainer sets up the role play using the logistics on the Relationship Care Worksheet 3 (p. 336).

Disclosure questions. "What was that exercise like for you?"; "What did you learn about Relationship Care?"

➡ *Orient to discussion.* "Before we finish for this week, I would like to ask a few more questions about some of the challenges in using Relationship Care."

Barrier questions. "What is difficult about doing Relationship Care with yourself?"; "What is difficult about doing Relationship Care with other people?"

Wisdom questions. "Is it important for you to do Relationship Care with yourself?"; "With other people?"

Commitment questions. "What Relationship Care will you do with yourself?"; "What Relationship Care will you do with other people?"

Coaching questions. "How can you coach yourself to do Relationship Care with yourself?"; "How can you coach yourself to do Relationship Care with other people?"

➡ *Orient to home study.* "This week we are going to practice using Relationship Care with ourselves and other people. Does that sound good? Also, if you want to study skills at home, review all the handouts we have gone over so far. You can also do Worksheets 1–5."

➡ *Orient to group ending.* "As you know, we ring the bell six times at the end of group. We do one ring for each of the Clear Picture Do's. It is a chance to notice what is happening inside and outside of us right now. We take a moment to get a Clear Picture as we go back to our activities. Who would like to ring the bell today?"

Relationship Care Handouts to Review in Future Cycles or for Home Study

✓ Relationship Care Summary Sheet (p. 324). The summary sheet can be used during the encoding phase to explain concepts as teaching points. It may be too boring to read in group, but having different group members read different sections can break it up. Summary sheets are helpful for home study and for teaching skills to skills coaches.

✓ Relationship Care Worksheet 1 (p. 328)

✓ Relationship Care Worksheet 2 (p. 332)

✓ Relationship Care Worked Example 1 (p. 335)
✓ Relationship Care Worked Example 2 (p. 338)
✓ Relationship Care Worksheet 4 (p. 339)

WEEK 12: SKILLS REVIEW

Preparing for Group

Handouts Needed

✓ Skills System Skill Master certificate (p. 342)

E-Spiral Phase 1. Exploring Existing Knowledge Base (Review)

➡ *Welcome group.* "Hello, everyone! We have made it to Week 12! How are you all doing today? Ready for the ringing of the bell?"

➡ *Orient to the mindfulness activity: passing the bell and getting a Clear Picture.* "We have to be able to get a Clear Picture in stressful situations, so we can use the rest of our skills. So, during this exercise, I am going to ask you to do more and continue to stay focused. Skill Masters stay focused even in a crisis."

Instructions for the mindfulness exercise. "We are going to make things a little harder! We will choose six people to ring the bell and to say one of the Clear Picture Do's. The first person will say, 'Notice the Breath,' then ring the bell. When the sound has finished, the task will pass to the next person. That person will say, 'Notice Surroundings,' and ring the bell. When the sound is gone, the bell is passed. The next person says, 'Do a Body Check,' and rings the bell. When the bell sound is finished, the the bell is passed. The next person says, 'Label and Rate Emotions,' and rings the bell. When the sound is gone, the next person gets the bell. That person says, 'Notice Thoughts,' and rings the bell. When the sound of the bell has disappeared, the bell is passed to the last person, who says, 'Notice Urges,' and rings the bell. While all this is happening, we focus on doing the Clear Picture Do that is being stated at that moment. If you get lost or your mind begins to drift, gently bring your mind back to the bell and the instructions we are being given. Any questions?"

Describe questions. "How did that exercise go for you?"; "Were you able to stay focused?"; "Were you able to bring your mind back?"

➡ *Orient to Skills System review.* "Ready to review our skills?"
Note: The skills trainer can choose a Basic Review Activity from Week 1 (p. 115) or an Advanced Review Activity from Week 3 on page 127 or create a new one.

➡ *Orient to skills practice.* "We are really learning our skills well! OK, it is time to go over our skills practice. Our homework this week was to practice Relationship Care. Who would like to start?"

Disclosure questions. "Who can share about Relationship Care that you did with yourself?"; "Who can tell us about Relationship Care that you did with other people?"

➡️ *Orient to new skills topic.* "Good job. Today is a review of all of our skills. We are going to talk for a few minutes about how you are doing learning your skills. OK?"

🗨️ **Discuss existing knowledge about the new topic.**

Assessment questions. "Which skills do you use the most?"; "For which skills do you need more practice?"
Note: Writing the answers on the board may be helpful.

Relevant context questions. "What is easy about learning skills?"; "What is hard about learning skills?"

Clarifying questions. "How is life different when people use skills?"; "How is life when we don't use skills?"

➡️ *Orient to relevant context of the new topic.* "It is hard to remember all of our skills, especially when we are upset. We have to practice our skills a lot to learn them. As we get to know our skills better, we learn how to put them together to handle tough life situations."

E-Spiral Phase 2. Encoding: New Learning

➡️ *Orient to new learning.* "Today we are going to fill out Skills System Skills Quiz 1, on page 340. None of us loves quizzes. This will help us find out the skills we understand and those with which ones we need more help. We will pass in the quizzes and go over the answers when we get done. I brought in sodas and cookies today to celebrate us finishing our 12 weeks. I am very proud of you all. Are we ready to get started?"

Instructions for the encoding activity. "If you have a hard time reading and writing, either I or your staff can help you. Let's take a few minutes to make a plan about how we can fill out this sheet. If you do not know the answer, you can guess or leave it blank. The good news is that once you hand in your quiz, get a soda and cookies. Any questions?" (The answers are provided on the Skills System Skills Quiz 1 Answer Sheet, page 341.)

➡️ *Orient to the end of the Encoding Phase.* "Great job! I think I saw a lot of people doing On-Track Actions here today."

E-Spiral Phase 3. Elaboration: Practice and Linking

➡️ *Orient to the elaboration activity.* "OK, let's go over the quiz together."

Instructions for the practice exercise. "I will ask the group the questions, and let's come up with the right answers together."

Disclosure questions. "How do you think you did on the quiz?"; "How do you think you are doing learning your skills?"

➡️ *Orient to discussion.* "We are going to talk a little more about how we are doing learning skills?"

Linking question. "Has it been hard for you to learn to control yourself in the past?"

Disclosure questions. "What are you doing now that works?"; "What are you doing that does not work as well?"

Expansion question. "What do you need to do to make skills work better for you?"

➡️ *Orient to the end of the Elaboration Phase.* "Great awareness. How about we talk more about how we use our skills together to handle tough situations?"

E-Spiral Phase 4. Efficacy: Bridge to Real Life

➡️ *Orient to efficacy activities: skills review activity.* "Let's talk together about the situations in our lives that are really hard to deal with. We can work together to see how our skills can help us in those situations."

Instructions for the efficacy activity. "We are going to begin by listing difficult situations that you have faced in the last few months. We are going to make a list of these stressful situations on the board. Then we are going to look at making a skill plan for each of the situations. When we make a skill plan today, we are going to use the number of the skill to show what the plan is. For example, if the situation is one where we think there is risk, we might use 1. Clear Picture, 2. On-Track Thinking, 3. On-Track Action, 4. Safety Plan, and 5. New-Me Activity. So, that skill cluster is a 12345. If we were bored and wanted to go watch TV, the skill would be a 1235; Clear Picture, On-Track Thinking, On-Track Action, and New-Me Activity. We talked last week about Relationship Care—Finding Middle Ground skills chains that need to include seven skills, 1236789, to solve relationship problems. Who would like to share a situation they handled using skills? We will all help you figure out the skills chain you used. Any questions?"

Disclosure questions. "How was it using the numbers to label skill chains?"; "Did it help you understand it better, or was it more confusing?"

➡️ *Orient to discussion.* "Before we end for the day, let's talk about some of the challenges that we face when we are learning skills. OK?"

Barrier question. "What is difficult about learning skills?"

Wisdom questions. "Do you think it is important for you to learn skills?"; "Why?"

Commitment question. "What are you going to do to keep practicing skills?"

Coaching question. "How can you coach yourself to practice your skills?"

➡ *Orienting to home study.* "This group has done an amazing job. I would like to hand out your certificates now. [The template for the Skills System Skill Master Certificate is on page 342.] I will announce your name and the number of cycles you have completed in the Skills System. This is like getting different belts in karate. The more cycles we get, the stronger Skills Masters we become. Fantastic, I am so happy that you are all here and have worked so hard. It is our favorite part: homework! Please practice putting your skills together in skills clusters this week. If you want to study skills at home, review all the handouts we have gone over so far. You can also do any worksheet that you have not completed yet. Thank you all!"

➡ *Orient to group ending.* "As you know, we ring the bell six times at the end of group. We do one ring for each of the Clear Picture Do's. It is a chance to notice what is happening inside and outside of us right now. We take a moment to get a Clear Picture as we go back to our activities. Who would like to ring the bell today?"

Note: Trainers may want to develop a graduation ceremony process for individuals who have completed a certain number of cycles through the Skills System curriculum. Creating a diploma, inviting friends/family members, providing refreshments, and having individuals share about how they integrated the skills are meaningful, transitional activities.

Skills Review Handouts to Review in Future Cycles or for Home Study

✓ Skills System Review Questions (p. 223)
✓ Skills System Quiz 1 (p. 340)
✓ Skills System: Quiz 1 Answer Sheet (p. 341)
✓ Skills System Skill Master Certificate (p. 342)

SUBSEQUENT CYCLES THROUGH THE SKILLS SYSTEM CURRICULUM

Once the group members complete a 12-week cycle through the skills curriculum, they have a much better understanding of the skills concepts. For example, the group will have done 12 different mindfulness activities. During each group session, prior learning is reviewed, new learning is introduced, and new learning is linked to all the previous skills that were addressed. Due to the variable strengths of participants, each group member will have integrated different amounts of information.

The skills trainers juggle many things at the same time. Trainers have to teach the group while individualizing interventions for the diverse levels of skills integration and cognitive abilities of each group member. Although certain group members may be able to generalize all nine skills, others may struggle to remember even three names of the skills. Skills trainers must make the group an effective learning experience for each participant or find an alternative group for a client who is significantly ahead or behind the rest of the group.

Throughout each cycle of the group, there are opportunities to return to fundamental Skills System concepts and basic commitment to learning and utilizing skills. In general, teaching progresses in the following ways through multiple cycles of the Skills System curriculum:

- Teaching moves from being more general to more specific. For example, as the individual learns about breathing, she learns to focus awareness specifically on the nose or belly.
- Teaching integrates more detailed information as the knowledge base increases. For example, as the individual understands On-Track Thinking, more of the steps of On-Track Thinking are integrated into the individual's behavior. Initially the person may take a second to think about a decision, while after repetition the client may Check It, Turn It Up, Cheerleading, and make a skills plan.
- Exercises become more realistic to replicate real-life forces in the participant's environment. For example, skills trainers may create distractions during a mindfulness breathing exercise so that the group must master focusing attention while experiencing interfering forces.
- The individual becomes more able to share helpful personal awareness and information related to skills discussions. For example, initially the participant may be hesitant to disclose that he has ever had difficulties related to overwhelming thoughts or emotions. As the individual gains competence managing emotions, he reduces his emotional vulnerabilities and increases his abilities to participate fully.
- Discussions become increasingly dialectical as group progresses through the curriculum. During preliminary cycles, the group focuses heavily on integrating concrete skill information. As a group develops a skills knowledge base, discussions become more lively and expansive. As capacities increase, alternative views are encouraged and managed in group.
- Discussions related to barriers for skills use become increasingly personal and detailed. As skills trainers become familiar with each participant and as group members get to know each other, barriers to integrating skills are clearer. For example, initially the leader may not know that a participant lives with an abusive housemate. Throughout the group experience, individual challenges become evident. It is crucial that group leaders understand the forces that impede generalization of skills in each participant's life. Skills trainers coach participants to manage challenging situations throughout the cycles of the Skills System curriculum.

Skills System group members learn crucial information from both the teaching and social aspects of the curriculum. The participant cycles through the program, building skills that enhance self-awareness, self-acceptance, self-value, and self-trust. As these factors increase, the individual improves her ability to manage relationships effectively. The Skills System helps the individual to navigate the human experience skillfully. Participants gain mastery that allows them to create fulfilling lives that include freedom and joy.

TRANSITION TO CHAPTER 8

Chapter 8 presents skills coaching techniques that can be used by support providers, family members, and/or other people in participants' lives to help them generalize skills in the natural environment. The chapter explores how extrinsic emotion regulation supports can help individuals manage even challenging emotions and situations. Having a skills coach who understands the Skills System and the skills coaching techniques can help participants reach personal goals in their lives.

CHAPTER 8

Skills Coaching Techniques

The section Clarifying Providers' Roles in the Introduction of the *DBT Skills Training Manual, Second Edition* (Linehan, 2015a, pp. 34–37) offers ways for the DBT skills trainer to manage relationships with collateral supports.

The Consultation-to-the-Client Strategies (pp. 97–98) are important to follow in all settings; these are particularly vital when working with individuals with ID. Factors such as disability, competence, and autonomy are crucial to balance to maximize learning. These guidelines help the Skills System skills trainers manage interactions with the individual and her support team in ways that maximize learning.

Information about the biosocial theory (pp. 5–11, 138–143) provides information about transactional relationships, which are relevant to skills coaching.

Validation strategies (Linehan, 2015a, pp. 88–90) are essential components in skills coaching. Information about the levels of validation help the practitioner have tangible tactics to validate the individual during a skills coaching interaction.

EMOTION REGULATION AND SKILLS COACHING

Zaki and Williams (2013) explain that interpersonal emotion regulation happens within social interactions. The presence of other people in stressful situations serves to help individuals modulate negative affect (Beckes & Coan, 2011). In addition to this implicit benefit, relationships can serve a more active role in the emotion regulation process.

Intrinsic interpersonal emotion regulation occurs when the individual can seek out support to regulate an emotion (Zaki & Williams, 2013). The individual engages in interactions to help her either up- or down-regulate emotions, depending on her goal in the situation. Extrinsic emotion regulation is not the individual (Person A) enacting strategies, but rather an external person (B) engaging in interpersonal behaviors that regulate the emotions of Person A. A skills coach engages in extrinsic emotion regulation strategies when he attempts to help someone regulate her emotions.

Within these two forms of interpersonal emotion regulation (intrinsic and extrinsic), there are two classes, "response-independent" and "response-dependent" (Zaki & Williams, 2013, p. 804). There are times when Person A can gain regulatory benefit just through an interaction regardless of Person B's responses (intrinsic response-independent). For example, when Person A labels an emotion during a conversation with Person B, it can serve as an emotion regulation function regardless of Person B's responses. Conversely, Person A's reactions can be response-dependent and impacted by Person B's responses during the same conversation. Response-dependent reactions can be risky, because if Person A seeks solace from Person B and he is unsupportive, Person A may feel worse.

Ideally, intrinsic interpersonal emotion regulation can make Person A feel more safe (less alone in times of stress). It offers Person A with an opportunity for combining psychological resources (A + B). When Person A shares an experience (i.e., being on the same page) with Person B it can communicate a sense of affiliation that can be rewarding for Person A. If Person A has an opportunity to label emotions and assess the causes of the emotion, there are emotion regulation benefits (Lieberman et al., 2011; Zaki & Williams, 2013).

INGREDIENTS WITHIN INTERPERSONAL EMOTION REGULATION

The core tenet of DBT, dialectics, is relevant in skills coaching in multiple ways. Linehan (1993a) explains that validation strategies, delivered as extrinsic emotion regulation strategies by a therapist, can help the clients decrease self-invalidation that undermines adaptive actions. This acceptance-based intervention is paired with change strategies that are designed to foster effective behaviors. Therefore, in DBT acceptance and change strategies are used to promote "the reconciliation of opposites in a continual process of synthesis" (Linehan, 1993a, p. 19). The combination of acceptance and change strategies provides key ingredients of growth.

Support staff members using the Skills System are encouraged to use both acceptance strategies (validation) and change strategies (skills coaching). Intertwining these strategies helps the individual both to co-regulate in the moment and experience longer-term intrapersonal development. The DBT validation strategies, presented in the text box below, are effective tools because they (1) expand Person A's self-awareness in the moment, (2) communicate acceptance from Person B to Person A, and (3) promote Person A's self-validation.

DBT Levels of Validation

1. The skills coach pays attention, listening carefully and observing the individual's behaviors to convey acceptance.

   • Examples: Consistent eye contact and staying on topic

2. The skills coach offers accurate reflection of what the individual is saying. Directly repeating and/or paraphrasing the individual's points (checking with

her to ensure accuracy of the assumptions) communicates an understanding of the individual's experience.

- Example: "So you are saying that you feel anxious?"

3. The skills coach labels unverbalized factors that may be impacting the individual. This strategy can help the individual deepen awareness of internal and external experiences.

- Example: "The way you are pacing makes me think you might be anxious."

4. The skills coach links the individual's responses to a precipitating event. Highlighting that a precipitating event caused an understandable reaction can serve to validate the response without necessarily reinforcing the action taken.

- Example: "I think that you being afraid of hearing your biopsy results makes complete sense."

5. The skills coach states that a behavior is a normal response to an event. Universalizing the experience can validate the individual's reaction as justified and human.

- Example: "Anyone who had those symptoms would be nervous."

6. The skills coach treats the person as an equal beyond the other roles of the relationship. The coach has a person-to-person, genuine response to the individual.

- Example: "That would really suck. I am going to keep my fingers crossed for you. Would you mind if I said a prayer for you?"

Validation strategies communicate to the Person A that (1) she is a valid person and (2) her responses make sense on some level. DBT validation strategies (i.e., communicating acceptance of the individual to promote self-acceptance) together with supports that are designed to improve the moment (e.g., skills coaching) provide extrinsic strategics that help Person A develop intrinsic emotion regulation capacities. Balancing may mean offering more acceptance than change comments, because of the sensitivity vulnerable individuals may have to guidance or feedback. Linehan recommends "surrounding negative feedback with positive feedback" (2015a, p. 337), to reduce negative reactions such as "stimulus overload or discouragement," which are both relevant to the ID population.

A + B = C SKILLS COACHING MODEL

The skills coach helps the individual move from early-stage to late-stage processing and responding (refer to the dual stage, two-phase model in Chapter 3 (p. 49). If Person A impulsively acts with first-phase responses, the effectiveness is likely to be low. Through interpersonal emotion regulation strategies (that include both validation and skills coaching) the coach can guide Person A through steps to deepen processing, hence improving accuracy, promoting learning, and increasing goal-directed behaviors.

A skills coaching conversation is not a regular dialogue between people. Person B is functioning to strategically help Person A effectively regulate emotions and reach her personal goals. Person B may be a parent, support staff, or a partner who is attempting to help Person A make mindful decisions for herself. Person B is not controlling Person A in their relationship, he is helping her reach her unique potential.

A coaching conversation can range from a relaxed chat (Person A and B are between a Level 0 and Level 3 emotion) to a more complicated interaction (Person A and/or B are at a Level 4–5 emotion). It is important that the skills coach have a simple framework to guide strategies due to the potentially high cognitive load demands that can accompany complex situations.

The A + B = C framework is a simple way to conceptualize how to structure interpersonal emotion regulation interventions. Column "A" represents effort made first to clarify the individual's perspectives. In this first phase (A), the focus is on awareness and acceptance. Column "B" represents the perceptions of the coach (Person B); this is the introduction of change strategies. Column "C" includes the synthesis interactions when Person A and Person B collaborate in executing adaptive behaviors strategies. Figure 8.1 presents an overview of the A + B = C concepts.

A: PERSON A'S PERSPECTIVE

Getting on the Same Page

Either Person A or Person B can initiate a coaching conversation. If Person A feels like she needs support, she may reach out to talk to Person B. Conversely, Person B may notice Person A's levels of emotion going up and/or behaviors changing and approach to offer skills coaching. In both of these circumstances, getting on the same page is an important first step. Person B asks questions and validates to help Person A with the goal of helping her get a Clear Picture of her internal and external experiences in the moment. The focus and scope of coaching questions and validation strategies change depending on Person A's level of emotion.

Adjusting the Skills Coaching Questions for the Level of Emotion

The coach has to make adjustments in the focus of the interaction to accommodate for the individual's level of affective arousal. For example, if the individual is well-regulated and experiencing relatively low levels of feeling (0–3), the coach can inquire about the details of the content related to the situation. At these levels, it is an opportunity to have an in-depth conversation with Person A about a complex situation, discussing details about content, reflecting on short- and long-term goals, and brainstorming about skills options (including Calm-Only skills).

Alternatively, if the individual is over a Level 3 emotion, the coach asks questions that supply the pair with key information about Person A's stressor, emotion, the level of the emotion, urges, and plan. The coach structures his part of the dialogue in ways that shift Person A's attention from emotional and cognitive triggers that are serving to escalate her feelings, toward

A	+	B	=	C
Person A's Perspective		Person B's Perspective		Both People Work Together

A. Person A's perspective—getting on her page:

Person B tries to get a Clear Picture of Person A's situation. Person B asks questions *and* uses validation strategies. The focus is Person A's awareness and acceptance. If Person A is at a 0–3 emotion, Person B can get more details about the situation.

Getting a Clear Picture of Person A:

- Ask a general question about what is going on to **find out the cause of the emotion**. (*"What's going on?"*)
- Elicit a **label and rating** for the emotion. (*"How are you feeling? What level?"*)
- Ask about the **breath**. (*"What do you notice about your breath?"*)
- Ask about the **urge**. (*"What do you want to do?"*)
- Expand awareness to other Clear Picture Do's, if possible. (*"Surroundings?"; " Body sensations?"*)

Explore her On-Track Thinking:

- Ask about her plan of action. (*"So, what is your plan?"*)
- Ask about the goal. (*"What is your goal in this situation?"*)
- Help Person A assess the plan with Check It. (*"Do you think that will help you get to your goal?"*)

Executing On-Track Actions:

- Review the plan. (*"So, your plan is to . . . ?"*) Confirm the first On-Track Action. (*"Your On-Track Action will be . . . ?"*)

B. Person B's perspective—Person B offers his two cents:

Person B asks Person A if she would like to hear Person B's thoughts about the situation. (*"Would you like to hear what I am thinking?"*)

Person B waits for consent:

- If Person A says "no," Person B explains that he will be available at a later time. (*"No problem; if you want to chat later, I will be around."*)
- If Person A says "yes," Person B asks if she is comfortable in that location. (*"Is here OK or do you want to move to a different place to talk?"*)
- Once settled, Person B offers an opinion about whether Person A's plan will effectively reach her stated goal.

FIGURE 8.1. A + B = C skills coaching model.

Assessment to On-Track Action:

- If Person B thinks it is an on-track plan to the expressed goal, he supports it and tries to promote Person A taking an On-Track Action. (*"I think that plan will work; what will be your On-Track Action? . . . Great job!"*)
- If Person B thinks the plan will not reach Person A's goal, he explains the problem. (*"I am concerned that if you . . . it might . . ., which is not your goal."*)
- Person B offers skills coaching support. (*"Do you want to take a few minutes to talk about options?"*)

C. Both people work together—plan skills chains together:

If "yes," Persons A and B chat about the situation and what skills may be helpful to link together.

- Remember the Categories of Skills (*0–3 emotion = all nine skills/4–5 = no Calm-Only skills*).
- Be sure to use enough skills (*Recipe for Skills*)!

Skills options:

- **On-Track Thinking:** Check It, Turn It Up, Cheerleading, and Make a Skills Plan.
- **On-Track Actions:** Take a Step to Your Goal, Switch Tracks, On-Track Action Plan, Accept the Situation, Turn the Page (All-the-Time skill).
- **Safety Plans help in risky situations:** Focus on a New-Me Activity, Move Away, and Leave (All-the-Time skill).
- **New-Me Activities:** Focus, Feel Good, Distraction, and Fun (All-the-Time skill).
- **Problem Solving:** Small problems—Quick Fix worksheet; medium and large problems— Clear Picture of the Problem, Check Options, Make Plans A, B, and C (Calm-Only skill).
- **Expressing Myself:** Communicating needs/concerns, etc; Expressing Myself Worksheet (Calm-Only skill).
- **Getting It Right:** Getting what he wants; Getting It Right Worksheet (Calm-Only skill).
- **Relationship Care:** Core Self; One- and Two-Way-Street relationships; Finding Middle Ground Worksheet; Steps of Responsibility Worksheet (Calm-Only skill).

Executing On-Track Actions:

- Review the plan. (*"So, your plan is to . . . ?"*)
- Confirm and support the first On-Track Action. (*"Your On-Track Action will be . . . ? Good job!"*)

FIGURE 8.1 (*continued*)

strategies that help her reregulate. Although Person A may want to focus on the content of the issue, over a Level 3, details (e.g., exploring all the factors that are annoying her) only serve to escalate feelings. If Person A is engaging in Expressing Myself while over a Level 3 emotion, Person B may need to be more assertive in asking questions that structure the focus of the conversation toward down-regulating versus up-regulating topics. Additionally, it is important to endorse valid behaviors versus off-track ones.

The Coach Self-Monitors and Makes Adjustments

Not only does the coach monitor the feelings rating of Person A, he self-monitors and makes necessary adjustments throughout the experience. The coach uses the Skills System guidelines to manage the immediate coaching situation that include him as part of the transactional equation. For example, if the coach is at a Level 4 emotion, he may need to Switch Tracks and do a Safety Plan—Move Away, rather than doing an in-depth coaching session at that time. At a Level 4 feeling, the coach will have difficulty managing effective Two-Way-Street Relationship behaviors. If it is not possible due to logistical constraints to withdraw from a coaching situation at that time, doing basic skills coaching of All-the-Time skills is preferred.

Getting a Clear Picture of Person A

Person Is a Level 3 Emotion or Below

The coach may choose to begin by eliciting information about what is generating the emotion or problem. A general inquiry such as "How are you doing?", "What's up?", or "Are you doing OK?" begins the process of increasing attention to the situation. More specific, clarifying direct inquiries (e.g., "What is bothering you?") may be helpful. Weaving in Validation Strategies (pp. 183–184; Linehan, 2015a, pp. 88–90) with other skills coaching tactics can improve the effectiveness of the coaching supports. Next, the coach may expand both Person A's and Person B's awareness of the situation by asking clarifying questions about the Clear Picture Do's. Technically, Person B helping Person A get a Clear Picture is implicitly a change strategy; " 'acceptance of what is' is itself change" (Linehan, 1993a, p. 99), yet the spirit of Column A, is to broaden awareness of the current moment without explicitly changing it.

Depending on the situation, the coach has to decide how to integrate skills language into the conversation. Some individuals may like (and benefit from) direct references to the Skills System language. For example, Person B may ask, "Can you help me get a Clear Picture of your situation?" and/or "Could we go through the Clear Picture Do's together so I really understand what going on with you?" Other individuals (e.g., an adolescent) may recoil when formal Skills System language is used. In this case, the skills coach must gain information that integrates Skills System concepts in a natural, jargon-free conversation. In these cases, it is important that the skills coach have a deep understanding of the Skills System framework, in order to weave in skills concepts easily rather than in a stilted way. It is difficult to "coolify" skills effectively unless the coach is well-versed in the model.

Whether using Skills System terms or a more conceptual approach, the coach strives to help expand Person A's (and Person B's) understanding of the experience. Eliciting Person A's awareness of the breath, surroundings, body sensations, emotion, rating of the emotion, thoughts, and urges facilitates late-stage, second-phase processing. (e.g., "What is an emotion you are having?"; "What level is it?"; "Do you notice any body sensations?"; "What are you thinking?"; and "Are you having any urges?"). When Person A is at a Level 3 emotion or below the conversation can meander in an exploratory way following a natural cadence.

Person A Is above a Level 3 Emotion

In a situation in which Person A is stressed, the coach may begin with a general inquiry about Person A's situation but progress in a more intentional way with follow-up questions. The coach may ask fewer clarifying questions about details of content, but rather target questions to understand what the stressor is and lead Person A through a process that will help her down-regulate versus continue to escalate. The coach needs to be mindful of not engaging in conversations that reinforce dysregulated emotions and expressing over a Level 3.

Once the coach has a sense of what the stressor is, he elicits the name of the feeling (e.g., "What is the feeling you are having?"). Additionally, he prompts Person A to rate the emotion (e.g., "What level is it, 0–5?"). The level of emotion gives Person A important information about which Category of Skills and the minimum number of skills necessary.

At some point in this initial part of the coaching conversation, Person B will want to help Person A focus attention on her breath. The coach may ask, "How is your breathing right now?" or "What do you notice about it?" It is a positive step when Person A strategically uses attentional deployment, shifting focus from the stressor to her breath (and other parts of Clear Picture). This simple action often serves to reduce triggering of the emotion and provides a cue for progressing through the Clear Picture Do's, engaging On-Track Thinking, and taking On-Track Actions.

Asking about Person A's urge (e.g., "What is your urge?" or "What do you feel like doing?") can help her separate the off-track urge from taking an off-track action. If Person A says, "I am going to punch him!", the coach will want to clarify whether that is her urge or her plan (e.g., "Is that what you would like to do or what you are going to do?"). Again, this helps the individual understand that (1) urges are not actions, and (2) just because she has an urge does not mean she has to act on it.

A coach's perspective may be that if he facilitates Person A in clarifying awareness in a situation, it will automatically lead her to act on the urges. The goal is to separate the awareness of the urge from the action. Without clarity about the urge, separate from the action, the individual may continue to link the urge and action, impulsively reacting without reflection. The coach may have to use his skills to tolerate the distress of engaging in a conversation with Person A that highlights her awareness of a high-intensity situation, without either Person A or Person B rushing to action.

Positively Reinforcing Clear Picture

Although it may be contrary to natural inclinations, the coach may want to reinforce an individual's Clear Picture. For example, if Person A says, "He is a jerk," the coach may want to say, "Good Clear Picture of your thought." This is different than reinforcing the content of the thought by saying, "Great thought." If Person A says, "I want to punch him in the face," the coach may say, "Good Clear Picture of the urge," which is different than saying "Good idea." Reinforcing the separation of awareness (Clear Picture) and a plan of action (On-Track Thinking and On-Track Action) is crucial. If the coach gloms it all together and is unable to elaborate the microtransitions, it may be more likely that Person A's reinforced patterns of emotional and behavioral dysregulation will be activated.

Similarly, if Person A says, "I want to punch him in the face!", and the coach says, "You can't do that, you will get arrested!" (change strategy) rather than "Good Clear Picture of your urge" (acceptance strategy), it may prematurely derail Person A's late-stage processing. Highlighting potential consequences and offering direct feedback about the course of action, beyond clarifying Person A's perspective are change strategies and happen in the second column of the A + B = C framework. Person B needs to be aware of not hijacking this process and undermining Person A's opportunity to engage in deeper levels of emotional learning due to the coach's own level of discomfort.

Shifting to On-Track Thinking

Whether Person A is at, above, or below a Level 3 emotion, once the pair has a Clear Picture of her perspectives, the coach guides Person A toward On-Track Thinking. It is important to note that Person A may be engaging in change strategies at this time, but Person B is not offering any explicit change-oriented feedback. This preliminary phase is all about Person A's perspectives as they are.

An easy transition question to On-Track Thinking is "What is your plan?" This implicitly communicates that (1) a plan is necessary, (2) the urge and plan are different, and (3) intentional behavior that executes the plan will follow. Referring to the generic word "plan" highlights her freedom to choose a course of action. Person B is still not offering personal commentary.

If it is not clear, the coach may want Person A to articulate her goal in the situation. Questions such as "What do you want to happen here?"; "How do you want this to turn out?"; "Do you want your emotions to go up or down?"; and "Do you want to feel better or worse?" can be useful. Asking without judgment or influence, strictly eliciting Person A's intentions first, is important.

Once the coach has elicited an expressed plan and goal, he helps Person A to elaborate this appraisal process. The coach and Person A reflect on whether the plan will get her effectively to her goal. The coach prompts Check It by asking, "Do you think your plan will get you to your goal?" The coaching strategies are expanding Person A's awareness of the situation, attention, and appraisal to increase the likelihood of responses that are on-track to her goals.

Teaching Opportunities

The skills coach listens to Person A and may highlight skillful *responses* and strategies she is planning or doing. For example, if Person A's plan is to go to her room and listen to music, the coach may ask, "What skill is it when you move away like that?" and/or "What skill is it when you listen to music?" If Person A does not know sufficient skills language to answer "Safety Plan" and "New-Me Activity," the coach may want to highlight that "Moving away from risk by going to your room is a Safety Plan" and "Listening to music is a New-Me Activity." Labeling and reinforcing skills language in context can facilitate learning.

Executing an On-Track Action

Person B's role as a coach is to help Person A activate On-Track Actions. Once there is a skills plan, then the coach can ask, "What is your On-Track Action going to be?" If Person A describes vague steps, the coach helps guide her to set a clear course of action; by asking her to summarize the plan and clearly state what she will do first, second, and third can help Person A consolidate efforts toward goal-directed behaviors.

+ B or Not

At this point, the coach may want to offer his perspective, although it is not necessary. If Person A is on-track, has a strong plan, and intends to execute a series of On-Track Actions, the coach may choose to say, "Great job, good luck. . . . I am here if you need me." There is no need for the coach to add his "2 cents." The individual was effective and self-reliant. This is a positive interaction for both Person A and Person B.

+ B: PERSON B'S PERSPECTIVE

There are times when Person B feels it would be either On-Track Relationship Care or effective skills coaching to offer a personal perspective to Person A. If the comments are going to highlight a different perspective from Person A's, it can be helpful to ask permission first. Getting informed consent (e.g., "Would you like to hear my thoughts?" or "Can I share my ideas about this with you?") establishes Person A as a viable, in-control entity. This simple strategy helps Person A experience a sense of identity; it is an even playing field. Person B's request for permission allows for reciprocity, collaboration, and respect, while simultaneously allowing for self-determination and independence of both parties. The partners are able to be together and separate at the same time, creating a dialectical synthesis that promotes personal and relationship growth.

Person B Waits for Consent

It is Person A's decision whether she wants to hear Person B's perspectives. It is important that the coach not push Person A into a coaching conversation. Therefore, if Person A says she does not want to hear Person B's opinions, it is fine. The coach can orient Person A to his availability at a later time, if coaching assistance is required. If Person A says "yes" about wanting to hear, then Person B can shared his thoughts. It is important for Person B to wait for consent prior to giving his "2 cents."

Finding a Mutually Agreed-Upon Location

It is important for the skills coach to be aware of the impact of the current environment on Person A's decision and participation in skills coaching conversations. The skills coach may want to make it clear to the individual that moving to another, perhaps more private, area to talk may be an option. Discussing the best location for the conversation is an important process. There are times when the vicinity reduces Person A's motivation to engage in a skills discussion.

Discussing options for where the pair can go to talk can be a process that reflects the coach's commitment to having a two-way-street relationship. If the coach dictates where the conversation happens, it may disempower Person A, creating a one-way street. When the coach collaborates with the individual to find a mutually agreed-upon location, it not only facilitates the pair finding the best location to talk but also establishes a strong relationship connection that may sustain an effective skills coaching session and promote future collaboration.

Assessment of On-Track Action

Once the pair is in a suitable location, Person B can clarify his points. It is important to note that when Person B functions as a skills coach, he assesses whether Person A's plan will help her reach her goal. The coach does not comment on what Person A should or should not do; it is about evaluating how the plan will function to get her to the stated outcome. Therefore, if the coach assesses that Person A's plan is on-track to her expressed goal, he supports the plan: "I think this plan will work to get you to your goal" or "It seems like a good plan." More personal disclosure could be more reinforcing, for example, "I really like your plan" or "That is exactly what I was thinking."

If the coach does not think the plan will help Person A reach her goal, he voices his concern to her (e.g., "I am concerned that if you go confront Jim in the break room, it might not work out well"). Prompting Person A to explore the coach's train of thought by asking questions can help her get a clearer Clear Picture (e.g., "If you confronted him in the break room, could there be any negative consequences?"). If the individual is unable to foresee problems, the coach can highlight his concerns (e.g., "I think it will drive Jim's and your own emotions up at work. You said your goal was to keep this job. I am worried that he or you will go over a Level 3, start yelling, and get in trouble with your supervisor"). The coach can offer to brainstorm with Person A, exploring other options that might help her manage the relationship problem and keep her job. He could say, "I know Jim is a problem, and we may want to figure out a way to deal with it that doesn't put your job at risk. You getting fired is not going to help. Can we talk about other options?" Person B waits for consent at every decision point, not assuming that Person A wants to continue the process. If Person A declines the offer to reevaluate the plan and look at other skills options, the coach can orient Person A to his availability at a later time.

C: BOTH PEOPLE WORKING TOGETHER

Planning Skills Chains Together

If Person A does want Person B's support in seeking alternatives, the pair explores options. It is important to outline clearly which skills are available for Person A to use. If she is over a Level 3, All-the-Time skills are available. If at or below a Level 3, all nine skills are accessible. Reviewing the Recipe for Skills can help as well. To this point, she has done Clear Picture and On-Track Thinking; the pair can figure out together how many and which additional skills will facilitate Person A in reaching her personal goal.

Skills Options

To find effective skills options, it may make sense to review each possible skill to discuss its applicability. There are various Skills System resources that can support this process. The Skills System Handout 2, How Our Skills Help Us (p. 200) highlights the functions of each skill. This can help the pair decide which skills may be effective in a given situation. Appendix C includes two worksheets (Using My Skills, Worksheets 1 and 2, pp. 346–350) that can be used to create a skills plan. These worksheets can guide Person A and B through a coaching conversation, once she has agreed to collaborate. Using My Skills Worksheet 1 is appropriate when Person A is at a Level 3 or below, whereas Using My Skills Worksheet 2 is appropriate when she is above a Level 3. Additionally, Table 8.1 highlights an assortment of common goals in situations and potential skills chains.

Complex situations may require addressing multiple goals; therefore, combined skills chains are necessary. For example, if the person is at a Level 5 emotion, multiple On-Track Actions and/or New-Me Activities will be necessary due to the requirement of using at least six skills (Recipe for Skills). When an individual is at or below a Level 3, integrating Calm-Only skills is often effective. For example, solving a problem may require the individual to use Expressing Myself and/or Getting It Right as part of the solution. This skills chain would be 123678.

Executing an On-Track Action

Once Person A has a plan that fits the situation, it may be time to help her take an On-Track Action. The plan may include several On-Track Actions; the coach focuses on the one that is a step toward her goal. For example, if Person A plans to go do a Focus New-Me Activity, getting the deck of cards to play solitaire may be the first On-Track Action.

The coach helps Person A understand the microtransitions that are ahead. It is helpful if he highlights any challenges or barriers that Person A may need to navigate (e.g., "Where is the deck of cards?", "Is your iPod charged?"). Troubleshooting and strategizing about how to overcome difficulties can ensure a higher rate of success. Additionally, the two discuss how to access additional coaching supports if necessary.

THE SKILLS COACHING RELATIONSHIP

Coaching conversations are not necessarily "normal" two-way-street conversations. The coach steps back, intentionally demonstrating relationship behaviors that aid Person A to regulate emotions. It is an opportunity for Person B to offer genuine feedback and opinions, but the format of the dialogue is strategically managed by the coach to maximize personal growth of Person A. This type of careful navigation between Person A and Person B can create opportunity for each individual to exist and flourish within the parameters of the relationship.

TABLE 8.1. Goals and Skills Chains

Factors	Skills chains: All-the-Time skills
Be aware of a situation.	1 (Clear Picture)
Make an on-track decision.	12 (On-Track Thinking)
Move toward my goal.	123 (On-Track Action—Take a Step toward My Goal)
Shift from off-track to on-track.	123 (On-Track Action—Switch Tracks to On-Track Action)
Keep my mind and body on-track.	123 (On-Track Action—On-Track Action Plans)
Tolerate a difficult situation.	123 (On-Track Action—Accepting the Situation)
Let go and move on from off-track TUFFs (Thoughts, Urges, Feelings, and Fantasies).	123 (On-Track Action—Turn the Page)
Manage inside and outside risks.	1234 (Safety Plan) and 12345 (Safety Plan and New-Me Activity)
Get more focused.	1235 (Focus New-Me Activity)
Be more comfortable.	1235 (Feel Good New-Me Activity)
Get my mind off of something that I can't change.	1235 (Distraction New-Me Activity: Distract my Mind and/or Distract My Body activities)
Increase positive emotions.	1235 (Fun New-Me Activity)
Solving small problems.	1236 (Problem Solving Worksheet—Quick Fix)
Solving medium and large problems.	1236 (Problem Solving Worksheets)
Sharing something that is on my mind and/or in my heart.	1237 (Expressing Myself Worksheets)
Getting something I want or need from someone.	1238 (Getting It Right Plan Worksheet)
Improving my relationship with myself.	1239 (Relationship Care Core Self Handouts)
Improving relationships with others.	1239 (Relationship Care Handouts)
Understanding how I should deal with different people in my life.	1239 (Relationship Care Handouts—Different Types of Relationships)

Factors	Skills chains: All-the-Time skills
Getting closer or further away from people in relationships.	1239 (Relationship Care Handout—Keeping Relationships On-Track)
Thinking about what type of relationship I have or want.	1239 (Relationship Care Handout—One-Way- and Two-Way-Street Relationships)
Changing off-track personal habits.	1239 (Relationship Care Handout—Getting On-Track with Myself)
Fixing relationship problems.	1236789 (Relationship Care Handout and Worksheets—Finding Middle Ground)
Repairing a relationship.	1239 (Relationship Care Handout and Worksheet—Steps of Responsibility)

TABLE 8.1 *(continued)*

Skills System Handouts and Worksheets

The Skills List

 1. Clear Picture

 2. On-Track Thinking

 3. On-Track Action

 4. Safety Plan

 5. New-Me Activities

 6. Problem Solving

 7. Expressing Myself

 8. Getting It Right

 9. Relationship Care

How Our Skills Help Us

There are NINE Skills in the Skills System.

Here is a list of the nine skills and how they help us.

All-the-Time Skills

 1. **Clear Picture:** Clear Picture helps me notice what is happening inside and outside of me *right now*. I see the situation as it is.

 2. **On-Track Thinking:** On-Track Thinking helps me think clearly about what I want and what will work to help me reach my goals.

 3. **On-Track Action:** Once I get a Clear Picture and have On-Track Thinking, I take an On-Track Action to do something positive to move toward my goals.

 4. **Safety Plan:** I use a Safety Plan to handle risky situations that are happening right now or may happen in the future.

 5. **New-Me Activities:** I do New-Me Activities to help me focus my attention, help me feel better, distract me, and to have fun.

Calm-Only Skills

 6. **Problem Solving:** I take time to solve problems in my life, so that I can be happier and reach my goals.

 7. **Expressing Myself:** I share what is on my mind and in my heart to help me stay on track with myself and other people.

 8. **Getting It Right:** Getting It Right helps me work with people to get what I want.

 9. **RelationSHIP Care:** Relationship Care helps me understand how to have on-track relationships with myself and others.

SKILLS SYSTEM

WORKSHEET 1

Name: ______________________________ Date: ______________

Please fill in the name of each skill.

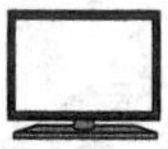

 1. ______________________________

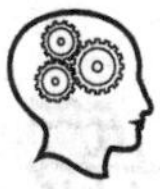

 2. ______________________________

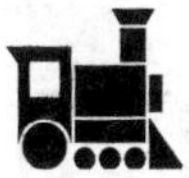

 3. ______________________________

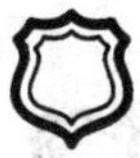

 4. ______________________________

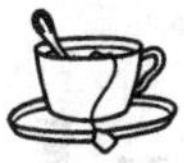

 5. ______________________________

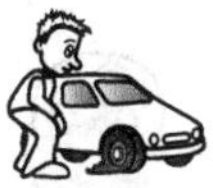

 6. ______________________________

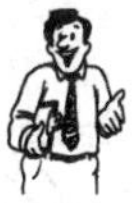

 7. ______________________________

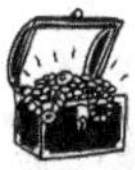

 8. ______________________________

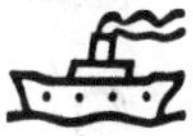

 9. ______________________________

Name: _____ Date: _____

Please draw a line from the number of the skill to the correct picture.

1. **CP**

2. **OTT**

3. **OTA**

4. **SP**

5. **NMA**

6. **PS**

7. **EM**

8. **GIR**

9. **RC**

Name: _____   Date: _____

Please fill in the name of each skill.

1. _____

2. _____

3. _____

4. _____

5. _____

6. _____

7. _____

8. _____

9. _____

How I Use the Skills System

A. The Feelings Rating Scale

The Feelings Rating Scale is a 0–1–2–3–4–5 scale I use to rate how strong my feelings are. The Feelings Rating Scale helps me know what skills and how many skills I link together in a situation.

B. Categories of Skills

 All-the-Time 0–5 Emotion   **Calm-Only 0–3 Emotion**

There are two Categories of Skills: All-the-Time skills and Calm-Only skills. I can use All-the-Time skills at any level of feeling: 0–1–2–3–4–5. I can only use Calm-Only skills when I am at a 0–1–2–3 feeling.

C. Recipe for Skills

The Recipe for Skills helps me know how many skills I need to link together in a skills chain. The recipe tells me to add one skill for every level of feeling (including 0). So, if I am at a 3 sad, I need to use four skills.

At a 5, I harm myself, others, or property.

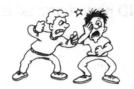

5

OVERWHELMING FEELING

At a 4, I have a hard time talking and listening and staying on-track.

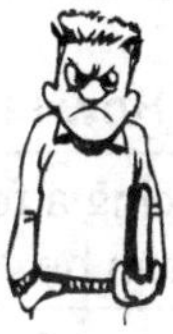

4

STRONG FEELING

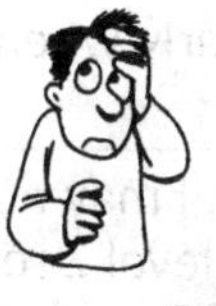

3

Medium feeling

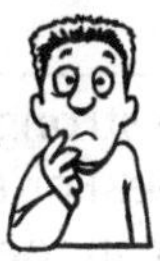

2

Small feeling

At 0–3 feelings, I can talk and listen and stay on-track.

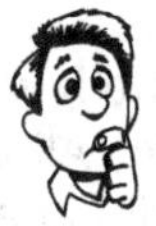

1

Tiny feeling

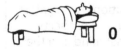

0

No feeling

Rating feelings using the 0–1–2–3–4–5 scale helps me to know which skills I should use AND how many skills I need to use.

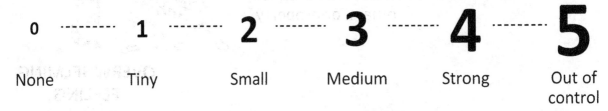

| 0 | 1 | 2 | 3 | 4 | 5 |
| None | Tiny | Small | Medium | Strong | Out of control |

Rating level	How I feel at different levels of emotion
0	A 0 is when I am not noticing a feeling. For example, a 0 anger means that I am not feeling angry at that moment. I can be a 2 sad and 0 angry.
1	A 1 is when I am having a tiny feeling. At a 1, I may notice just enough body sensations to label the emotion. The situation may make me feel a 1 or it may mean that a stronger emotion is beginning to happen. It may also mean that a stronger feeling is reducing to a 1. In all of these cases, at a 1, I am able to think clearly and control my urges, impulses, and actions. Because I am able to think clearly when I am at a 1 feeling, I can use all of my skills, even the Calm-Only ones!
2	A 2 is when I am having a small feeling. I may notice more body sensations than at a level 1. My thinking may be affected by the level 2 reaction. For example, at a 2 angry I may feel my heart beating faster and my thoughts may speed up. I am still able to think clearly, so I can use all of my skills at a 2, even the Calm-Only ones. This may be a good time to use Expressing Myself rather than at a 3 feeling or above.
3	A 3 is a medium feeling. This level of reaction will cause stronger body sensations. At a 3, these body sensations may make me feel uncomfortable. For example, at a 3 angry, my heart might pound and my breathing may be heavier. I can focus, talk, and listen, and stay on-track, even though I am stressed. I can still use my Calm-Only skills at a 3 feeling. If I am unable to focus, stop listening, or raise my voice, I am going over a 3. I create problems for myself when I try to use Calm-Only skills over a 3.
4	A 4 is a strong feeling. At a 4 there will be strong body sensations, and it will be harder to control my thinking. When I notice I am at a level 4, I use all five of my All-the-Time skills to help me become calmer. If I don't use enough of the All-the-Time skills at a level 4, I may try to use Expressing Myself and yell or do Problem Solving and make things worse! I have to wait to use my Calm-Only skills until I have gone down below a 3. I know I am at a 4 (rather than a 5) when I have strong emotions but do not hurt myself, others, or property.
5	A 5 is an overwhelming feeling. At a 5 I am not in control. The body sensations, thoughts, and urges are overwhelming. At a 5, I take actions that hurt myself, others, or property. For example, at a 5 anger I may break a window on purpose. My emotional mind is in the driver's seat (rather than my skills) and I do things that I regret. I have to use *all* of my All-the-Time skills and double up on New-Me Activities or On-Track Actions to get back on-track.

Name: _____ Date: _____

Please list events and feelings for each level 0–5.

_____ I blink my eyes. _____ **0** Anger

When this happens, I don't feel. _____ No feeling

_____ My stomach growls. _____ **1** Hungry

When this happens, I feel → _____ Tiny feeling

_____ There is no good food in the house. _____ **2** Frustrated

When this happens, I feel → _____ Small feeling

_____ I order a pizza to be delivered. _____ **3** Excited

When this happens, I feel → _____ Medium feeling

The pizza man yells at me and I am frozen. _____ **4** Nervous

When this happens, I feel → _____ Strong feeling

_____ The pizza man grabs my arm. _____ **5** Fear

When this happens, I feel → _____ Over-whelming feeling

Name: _____ Date: _____

Please list events and feelings for each level 0–5.

_____ **0**
                                    No feeling
When this happens, I don't feel.

_____ **1**
                                    Tiny
When this happens, I feel →   feeling

_____ **2**
                                    Small
When this happens, I feel →   feeling

_____ **3**
                                    Medium
When this happens, I feel →   feeling

_____ **4**
                                    Strong
When this happens, I feel →   feeling

_____ **5**
                                    Over-
When this happens, I feel →   whelming
                                    feeling

Name: _____ Date: _____

Please list events and feelings that may lead you to feel each level of that emotion.

Feeling: __Fear_____

_____I wake up in the morning._____ 0 Fear

When this happens, I don't feel. No feeling

_____I hear the wind blowing hard._____ **1** Fear

When this happens, I feel → Tiny feeling

_____I look outside and see it's snowing._____ **2** Fear

When this happens, I feel → Small feeling

_____I have to drive to work._____ **3** Fear

When this happens, I feel → Medium feeling

_____I skid and hit another car._____ **4** Fear

When this happens, I feel → Strong feeling

_____I'm trapped and can't get out._____ **5** Fear

When this happens, I feel → Over-whelming feeling

Name: _____   Date: _____

Please list events and feelings that may lead you to feel each level of that emotion.

Feeling: _____

_____   **0**   No feeling

When this happens, I don't feel.

_____   **1**   Tiny
                                                           feeling
When this happens, I feel →

_____   **2**   Small
                                                           feeling
When this happens, I feel →

_____   **3**   Medium
                                                           feeling
When this happens, I feel →

_____   **4**   Strong
                                                           feeling
When this happens, I feel →

_____   **5**   Over-
                                                           whelming
When this happens, I feel →   feeling

Once I know my level of emotion (0–1–2–3–4–5), I know what Category of Skills I can use:

   1. Clear Picture

   2. On-Track Thinking

   3. On-Track Action

   4. Safety Plan

   5. New-Me Activities

All-the-Time skills

0–5 emotions

   6. Problem Solving

   7. Expressing Myself

   8. Getting It Right

   9. Relationship Care

Calm-Only skills

Only 0–3 emotions!

Name: _____ Date: _____

Please fill in the Skills List and Categories of Skills.

_____

_____

_____

_____

_____

0–1–2–3–4–5

_____

_____

_____

_____

0–1–2–3

Name: _____ Date: _____

Please circle the skills that can be used when you are having these emotions.

_3_	Frustrated	🕐 (All-the-Time skills)	**Calm-Only skills**
_5_	Anger	🕐 (All-the-Time skills)	Calm-Only skills
_4_	Scared	🕐 (All-the-Time skills)	Calm-Only skills
_2_	Joy	🕐 All-the-Time skills	(Calm-Only skills)
_4½_	Sad	🕐 (All-the-Time skills)	Calm-Only skills
_1_	Envy	🕐 All-the-Time skills	(Calm-Only skills)
_3_	Happiness	🕐 All-the-Time skills	(Calm-Only skills)
_3½_	Shame	🕐 (All-the-Time skills)	Calm-Only skills

Name: _____   Date: _____

Please circle the skills that can be used when you are having these emotions.

_3_	_Sad_	🕐 All-the-Time skills	Calm-Only skills
_5_	_Fear_	🕐 All-the-Time skills	Calm-Only skills
_4_	_Disgusted_	🕐 All-the-Time skills	Calm-Only skills
_2_	_Happy_	🕐 All-the-Time skills	Calm-Only skills
_4½_	_Jealous_	🕐 All-the-Time skills	Calm-Only skills
_1_	_Mad_	🕐 All-the-Time skills	Calm-Only skills
_3_	_Love_	🕐 All-the-Time skills	Calm-Only skills
_3½_	_Guilty_	🕐 All-the-Time skills	Calm-Only skills

Name: _____   Date: _____

Please write feelings and rating levels in the blanks. Then circle the skills that can be used when at those levels.

Rating and Feeling

_____ _____   🕐 All-the-Time skills   Calm-Only skills

_____ _____   🕐 All-the-Time skills   Calm-Only skills

_____ _____   🕐 All-the-Time skills   Calm-Only skills

_____ _____   🕐 All-the-Time skills   Calm-Only skills

_____ _____   🕐 All-the-Time skills   Calm-Only skills

_____ _____   🕐 All-the-Time skills   Calm-Only skills

_____ _____   🕐 All-the-Time skills   Calm-Only skills

_____ _____   🕐 All-the-Time skills   Calm-Only skills

Once I know my level of feeling (0–1–2–3–4–5), I use the Recipe for Skills to decide how many skills I link together in a skills chain. Skills masters use more!

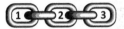 **Combine one skill for EVERY level of emotion:**

Level 0 feeling = At least one skill

Level 1 feeling = At least two skills

Level 2 feeling = At least three skills

Level 3 feeling = At least four skills

Level 4 feeling = At least five skills

Level 5 feeling = At least six skills

Helpful Hints:

Bigger feelings need more skills.

Smaller feelings can pass in a few moments. Larger feelings are more intense and last longer. I use more skills one after another in skills chains to deal with larger feelings.

Double up on All-the-Time skills at a level 5 feeling.

At a Level 5 feeling, I need six skills. If I can't use my Calm-Only skills over a 3, what is the sixth skill I use? I do more All-the-Time skills such as On-Track Actions and New-Me Activities.

Name: _____ Date: _____

Please circle the minimum numbers of skills that should be linked at these levels.

_3_	Frustrated	1	2	3	④	5	6
_5_	Anger	1	2	3	4	5	⑥
_4_	Scared	1	2	3	4	⑤	6
_2_	Joy	1	2	③	4	5	6
_4½_	Sad	1	2	3	4	5	⑥
_1_	Envy	1	②	3	4	5	6
_3_	Happiness	1	2	3	④	5	6
_3½_	Shame	1	2	3	4	⑤	6

Name: _____   Date: _____

Please circle the minimum numbers of skills that should be linked at these levels.

_3_	Sad	1	2	3	4	5	6
_5_	Fear	1	2	3	4	5	6
_4_	Disgusted	1	2	3	4	5	6
_2_	Happy	1	2	3	4	5	6
_4½_	Jealous	1	2	3	4	5	6
_1_	Mad	1	2	3	4	5	6
_3_	Love	1	2	3	4	5	6
_3_	Guilty	1	2	3	4	5	6

Name: _____ Date: _____

Please write rating levels and labels for the feelings in the blanks (like 4 sad). Circle the numbers of skills you need to link together.

Rating and Emotion

____ _____   1   2   3   4   5   6

____ _____   1   2   3   4   5   6

____ _____   1   2   3   4   5   6

____ _____   1   2   3   4   5   6

____ _____   1   2   3   4   5   6

____ _____   1   2   3   4   5   6

____ _____   1   2   3   4   5   6

____ _____   1   2   3   4   5   6

Name: _____   Date: _____

Instructions: Think of a challenging situation that happened recently. Answer the questions using the System Tools.

Briefly describe a situation when you felt stressed this week.

_I heard my best friend lost her job._____

_____

Feelings Rating Scale:

I felt __Sad_____ at a level __2__.

Categories of Skills:

I use my All-the-Time skills when I am at a __0__ to a __5__ emotion.

Could I use my All-the-Time skills in the stressful situation?   (YES) or NO

I use my Calm-Only skills when I am at a __0__ to a __3__ emotion.

Could I use my Calm-Only skills?   (YES) or NO

Recipe for Skills:

I was at a __2__ emotion, so I needed to use __3__ skills.

Name: _____ Date: _____

Instructions: Think of a challenging situation that happened recently. Answer the questions using the System Tools.

Briefly describe a situation when you felt stressed this week.

_____

_____

Feelings Rating Scale:

I felt _____ at a level _____.

Categories of Skills:

I use my All-the-Time skills when I am at a _____ to a _____ emotion.

Could I use my All-the-Time skills in the stressful situation?   YES or NO

I use my Calm-Only skills when I am at a _____ to a _____ emotion.

Could I use my Calm-Only skills?   YES or NO

Recipe for Skills:

I was at a _____ emotion, so I needed to use _____ skills.

A Skills Chain I Used Today

Name: _____ Dates: _____

Mon.	
	Situation: _____ Feeling: 0 1 2 3 4 5
Tue.	
	Situation: _____ Feeling: 0 1 2 3 4 5
Wed.	
	Situation: _____ Feeling: 0 1 2 3 4 5
Thur.	
	Situation: _____ Feeling: 0 1 2 3 4 5
Fri.	
	Situation: _____ Feeling: 0 1 2 3 4 5
Sat.	
	Situation: _____ Feeling: 0 1 2 3 4 5
Sun.	
	Situation: _____ Feeling: 0 1 2 3 4 5

SKILLS SYSTEM REVIEW QUESTIONS

1. What is skill 1?

2. What is skill 2?

3. What is skill 3?

4. What is skill 4?

5. What is skill 5?

6. What is skill 6?

7. What is skill 7?

8. What is skill 8?

9. What is skill 9?

10. Who can tell us about the Feelings Rating Scale?

11. What are the Categories of Skills?

12. Which skills are All-the-Time skills?

13. At what level of emotion can we use the All-the-Time skills?

14. Which skills are the Calm-Only skills?

15. At what level of emotion can we use the Calm-Only skills?

16. What is the Recipe for Skills?

17. What are the six Clear Picture Do's?

Getting a Clear Picture

Clear Picture is an All-the-Time skill. I use my Clear Picture skill at all levels of feeling, 0–1–2–3–4–5. When I notice my feelings or situation change, I take a moment to get a Clear Picture of what is happening inside and outside of me. I guide my attention to be mindful of the six different parts of this one moment.

1. I **Notice My Breath.** I notice the air going in and out. I notice my breath, as it is. I can notice the coolness of the breath in my nose. I can also notice the air filling my chest and belly. Bringing my attention to the breath, focusing 100% on it, helps me be aware of myself in my present moment. In the breath, I handle *this one moment*, which is easier than managing my past and future moments.

2. I **Check My Surroundings.** I notice what is going on around me using my senses (see, hear, smell, taste, and touch). I notice what is happening in the situation right now. I may not like what is happening and I have to see it clearly to deal with it. I see what is real; I check the facts. When I focus on how things should be, rather accepting the moment as it is, my emotions can go up.

3. I do a **Body Check.** I notice my body sensations. Emotions and thoughts may cause body sensations. The different body sensations help me be mindful of how I am feeling. Body sensations come and go, even intense ones. I notice the responses as they are.

4. I **Label and Rate** my feelings. I notice emotions such as sadness, happiness, hurt, fear, jealousy, guilt, and anger. I notice other feelings such as hunger, tiredness, and stress that affect my mood. I may have more than one emotion or feeling at one time. Once I label a feeling, I rate how strong it is, using my 0–1–2–3–4–5 scale. Feelings, both pleasant and uncomfortable ones, come and go. I allow the emotions to pass like clouds, without holding on to them or pushing them away.

5. I **Notice My Thoughts.** My brain is active and creates many thoughts all day long. Noticing thoughts in my mind is like watching my thoughts moving across a TV screen. I notice some are automatic thoughts that pop into my mind. Others I create in my mind like self-talk. I watch all these thoughts come and go, like watching city buses pass by. Some thoughts are helpful, others are not. Some buses are going where I want to go and others do not. Just because I have a thought doesn't mean it is true; it is not who I am. I observe and accept thoughts in Clear Picture. Off-track thoughts can be challenging, but I remember that just because I notice a thought doesn't mean it is my plan. (I make plans in On-Track Thinking.)

6. I **Notice My Urges.** Urges make me feel like taking actions. Some of the urges are small; others are powerful. Urges can make me want to act on impulse. I have to remember that urges, like feelings and thoughts, come and go. This means that I can have powerful off-track urges and not take action on them. I don't ignore urges, instead I use Clear Picture and On-Track Thinking, and take On-Track Actions to manage them.

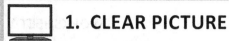

Focus 100% on the Clear Picture Do's

1. Notice my breath

2. Check my surroundings

3. Body check

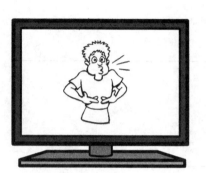

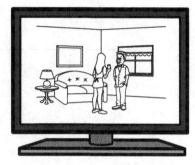

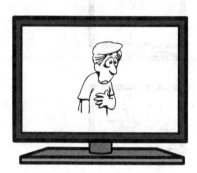

4. Label and rate my feelings

5. Notice my thoughts

6. Notice my urges

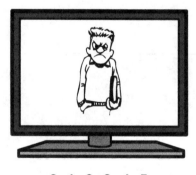

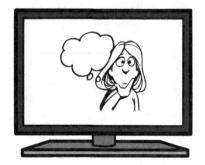

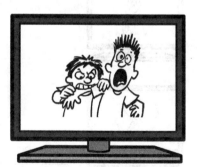

0 1 2 3 4 5

Name: _____ Date: _____

Please write the name of the Clear Picture Do next to the picture.

_____

_____

_____

_____

_____

_____

Name: _____   Date: _____

Situation: <u>I am opening the door on the first day of my new job.</u>

<u>I notice my breath is shallow.</u>

The lights are on inside.
<u>I don't see anyone I know.</u>

I have a pit in my stomach.
<u>My heart is beating fast.</u>

<u>I feel anxious at a Level 3.</u>

<u>I hope I like this job.</u>

<u>Go home.</u>

1. CLEAR PICTURE

Name: _____   Date: _____

Please write what you are noticing in this one moment.

Situation: _____

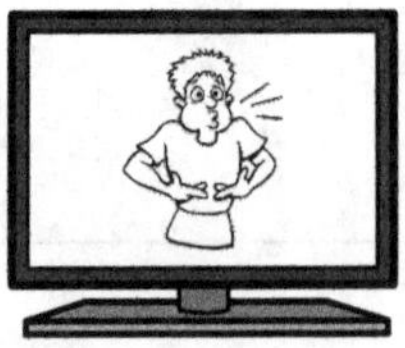

_____

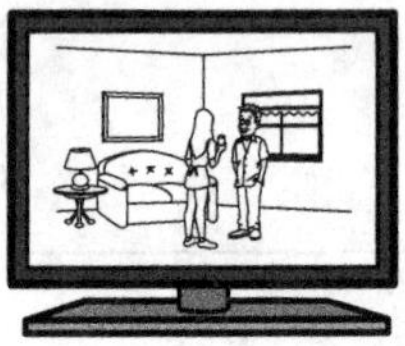

_____

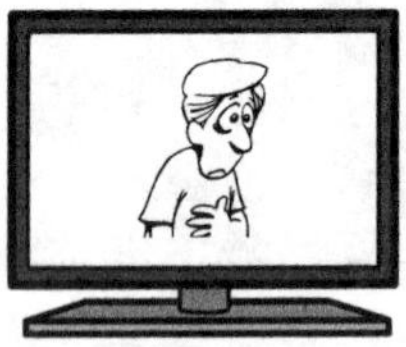

_____

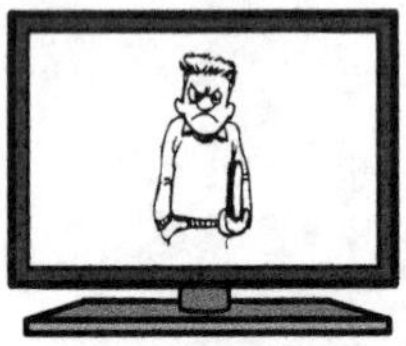

_____

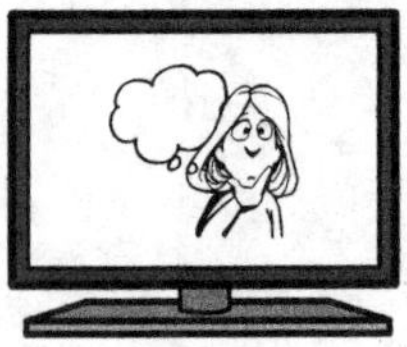

_____

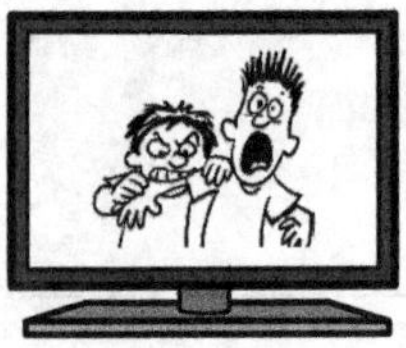

_____

Notice My Breath

 I turn my attention to my breathing.

Where do I notice my breath?

 I can feel the air going in and out of my nose.

 I can feel my chest rise and fall.

 I bring the air in and out of my belly.

What do I notice about my breathing?

Is it shallow or deep?

Is it fast or slow?

I use my senses to get a Clear Picture of my surroundings.

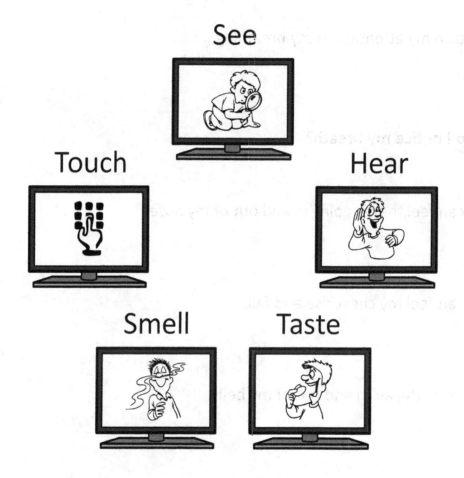

1. CLEAR PICTURE: NOTICE SURROUNDINGS

Name: _____   Date: _____

Please check your surroundings and write down what you notice.

Situation: _I am sitting in my living room._ _____

I see _the TV, the furniture._ _____

I hear _the TV, a dog barking outside._ _____

I taste _the tea I am drinking._ _____

I smell _the lemon in my tea._ _____

I touch _the warm cup, the soft couch._ _____

1. CLEAR PICTURE: NOTICE SURROUNDINGS

Name: _____ Date: _____

Please check your surroundings and write down what you notice.

Situation: _____

I see _____

I hear _____

I taste _____

I smell _____

I touch _____

1. CLEAR PICTURE: BODY CHECK

Add to this list of different body sensations.

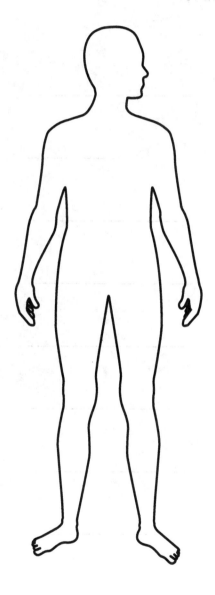

Head	Ache
Neck	Tight Muscles
Shoulders	Pain
Arms	Shaky
Hands	Sweaty
Belly	Butterflies
Bottom	Tired
Legs	Restless
Feet	Sore

Name: _____ Date: _____

What sensations do you feel in each part of your body?

Head _____

Neck _____

Shoulders _____

Arms _____

Hands _____

Belly _____

Bottom _____

Legs _____

Feet _____

1. CLEAR PICTURE: BODY CHECK

Name: _____ Date: _____

Please choose a feeling. List body sensations for each level of that feeling.

Emotion: _____Anger_____

0 _____ I am smiling. _____

1 _____ I stop smiling, I squint my eyes a little. _____

2 _____ I tighten my lips, I make a frown. _____

3 My jaw muscle tightens,
_____ my heart beats faster. _____

4 My fists tighten,
_____ my chest is exploding inside. _____

5 _____ My mind and body feel like a tornado. _____

1. CLEAR PICTURE: BODY CHECK

Name: _____ Date: _____

Please choose a feeling. List body sensations for each level of that feeling.

Emotion: _____

0 _____

1 _____

2 _____

3 _____

4 _____

5 _____

1. CLEAR PICTURE: BODY CHECK

EXERCISE 1

Name: _____ Date: _____

Body Check as a Focus New-Me Activity

Please sit or lie down. Starting at your feet, tighten and then relax the muscles in each part of your body. This exercise really helps when YOU are at high emotion and want to lower it.

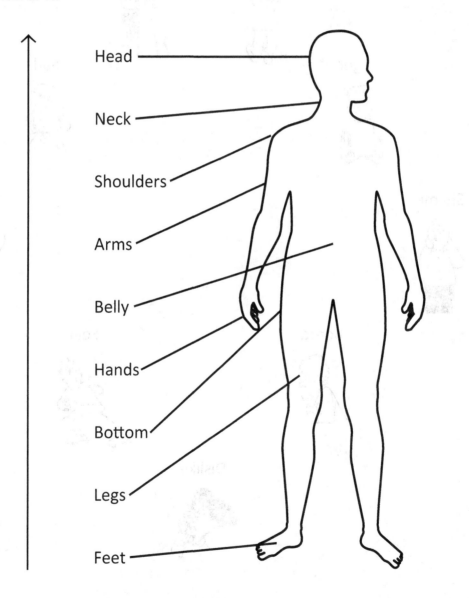

Head

Neck

Shoulders

Arms

Belly

Hands

Bottom

Legs

Feet

Please brainstorm a list of all possible emotions and feelings.

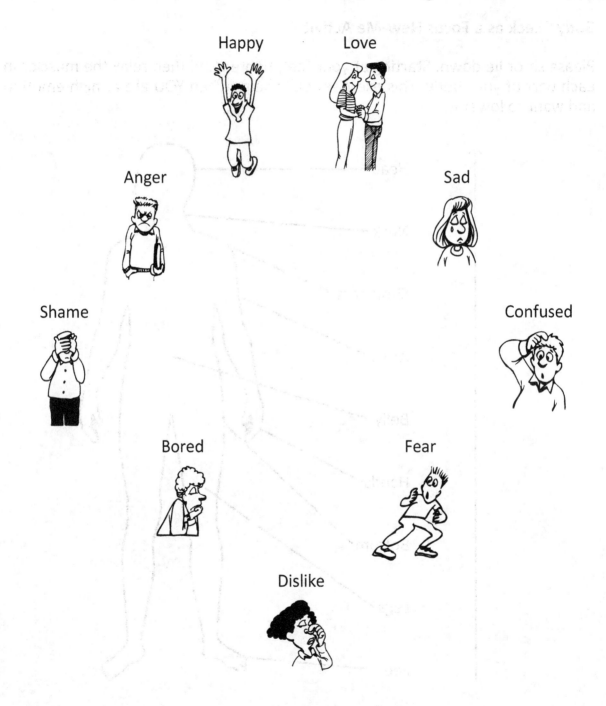

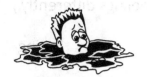 I react to situations with emotions.

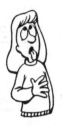 Emotions can affect how my body feels.

 Emotions can affect how my face looks.

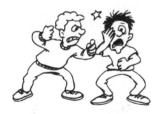 When I have an emotion, I may feel like doing something.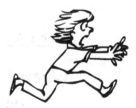

Name: _____   Date: _____

Please list situations when you feel each emotion. (We all rate feelings differently.)

		Rating
Going out to dinner with my friends	Happy	2
When I think about my best friend	Love	3
Thinking about family I miss	Sad	4
When my doctor told me about my medications	Confused	3
On the first day of a new job	Fear	2
When my boyfriend cheated on me	Dislike	4
When I have nothing to do	Bored	2
When I think about hurting people in the past	Shame	3
When someone steals my stuff	Anger	4

Name: _____   Date: _____

Please list situations when you feel each emotion.

		Rating
	Happy	_____
	Love	_____
	Sad	_____
	Confused	_____
	Fear	_____
	Dislike	_____
	Bored	_____
	Shame	_____
	Anger	_____

Name: _____　Date: _____

Noticing My Thoughts

2. My mind makes lots of thoughts, like a popcorn machine. Some thoughts are helpful and others are not.

1. I turn my attention to my thoughts.

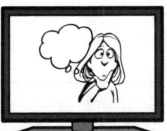

3. Thoughts go through my mind like city buses pass by on the street.

4. Some will take me to my goal and some will not.

5. I can allow off-track thoughts to pass like a cloud through the sky.

1. CLEAR PICTURE: NOTICE THOUGHTS

Name: _____   Date: _____

Please list thoughts that may go with each emotion. (We all rate thoughts differently.)

		Rating
I am doing a good job!	Happy	2
My brother is my best friend.	Love	3
I miss my family.	Sad	3
I don't know what I am doing.	Confused	2
That man is going to yell at me.	Fear	4
That woman was mean to me.	Dislike	4
I am sick of just watching TV.	Bored	1
I am ugly.	Shame	3
I hate how she looks at me.	Anger	4

Name: _____ Date: _____

Please list thoughts that may go with each emotion.

		Rating
_____	Happy	_____
_____	Love	_____
_____	Sad	_____
_____	Confused	_____
_____	Fear	_____
_____	Dislike	_____
_____	Bored	_____
_____	Shame	_____
_____	Anger	_____

Name: _____ Date: _____

Thoughts and feelings lead to action urges.

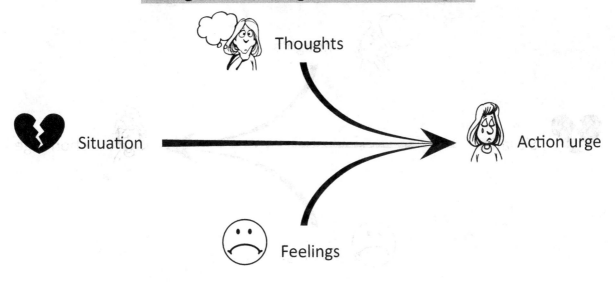

Thoughts

Situation

Feelings

Action urge

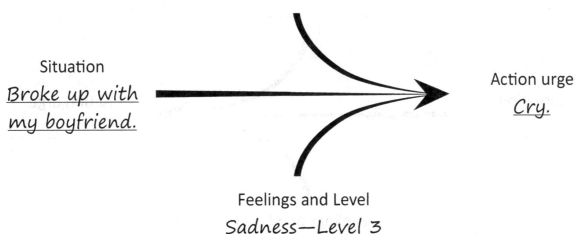

Thoughts
I really liked him.

Situation
Broke up with
my boyfriend.

Action urge
Cry.

Feelings and Level
Sadness—Level 3

Name: _____ Date: _____

Thoughts and feelings lead to action urges.

Thoughts

Situation ──────────────▶ Action urge

Feelings

Thoughts

_____

Situation ──────────────▶ Action urge

_____

Feelings and Level

_____

1. CLEAR PICTURE: NOTICE URGES

Name: _____   Date: _____

Please list action urges that each emotion gives you.

	Emotion	Urge
	Happy	Clap my hands
	Love	Hug
	Sad	Look down
	Confused	Avoid
	Fear	Scream
	Dislike	Move away
	Bored	Complain
	Shame	Hide
	Anger	Yell

Name: _____ Date: _____

Please list action urges that each emotion gives you.

Happy _____

Love _____

Sad _____

Confused _____

Fear _____

Dislike _____

Bored _____

Shame _____

Anger _____

1. CLEAR PICTURE: NOTICE URGES

Please choose a feeling and list an action urges for each level.

Emotion: ___Anxiety___

 0 _____ Relaxed _____

 1 _____ Get fidgety _____

 2 _____ Talk a lot _____

 3 _____ Get out of here _____

 4 _____ Run and find a safe place _____

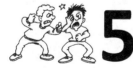 **5** _____ Gasp for breath _____

Please choose a feeling and list an action urges for each level.

Emotion: _____

 0 _____

 1 _____

 2 _____

 3 _____

4 _____

5 _____

On-Track Thinking is an All-the-Time skill. I use On-Track Thinking at every level of emotion, 0–5.

Once I get a Clear Picture and notice my thoughts and urges in a situation, I begin to do On-Track Thinking. The first step in On-Track Thinking is to **stop** and **Check It.** I *Check the urge* before I take any action to be sure it will help me reach my goals. I give it a *thumbs-up* if it is a helpful urge. Helpful urges help me to be on-track to my goals. I give the urge a *thumbs-down* if the urge is off-track. Off-track urges do not help me reach my goals. I try to balance my short-term and long-term needs when I check if something is helpful or not. Thoughts and urges are like city buses; I only get on those that will take me where I want to go.

If the urge is off-track, I **Turn It Up** to on-track thinking. Instead of having more off-track thoughts, I create on-track thoughts in my mind. I coach myself to head in the right direction. I allow off-track thoughts to pass. If an off-track thought pops back in, I notice it, Turn It Up, and don't get on that bus!

Once I start on-track thinking, I **Cheerlead.** Off-Track thoughts can come back, so I cheer myself on to stay on-track to my goal even when is it difficult. I tell myself about how I want to stay on-track and not act on urges that would cause negative consequences. I also use Cheerleading to give myself the strength and motivation to get where I want to go. The stronger the off-track urges are, the more I need to do Check It, Turn It Up, and Cheerleading thinking while I make and do my Skills Plan. I get on and stay on the right buses all the way to my goal!

Then I make a Skills Plan.

• My level of feeling 0–1–2–3–4–5 helps me know which skills and how many I need to use.
• I use the Categories of Skills to help me decide which skills I can use. If I am at or below a 3 emotion, I can use all nine skills—even the Calm-Only ones. I have to be focused and thinking clearly when using Problem Solving, Expressing Myself, Getting It Right, and Relationship Care. When I am at or below a 3, I am better able to interact with people in positive ways. I have to be able to talk and listen to use my Calm-Only skills.

If I or the other person are over a 3, even a little bit, I use my All-the-Time skills. My All-the-Time skills are Clear Picture, On-Track Thinking, On-Track Action, Safety Plan, and New-Me Activity. I might be ready to interact using Calm-Only skills, but if the other person is over a 3, the situation is likely to go off-track for both of us. I wait until we are both below a 3 to fix problems, express ourselves, use Getting It Right, or do Relationship Care.

• Then I use the Recipe for Skills. The recipe tells me how many skills I need to use. I add one skill to my level of emotion. So, at a 3 emotion, I need to use at least four skills. The higher the feeling level, the more skills I need to chain together, because stronger feelings tend to last longer. The recipe tells me the minimum number of skills to use in a situation. A Skills Master uses more than just the minimum! It is important to remember that if I am at a level 5 feeling, I can't use my Calm-Only skills. In that situation I have to double-up on All-the-Time skills such as On-Track Actions and New-Me Activities.

• Next, I think about which skills I will use in a situation. I always start with Clear Picture and do On-Track Thinking to be sure I take On-Track Actions. If I have a fuzzy picture or off-track thinking, I am likely to take off-track actions. Using skills 123 together helps me be in Wise Mind. The skill 123 Wise Mind is for when I am thinking *and* feeling *and* moving toward my goals.

Building Strong Skills Chain

• Wise Mind skills chains start with Skills 1 (Clear Picture), 2 (On-Track Thinking), and 3 (On-Track Action) as the first three links. I add other skills as needed. For example, I add Safety Plan if there is risk. That chain would be a 1234. I add New-Me Activities to help me focus, feel good, distract myself, and to have fun. That chain would be a 1235 if I did one New-Me Activity and a 12355 if I did two New-Me Activities. If I do a Safety Plan and go do two New-Me Activities, it would be a 123455 skills chain. If I am at or below a 3, I may add Problem Solving, Expressing Myself, Getting It Right, and/or Relationship Care as needed to best reach my goals. A Problem Solving skills chain would be a 1236.

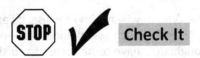

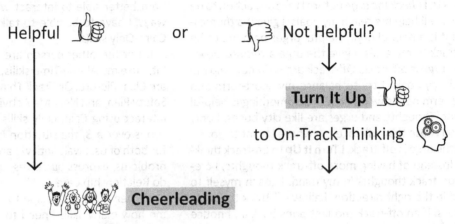

STOP ✔ **Check It**

Does the urge help me reach my goal?

Helpful 👍   or   👎 Not Helpful?

Turn It Up 👍

to On-Track Thinking

Cheerleading

Cheerleading thoughts coach me to Do What Works to get me to my goal.

"I don't want to go off-track."

"I want to reach my goal."

"I will make the best of it."

"I can handle this."

Make a Skills Plan

- Can I use Calm-Only Skills?

- How many skills do I need?

- What skills will I link together to help me reach my goal?

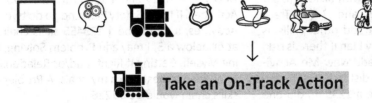

Take an On-Track Action

2. ON-TRACK THINKING

Name: _____ Date: _____

Situation: _I am at work and I feel sick._

✔ Check It

I have the urge to _quit my job._

Is the urge HELPFUL? 👍 or 👎 NOT HELPFUL to reach my goal?

👍 Turn It Up to On-Track Thinking

I need this job!

Cheerleading

I quit my last job and that didn't work out well.

I can deal with this even though I am miserable.

Make a Skill Plan

I am at a: 0–1–2–③–4–5

Can I use Calm-Only skills now?   ⟨YES⟩ or NO

How many skills do I need to use (at least)? _4_

What skills will I link together to help me reach my goal?

My plan: _I will use Clear Picture to know what is going on inside and out._

I will use On-Track Thinking to make a skills plan.

I will use Getting It Right to see if I can go home early.

On-Track Action

I will go talk to my boss.

---

2. ON-TRACK THINKING

Name: _____   Date: _____

Situation: _____

✔ **Check It**

I have the urge to_____

Is the urge HELPFUL? 👍 or 👎 NOT HELPFUL to reach my goal?

👍 **Turn It Up to On-Track Thinking**

_____

_____

🙌 **Cheerleading**

_____

_____

🔗 **Make a Skill Plan**

I am at a: 0–1–2–3–4–5

Can I use Calm-Only skills now?   YES or NO

How many skills do I need to use (at least)? _____

What skills will I link together to help me reach my goal?

🖥️ ⚙️ 🚂 🛡️ ☕ 🚗 🧑 💰 🚢

My plan: _____

_____

_____

🚂 **On-Track Action**

_____

Name: _____   Date: _____

✔ **Check It**

Does the urge help me reach my goal?

👍 = 🚂 On-Track Urges

👎 = 🚂💥 Off-Track Urges

Please think about your personal goals.

Circle whether the urge is helpful 👍 or not helpful. 👎

1. I feel like hitting that girl.   👍   👎

2. I want to focus in group.   👍   👎

3. I want to drive too fast.   👍   👎

4. I want to steal a CD.   👍   👎

5. I want to be healthy.   👍   👎

6. I want to put myself down.   👍   👎

7. I want to make some new friends.   👍   👎

8. I want to scream at my boss.   👍   👎

Name: _____ Date: _____

👍 **Turn It Up** 👎

🚂 **From Off-Track to On-Track Thinking** 🚂

To Check It and Turn It Up, I have to take a second to think about my goal in the situation.

> **Goal:** *I want my own apartment.*

Urge:

I don't want to do my laundry.

Check It

👍 or 👎

👍 **Turn It Up** *I need to do my laundry.*

🙌 **Cheerleading** *If I wear dirty clothes I will look terrible.*

I want to be a clean person and look good.

I want to be independent and responsible.

I will feel better when it is done.

Name: _____ Date: _____

👍 **Turn It Up** 👎

🚂 **From Off-Track to On-Track Thinking** 🚂

To Check It and Turn It Up, I have to take a second to think about my goal in the situation.

Goal:

Urge: **Check It**

_____ 👍 or 👎

👍 **Turn It Up**   _____

🙌 **Cheerleading**   _____

_____

_____

_____

Instructions: Please work together to fill in the blanks in this story.

Situation: Jill has a meeting with her boss this morning and she is running 10 minutes late for work. She gets in her car and . . .

She noticed her breathing was _____.

She did a body check and noticed _____

She noticed her surroundings _____

_____

She was feeling _____ at a level _____.

She was thinking _____.

She had the urge to _____.

Jill checked her urge and it was ON-TRACK or OFF-TRACK to her goal?

(If off-track) What was Jill's Turn It Up thought? _____

_____

Cheerleading thoughts: _____

_____

Jill made a Skills Plan. Because Jill was at a level _____ of feeling, she could use her

All-the-Time Skills   Calm-Only Skills

How may skills did she have to use? _____

What skills could Jill link together in this situation?

Instructions: Please create your own story.

Situation: _____

_____

I noticed my breathing was _____.
I did a body check and noticed _____.
I noticed my surroundings _____
_____

I was feeling _____ at a level:_____.
I was thinking _____
I had the urge to _____.

I checked my urge and it was ON-TRACK or OFF-TRACK to my goal?
(If off-track) What was my Turn It Up thought: _____
_____

Cheerleading thoughts: _____
_____

I made a Skills Plan. Because I was at a level _____ of feeling, I could use my

All-the-Time Skills   Calm-Only Skills

How many skills did I have to use? _____

What skills could I link together in this situation?

💻 🧠 🚂 🛡️ ☕ 🚗🧍 🧍 💰 🚢

On-Track Action is an All-the-Time skill. This means that I can use On-Track Action at any level of emotion, 0–1–2–3–4–5. First, I get a Clear Picture, then I do On-Track Thinking. I Check It, Turn It Up, Cheerlead, and make a Skills Plan. Once I have made an On-Track Skills Plan, I decide what my On-Track Action will be. When I do skills 123 it helps me be in Wise Mind.

I use On-Track Action when I **Take a Step toward My Goal.** I do something positive to be on-track. For example, I may move to my room as part of a Safety Plan or turn on my radio when I want to do a New-Me Activity. I choose to do an On-Track Action to stay on-track.

I **Switch Tracks** when I need to use a different skill. For example, if I go over a 3 using a Getting It Right, I will have to switch tracks to use an All-the-Time skill instead. I also use Switch Tracks when I have urges to go off-track but do something on-track instead. We all go off-track, and it is important to get back on-track as soon as possible—ASAP! The longer I wait, the more difficult it may be! I realize when I am off-track and do several On-Track Actions to be sure that I am on the right road to my goals!

I give 100% effort to an On-Track Action. I **Jump in with Both Feet** to an On-Track Action rather than going halfway. When one foot is on-track and the other is off-track, I am still off-track. Sometimes I do the opposite of off-track urges to make sure I am really on-track. For example, I do **Opposite Action** if I feel like avoiding work; instead, I give work 100% effort. Even though it might be hard, I give 100% effort and focus to the On-Track Action.

I make and follow **On-Track Action Plans** to help myself stay on-track. I do things to keep myself and my life in balance. When my body is in balance, I am able to manage life and relationships better. I balance my eating, exercise, health, work, and have fun. For example: I take walks, get enough sleep, eat healthy food, take proper medications, go to work, and talk to friends as part of my On-Track Action Plan each day.

There are times when I do On-Track Action—**Accept the Situation.** When I have done all I can and I have to wait for the situation to change, I may have to Accept the Situation. For example, if I start fixing a problem and my feelings level goes up, I may have to step back and do On-Track Action—Accept the Situation. I may have to accept when I am over a 3 feeling and need to wait before using Calm-Only skills. It may be important to fix the problem, but waiting until a time when I can do it in an on-track way is best. Also, there are times when I have to do things I don't want to do. I may have to accept the situation and jump in with both feet to get it done. Plus, sometimes it isn't possible to change difficult situations. People may say things to me or things may happen to me that I don't like. I have to do what I can to make it better and then maybe do On-Track Action—Accept the Situation. Life gives us plenty of lemons, I have to make lots of lemonade.

There are times when I have to **Turn the Page,** let it go, and move on. I may have the urge to hang on to certain thoughts, feelings, memories, and urges to the point where it begins to cause me a problem. I have to pay attention to when "enough is enough." I have to be careful to focus on things that help me and to notice when it is no longer helpful. At that point, I may need to do On-Track Action—Turn the Page and move on toward my goals.

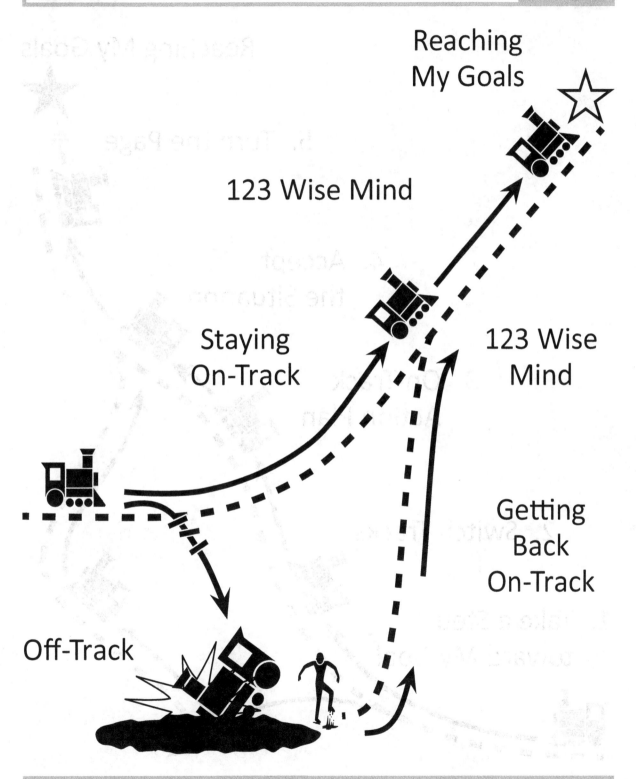

Reaching
My Goals

123 Wise Mind

Staying
On-Track

123 Wise
Mind

Getting
Back
On-Track

Off-Track

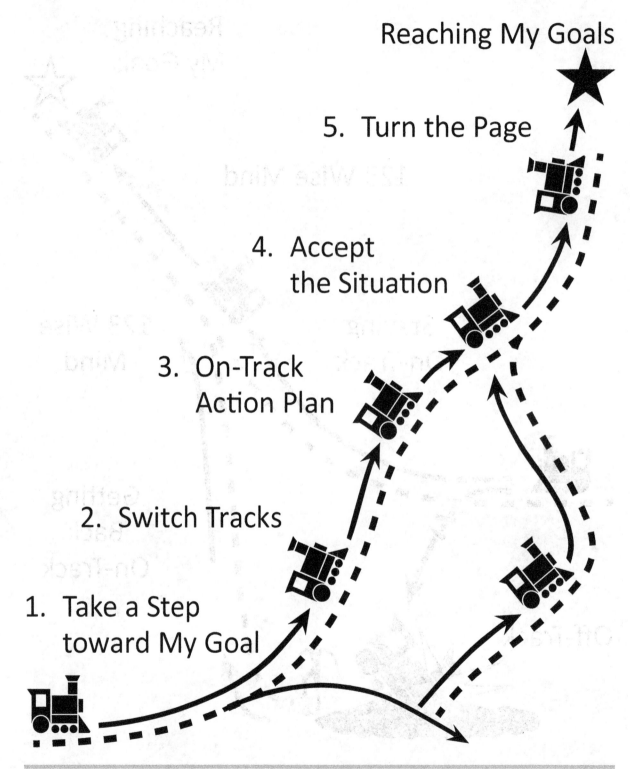

Reaching My Goals

5. Turn the Page

4. Accept the Situation

3. On-Track Action Plan

2. Switch Tracks

1. Take a Step toward My Goal

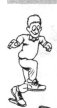

Take a Step toward My Goal in Wise Mind

0–1–2–3

I can also step to:

 6. Problem Solving

 7. Expressing Myself

 8. Getting It Right

 9. Relationship Care

0–1–2–3–4–5

I can step to:

 3. On-Track Action

 4. Safety Plan

 5. New-Me Activity

Goal:
"I want to be safe"

5. New-Me Activity:
Play solitaire

3. On-Track Action

4. Safety Plan—
Move away

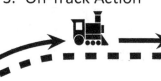

2. On-Track Thinking

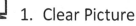

1. Clear Picture

On-Track Action—Take a Step toward My Goal in Wise Mind

Switch Tracks to On-Track Action

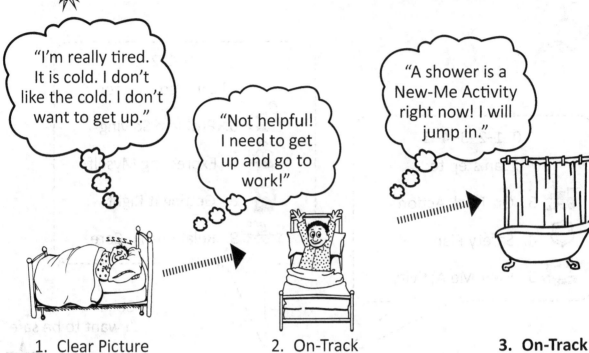

"I'm really tired. It is cold. I don't like the cold. I don't want to get up."

"Not helpful! I need to get up and go to work!"

"A shower is a New-Me Activity right now! I will jump in."

1. Clear Picture

2. On-Track Thinking

3. On-Track Action!

Helpful Hints:

Jump On-Track with Both Feet!

I give 100% effort and focus to my On-Track Action.

One foot off-track and one on-track is still off-track!

Do the Opposite Action of Off-Track Urges!

Doing an Opposite Action can help me get used to things I want to avoid. If I would like to dance but avoid it because I am afraid, I do the opposite. I take lessons and ask people to dance. Opposite Action can make me feel good things I tend to avoid!

On-Track Action Plans

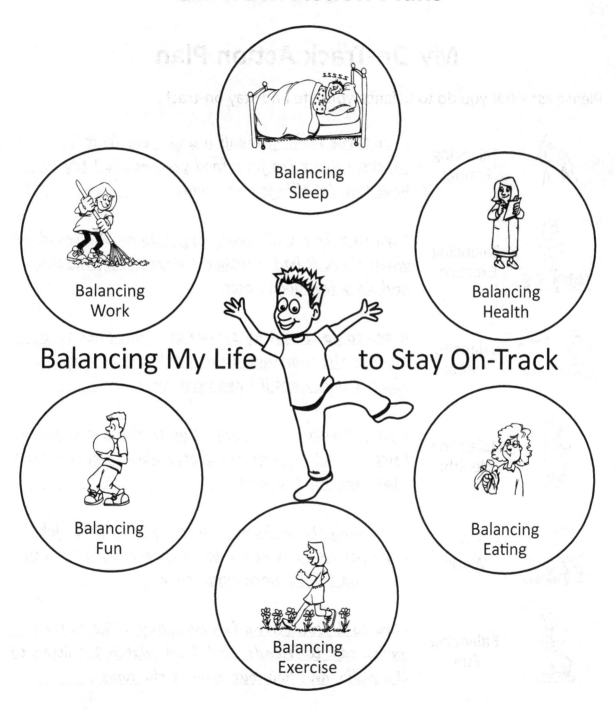

Name: _____ Date: _____

My On-Track Action Plan

Please list what you do to balance your life and stay on-track.

Balancing Eating: I eat three healthy meals a day. I eat fruit for snacks. I don't eat junk food very much. I try to have low-fat things and salads.

Balancing Exercise: I try to take a walk every day. I go on the treadmill when there is bad weather. I stretch my muscles and do a few yoga poses.

Balancing Sleep: It try to go to bed by 10:00 at night. I get up at 6:00 in the morning. That is 8 hours of sleep per night. I take naps if I am very tired.

Balancing Health: I get a checkup every year. I go to the doctor when I need to. I talk with my doctor about my concerns. I take my medications.

Balancing Work: I do many chores in my house. I put in three job applications per week. I do volunteer work to keep busy and to get work experience.

Balancing Fun: I try to do something fun everyday. I like to take walks, talk to friends, cook food, watch TV, listen to the radio, and help out around the house.

Name: _____   Date: _____

My On-Track Action Plan

Please list what you do to balance your life and stay on-track.

Balancing
Eating: _____
_____
_____

Balancing
Exercise: _____
_____
_____

Balancing
Sleep: _____
_____
_____

Balancing
Health: _____
_____
_____

Balancing
Work: _____
_____
_____

Balancing
Fun: _____
_____
_____

Accepting the Situation

When do I practice acceptance?

When I have done all I can and have to wait for the situation to change.

When I have to move away from something because it is making my feelings level go up too high.

When I have to give my feelings time to go down below a Level 3 until I can use my Calm-Only skills.

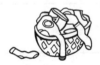

When there are things I don't want to do and have to anyway.

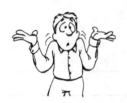

When there is nothing I can do to change the situation right now.

When life gives me lemons, I accept and make lemonade.

Turn the Page

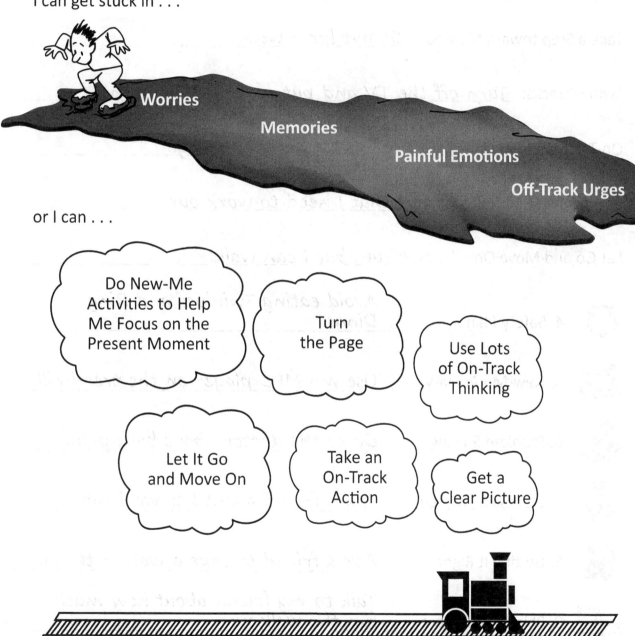

I can get stuck in . . .

Worries

Memories

Painful Emotions

Off-Track Urges

or I can . . .

Do New-Me Activities to Help Me Focus on the Present Moment

Turn the Page

Use Lots of On-Track Thinking

Let It Go and Move On

Take an On-Track Action

Get a Clear Picture

3. ON-TRACK ACTION

Name: _____   Date: _____

Please list examples of On-Track Actions.

Take a Step toward My Goal: *Go out for a walk.* _____

Switch Tracks: *Turn off the TV and put on work out clothes.* _____

On-Track Action Plan: *Exercise for 30 minutes a day.* _____

Accept the Situation: *Accept that I need to work out.* _____

Let Go and Move On: *I can't run, but I can walk.* _____

	4. Safety Plan	*Avoid eating Twinkies and Ring Dings.*
	5. New-Me Activity	*Use my MP3 player on the treadmill.*
	6. Problem Solving	*Go to the doctor about back pain.*
	7. Expressing Myself	*Ask a friend about her workout.*
	8. Getting It Right	*Ask a friend to take a walk with me.*
	9. Relationship Care	*Talk to my friend about how much fun the walk was.*

Name: _____   Date: _____

Please list examples of On-Track Actions.

Take a Step toward My Goal: _____

Switch Tracks: _____

On-Track Action Plan: _____

Accept the Situation: _____

Let Go and Move On: _____

4. Safety Plan   _____

5. New-Me Activity   _____

6. Problem Solving   _____

7. Expressing Myself _____

8. Getting It Right _____

9. Relationship Care _____

123 Wise Mind

Name: _____ Date: _____

1. What are the three skills in the 123 chain?

   _____

   _____

2. What are the initials of these three skills? _____

3. Write the initials for these skills:

4. **S**afety **P**lan: _____   5. **N**ew-**M**e **A**ctivity: _____

6. **P**roblem **S**olving: _____   7. **E**xpressing **M**yself: _____

8. **G**etting **I**t **R**ight: _____   9. **R**elationship **C**are: _____

10. Using initials, list the skills in these skills chains:

    1234: _____, _____, _____, _____

    1235: _____, _____, _____, _____

    12345: _____, _____, _____, _____, _____

    1236: _____, _____, _____, _____

    1237: _____, _____, _____, _____

    1238: _____, _____, _____, _____

    1239: _____, _____, _____, _____

Safety Plan is an All-the-Time Skill. That means that I can use Safety Plan when I am at any level of emotion, 0–1–2–3–4–5.

First, I use Clear Picture and On-Track Thinking. If I notice any risks, my On-Track Action may be a Safety Plan. For example, if I am near a certain person that causes me to have stress, problems, or danger, I use a Safety Plan to handle the situation. It is best to do a Safety Plan before there is a bigger problem. If I do take an off-track action, go near risk, or do something dangerous, Safety Plans can help me get back on-track.

The first step in Safety Plan is to get a **Clear Picture of the Risk.** There are Inside Risks, such as off-track Thoughts, Urges, Feelings and Fantasies (TUFFs). There are also Outside Risks, such as people who are a risk or places or things that are dangerous. I handle Inside and Outside Risks before I do things that are off-track.

Next, I rate Level of Risks as either **Low, Medium,** or **High.**

- In *low-risk* situations the problem is far away or contact may cause stress.
- In *medium-risk* situations the danger is in the area or contact may cause problems.
- In *high-risk* situations the danger is close or contact may cause serious damage.

It is important not to **overrate** or **underrate** risk. *Overrating risk* means that I think that a low-risk situation is high-risk instead. This can cause me to avoid activities that are helpful to do. For example, if I rate my first day of work as a high risk, I will not go and may get fired before I even start. *Underrating risk* means that I rate a high-risk situation as low risk. This can lead me into danger and harm because I stay in the area rather than moving away or leaving.

Once I have a Clear Picture and know if it is low, medium, or high, I think about what kind of Safety Plan is best. There are three Types of Safety Plans: **Thinking, Talking,** and **Writing.**

- A *Thinking Safety Plan* is when I think about how I am going to handle the risk and take an On-Track Action to handle the risk. I usually use Thinking Safety Plans in *low-risk* situations.
- A *Talking Safety Plan* is when I tell someone about the risk. When I tell someone what could happen, what I have the urge to do, or how I am going to handle the risk, it helps me stay on-track in tricky situations. The other person can help me think through my skills plans. I usually use Talking Safety Plans in *medium-* and *high-risk* situations.
- A *Written Safety Plan* is when I write down the possible risk and dangers that are happening or may happen in the future. I write down plans to handle the risk in safe ways. I usually use Written Safety Plans in *high-risk* situations or when I know I will be heading into a difficult situation. It helps to review how I will keep myself safe! I can give people who are trying to help me the plan, so that we can be on the same page about what will help me.

There are three Ways to Handle Risk: **Focus on a New-Me Activity, Move Away,** and **Leave the Area.**

- *Focus on a New-Me Activity*: This means that I focus my attention on what I am doing or another New-Me Activity, rather than being distracted by the risk. I only pay enough attention to the risk to be sure I am safe and that the situation is not getting worse. I Focus on a New-Me Activity in a low-risk situation and Move Away or Leave the Area as the risk goes up.
- *Move Away*: This means that I go to a safer area or get distance between myself and the risk. After I move and Focus on a New-Me Activity. I move away in *medium-risk* situations.
- *Leave the Area*: In *high-risk* situations, I need to leave the area and go where I cannot hear, see, talk to, or touch the risk. I should go to a safer area and do a Focus New-Me Activity. If I am in the community, it may be helpful to return home. I have to be sure that where I go is not risky. It isn't helpful to leave one risky situation and jump right into another one.
- *Safety Pickle*: A Safety Pickle is when we are in a medium- or high-risk situation and it is not possible to move away or leave. We do the best we can to Focus on a New-Me Activity until moving away or leaving is possible.

Safety Plans help us handle risks that come from inside and outside of us.

Inside Risks   # Outside Risks

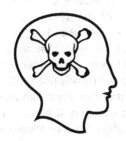   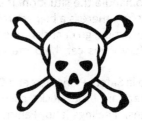

 Thoughts   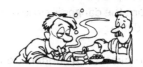 People

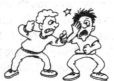 Urges   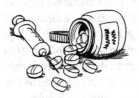 Places

Feelings   Things

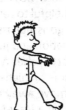 Fantasies

4. SAFETY PLAN

Name: _____ Date: _____

Please list a few of your inside risks.

Thoughts: _He needs to be taught a lesson._

Urges: _I want to smack him._

Feelings: _I hate him._

Fantasies: _I would like to throw him off the bridge._

List things in your surroundings that are outside risks.

People: _That man stole my girlfriend._

Places: _The guy who sells me drugs lives on Main St._

Things: _When I hear "our song," I get mad._

Name: _____ Date: _____

Please list a few of your inside risks.

Thoughts: _____

Urges: _____

Feelings: _____

Fantasies: _____

List things in your surroundings that are outside risks.

People: _____

Places: _____

Things: _____

Getting a Clear Picture of the Risk:
Three Levels of Risk

 Contact with the risk will cause serious damage,

HIGH RISK ➡️

 and/or

the danger is **close.**

 Contact will cause problems,

Medium risk ➡️

and/or

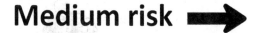 the danger is in the area.

 Contact will cause stress,

Low risk ➡️

and/or

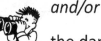 the danger is far away.

Helpful Hints:

Be careful to not to rate high risks as low risks.

> This is a problem, because I might not move away from the risk.

Be careful to not to rate low risks as high risks.

> This is a problem, because I might avoid a situation when it is more on-track to stay and Focus on a New-Me Activity.

Name: _____ Date: _____

Please list your high-, medium-, and low-risk situations.

High-risk situations (close by and/or will cause serious damage)

I am drunk and want to drive.

_____

_____

_____

Medium-risk situations (in area and/or will cause problems)

I am in a restaurant waiting for a table before dinner and

the bartender asks if I want a drink.

_____

_____

Low-risk situations (far away and/or will cause stress)

I am an alcoholic and I hear a beer ad on TV.

_____

_____

Name: _____   Date: _____

Please list your high-, medium-, and low-risk situations.

High-risk situations (close by and/or will cause serious damage)

_____

_____

_____

_____

Medium-risk situations (in area and/or will cause problems)

_____

_____

_____

_____

Low-risk situations (far away and/or will cause stress)

_____

_____

_____

_____

Three Types of Safety Plans

Thinking Safety Plans

A Thinking Safety Plan is when I think about how to handle risky situations. I think about whether I should Focus on a New-Me Activity, Move Away, or Leave the Area. Thinking Safety Plans are helpful in low-risk situations.

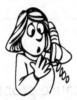

Talking Safety Plans

In Talking Safety Plans I talk to someone and let him know about my safety concerns. When I tell him about my risks, he can help me make safe decisions. I talk about whether it is best to Focus, Move Away, or Leave the Area. It is important to be honest and get support in medium- and high-risk situations.

Written Safety Plans

In Written Safety Plans I write down any possible risks that I am concerned about and make a plan to handle each of the risks. In low-risk situations, I plan to Focus on a New-Me Activity. For medium risks, I Move Away, and in high-risk situations, I Leave the Area. If I think that a situation may be medium or high risk, I may want to do Thinking, Talking, and Written Safety Plans to be sure I will be safe.

Three Ways to Handle Risk

Focus on a New-Me Activity in low-risk situations

In low-risk situations, I can focus my attention on a New-Me Activity. By focusing on what I need to do, I am able to stay on-track AND keep my feelings from going higher. When I stare at the risk, I may become more unsafe and emotional. When I focus on a New-Me Activity, I am able to think more clearly.

Move away in medium-risk situations

In a medium-risk situation, I move away from the risk. For example, if I am having a problem with a person I live with, I should go to my room. Focusing on a New-Me Activity when I get there can help me stay on-track.

Leave the area in high-risk situations

In a high-risk situation, I leave the area or activity. I go to a safer place. It is important to go where I can't hear, see, talk to, or touch the risk. Leaving, talking to someone, and focusing on a New-Me Activity in a safe area will help me be on-track.

Safety Pickles

A Safety Pickle is when I am in a medium- or high-risk situation and I can't move or leave. I use lots of On-Track Thinking and Focus on a New-Me Activity until I can move or leave.

Name: _____   Date: _____

Instructions: Please write in a risk. Then circle the type of risk, level of risk, type of Safety Plan, and how you would handle the risk.

	Type of Risk	**Level of Risk**	**Type of SP**	**Handle the Risk**
Risk:	Inside Outside	Low Medium High	Thinking Talking Writing	Focus Move away Leave
Risk:	Inside Outside	Low Medium High	Thinking Talking Writing	Focus Move away Leave
Risk:	Inside Outside	Low Medium High	Thinking Talking Writing	Focus Move away Leave
Risk:	Inside Outside	Low Medium High	Thinking Talking Writing	Focus Move away Leave
Risk:	Inside Outside	Low Medium High	Thinking Talking Writing	Focus Move away Leave

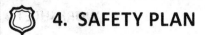

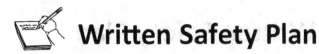

Written Safety Plan

Name: _____   Date: _____

Getting a Clear Picture of the risk:

What is the risk? *I feel like yelling at my coworker.*

Who is involved? *Me and Joe*

Where is the risk? *In the break room*

When is the risk happening? *10:00 a.m. tomorrow morning*

Is the risk   LOW   (MEDIUM)   HIGH

Making a Safety Plan:

Low risk = focus in New-Me Activities.

What activity will I focus on? _____

Who can I talk to ? _____

Medium risk = I move away and focus on an activity.

Where will I go? *I will go outside instead.*

Who can I talk to? *I will ask my friend to help me.*

What activity will I do? *I will take a walk and get some fresh air.*

High risk = I leave the area, talk to someone, and do an activity.

Where will I go? _____

Whom will I talk to? _____

What activity will I do? _____

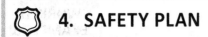

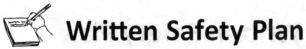 # Written Safety Plan

Name: _____ Date: _____

Getting a Clear Picture of the risk:

What is the risk? _____

Who is involved? _____

Where is the risk? _____

When is the risk happening? _____

Is the risk   LOW   MEDIUM   HIGH

Making a Safety Plan:

Low risk = focus in New-Me Activities.

What activity will I focus on? _____

Who can I talk to? _____

Medium risk = I move away and focus on an activity.

Where will I go? _____

Who can I talk to? _____

What activity will I do? _____

High risk = I leave the area, talk to someone, and do an activity.

Where will I go? _____

Whom will I talk to? _____

What activity will I do? _____

New-Me Activities are All-the-Time skills. This means that I can use New-Me Activities at any level of emotion, 0–1–2–3–4–5.

New-Me Activities are the on-track activities that I do during each day. Different New-Me Activities help me in different ways. It is important to choose the right activities at the right time to help me reach my long-term goals. There are four types of New-Me Activities:

- **Focus Activities:** Focus activities improve my attention and focus in the moment. When I do sorting, organizing, following step-by-step instructions, and/or counting, my mind becomes more focused. Examples: Solitaire, following a recipe, counting money, folding clothes, cleaning, and playing video games.
- **Feel Good Activities:** I do Feel Good New-Me Activities when I want to soothe myself. I use my senses to enjoy pleasant things. I see, listen to, smell, taste, and feel things that help me feel good. I also may do self-care to feel better. A few examples are walking in a pretty area, using hand lotions that smell good, listening to nice music, drinking a cup of tea, washing my face, taking a bath, and eating chocolate.
- **Distraction Activities:** I do New-Me Activities to *distract my mind* when I want to get my mind on something else (Switch Tracks). A few examples are watching TV and movies, playing video games, and reading. I focus 100% on the New-Me Activity and Turn the Page from the things that are bothering me. I want to be sure I have done all of the other skills I need to, before I choose to distract myself. For example, it is often on-track for me to do my chores rather than avoid them by watching TV. Sometimes, though, if I have had a hard day, TV is perfect before my chores. I use Clear Picture and On-Track Thinking to decide what my On-Track Action will be.

I do *distract my body* New-Me Activities when I want to change how my body is feeling. Changing my body can help my feelings and thoughts Switch Tracks. I can distract with cold by holding ice cubes or using an ice pack. I can distract with tastes by eating spicy food or having strong flavored candies or gum (super sour, cinnamon, or minty). I can distract

through exercise by doing activities that get my heart pumping and make me sweat. I can walk, jog, run, do yoga, stretch, lift weights, do sit-ups, and use an exercise ball or DVD to get back or stay on-track. Even though these activities distract me from other things, I have to be focused 100% on the activity. If I am mindless rather than mindful, I could go off-track. It is important that I do these activities in on-track ways to be sure I do not harm myself. For example, ice can burn if I hold it too long, and I can injure myself during a workout if I push my body too far, too fast.

- **Fun Activities:** Fun Activities help me feel happiness and joy. I try to do different things, and that is the spice of life! Examples are drawing, playing sports and video games, working, cooking, cleaning, reading, watching TV, listening to music, talking to friends, going out, studying skills, and so forth. Sometimes I hold back from trying new activities. I do an On-Track Action when I jump in and try something new.

I want to pick New-Me Activities that help me most in the moment. For example:

- If I am getting confused, I choose a Focus New-Me Activity to increase focus and to think more clearly.
- If I am feeling uncomfortable or stressed, I do Feel Good New-Me Activities that help me relax and feel better.
- If I have to wait for a few hours and I want to keep my mind off of it, I use a Distraction New-Me Activity.
- If I want to feel good about myself and my life, I do Fun New-Me Activities.

Some New-Me Activities do more than one thing for me. For example, video games may help me focus or distract me from my worries, and they are fun! A phone call to a friend may make me feel good and be fun at the same time.

I like to do New-Me Activities with people. I have to remember that when I interact with people, I and the other person should be at or below a level 3 emotion. If we are both over a 3, I should do New-Me Activities by myself.

5. NEW-ME ACTIVITIES

HANDOUT 1

New-Me Activities help me to:

Focus

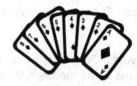

Feel good

Distract myself

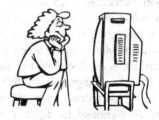

Have **fun**

Doing Focus New-Me Activities helps me have clear thinking.

They can help me go from feeling:

 Confused to **Focused**

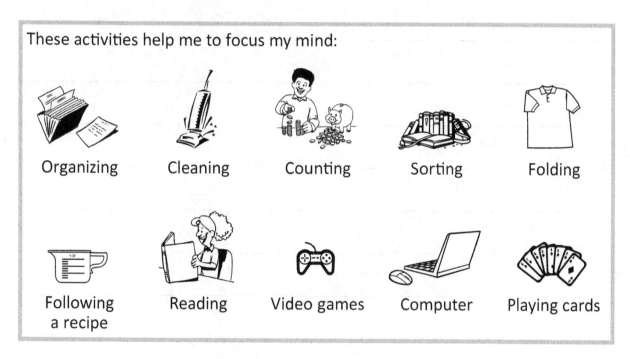

These activities help me to focus my mind:

| Organizing | Cleaning | Counting | Sorting | Folding |
| Following a recipe | Reading | Video games | Computer | Playing cards |

Helpful Hints:

Have a few Focus New-Me Activities to do when feelings are high.

Playing solitaire, doing a word search, making a puzzle, and cleaning help me focus and stay on track.

5. NEW-ME ACTIVITIES

Name: _____ Date: _____

Please list New-Me Activities that help you focus your mind.

My Focus New-Me Activities

_____

_____

_____

_____

_____

_____

_____

_____

_____

_____

_____

Doing Feel Good New-Me Activities helps me to relax and be more comfortable.

They help me go from

 Feeling stressed   to   **Feeling better**

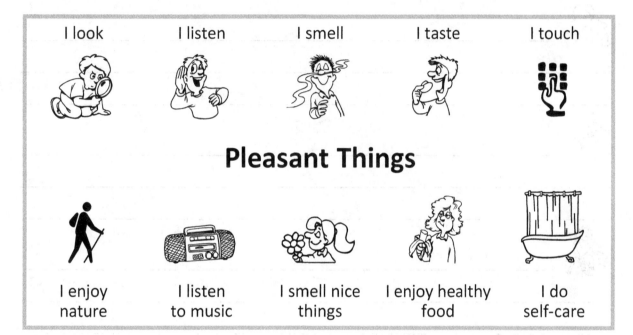

I look	I listen	I smell	I taste	I touch

Pleasant Things

I enjoy nature	I listen to music	I smell nice things	I enjoy healthy food	I do self-care

Helpful Hints:

Have a few Feel Good New-Me Activities to do when feelings are high.

Changing into cozy clothes, sitting in the sun, eating chocolate, and belly breathing help me feel better when I am uncomfortable.

Name: _____   Date: _____

Please list New-Me Activities that help your body feel good.

My Feel Good New-Me Activities

_____

_____

_____

_____

_____

_____

_____

_____

_____

_____

_____

_____

_____

Doing Distraction New-Me Activities help me to take a break and turn my mind away from off-track things.

They can help me go from feeling

 Frustrated   to   **Calmer**

These activities help me distract my mind:

Listening to
the radio, CDs,
and MP3s

Watching TV,
sports
and movies

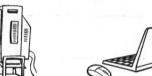

Play video games
or going online

Reading
magazines
or books

Cold—hold ice
cubes/ice packs

Strong flavors:
spicy food, sour
candy, fire balls,
gum, and mints

Exercise large muscles:
running, yoga, workout DVDs,
exercise balls, weights, and
walking—Do what you can!

Helpful Hints:

Watching TV, cold water on my face, listening to head phones, and walking outside help distract me while feelings go down.

Name: _____   Date: _____

Please list New-Me Activities that help you get your mind off of things.

Distraction New-Me Activities

_____

_____

_____

_____

_____

_____

_____

_____

_____

_____

_____

Doing Fun New-Me Activities to add joy and happiness to my life!

They can help turn my mood from

 Grumpy to **Happy**

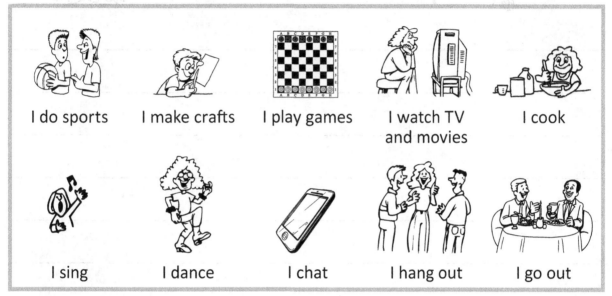

Helpful Hints:

Do Fun New-Me Activities each day.

> I go to the park, call friends, watch TV, and drink tea.

Have Fun activities that are free and easy to do.

> I take a walk, listen to the radio, and pet my neighbor's dog.

Try new Fun New-Me Activities.

> I sometimes need to do an On-Track Action to try new activities. I get nervous at first but then jump in with both feet! Maybe I go to the library, take a bus somewhere new, or go on a picnic!

Name: _____ Date: _____

Please list New-Me Activities that help you have fun!

My Fun New-Me Activities

_____

_____

_____

_____

_____

_____

_____

_____

_____

_____

_____

_____

Problem Solving is a Calm-Only skill. This means that I can use Problem Solving when I am at or below a level 3 emotion. When I try to do Problem Solving when I am over a level 3 emotion, I usually make things worse for myself. I fix problems when I am in Wise Mind; I use 1236 to solve problems in on-track ways.

1. When I notice that something is bothering me in my life, I try to get a **Clear Picture of the Problem.** I think about what I want and what is getting in the way of reaching that goal. For example, if I want to go out to dinner and I have no money, that is a problem. When I have a problem I can handle it in four ways: (1) fix it; (2) not fix it, but change how I think about it so it bothers me less; (3) not fix it, but Accept the Situation as it is; and (4) do none of these and suffer. I use a 1236 skills chain to figure out which of these I want to do. Doing a Quick Fix and Problem Solving helps me change situations and fix problems.

Size of the Problem: There are different size problems. Small problems are often not too serious and cause low-level feelings. For example, I lost my favorite hat. It makes me a level 2 sad, but it will not really cause other harm. Small problems usually get fixed with a few simple steps and can be solved more quickly; I can save $15 and buy another hat. I can do a Quick Fix worksheet to help me solve simple problems. Medium-size problems cause higher feelings (levels 3 and 4) and take more steps and time to fix. For example, I lost my car keys. Now I have to call a taxi, be late for work, miss my meeting, find out how to get a new key, and get a ride to get a new key. Large or overwhelming problems are very serious, for example, if I lost my job or someone I love passed away. Large problems often cause me to have level 4–5 feelings, may take weeks–months–years to fix, and change our lives in serious ways.

Fuzzy and Clear: It is important to be clear about the size of problem, so I deal with it in an on-track way. I have a *Fuzzy Picture of the Problem* when I *think a small problem is a large one.* Rather than focusing in the present moment and seeing it as it is (Clear Picture of the Problem), I worry about the future, assume that the worst will happen, think I can control things I can't, and drive my feelings level up. My mind and body can react to some nonemergency situations with a 911 response, so using the skills chain 1236 is important to help me be clear. I can also have a fuzzy picture when I *think a medium or large problem is small.* Doing this

can make me not do enough to fix the problem. Sometimes it is hard to know how big a problem is when I first notice it. Taking time to Get a Clear Picture of the Problem helps me stay on-track to my goals.

2. Once I have a Clear Picture of the Problem and decide the solution is not clear enough for just a Quick Fix, I **Check All Options.** I think about a few different things I could do to fix the problem. Each option might lead to some helpful and not helpful results for me. When I Check All Options, I *fast-forward* each option to see what will happen if I take that action. I check the fit of each option to see whether the action would be on-track (thumbs-up) or off-track (thumbs-down) to my goal. With medium and large problems, it may be useful to list out the *pros and cons* of each option. Pros are the possible on-track or helpful results of an action; cons are the not helpful or off-track results. For example, Option 1—Yell at my boss. Pro: I will feel better. Con: I will get fired. Option 2—Use Getting It Right to get my hours changed. Pro: I might get my hours changed. Con: I will have to be polite to someone I don't like. I choose the option that has the most pros and helps me reach my goals.

3. Next, I make **Plans A, B, and C.** *Plan A* is the plan that I think will work best to fix the problem. I put 100% effort and focus into my plan. I think about all the steps that I need to take. I think about all the people I need to talk to, what I need to say, and how I will say it. I think about all the other skills I need to use to solve the problem.

After I make Plan A, I think about the fact that sometimes Plan A doesn't work. Sometimes I have to be ready to compromise with the person. I make *Plan B* to have a backup plan that will help me get part of the problem solved. Plan B may help me make the situation better, at least for now, until I can figure out another Plan A that will work better.

I realize that even Plan B doesn't work out sometimes, so I need *Plan C*, which is my fallback plan. I might have another tactic to get what I want. I might plan on Accepting the Situation until I can regroup to make another plan. I might plan to do a New-Me Activity to help me stay on-track as plans fall apart. A Safety Plan might be necessary if I am having urges to take my frustration out on other people.

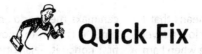 # Quick Fix

Name: _Jane_ _____ Date: _____

Problem: _My room is a mess._ _____

What do I want? _My room to be clean._ _____

What is in my way? _Boxes are all over the room._ _____

What is the fix? _Put the boxes away._ _____

What is in the way of the fix? _There are no shelves in the closet._ ____

How big a problem is this? (circle) (Small) Medium Large

Now that I have a Clear Picture of the problem, what do I want to do? (circle)

(Fix it) **Make Lemonade** **Accept the Situation** **Suffer**

(Change how I think about the problem) (Accept it as it is) (Do nothing different)

If I choose, fix it, what am I going to do? _Put up shelves in the closet._

_____

What makes the fix difficult? _I don't know how._ _____

Plan: _Ask Jim to help me put up shelves in the closet._ _____
  Use Getting It Right with Jim. _____

_____

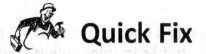 **Quick Fix**

Name: _____   Date: _____

Problem: _____

What do I want? _____

What is in my way? _____

What is the fix? _____

What is in the way of the fix? _____

How big a problem is this? (circle)   Small   Medium   Large

Now that I have a Clear Picture of the problem, what do I want to do? (circle)

Fix it	**Make Lemonade**	**Accept the Situation**	**Suffer**
	(Change how I think about the problem)	(Accept it as it is)	(Do nothing different)

If I choose, fix it, what am I going to do? _____

_____

What makes the fix difficult? _____

Plan: _____

_____

Problem Solving is a Calm-Only skill. I have to be at a 0–3 emotion to do Problem Solving. I have to be focused, so that I can think things through to reach my goals. Problem Solving:

Problem Solving

 Clear Picture of the Problem

What's my goal and what's in my way?

Size of the problem: small, medium, and large

⬇

 Check All Options

Fast forward each option.

Check the pros and cons.

⬇

 Make Plans A, B, and C

Plan A is the best option.

Plan B is a back-up or second favorite option.

Plan C is the option if A and B don't work.

Helpful Hints:

Fix Problems in Wise Mind.

I want to see small problems as small problems, so I don't overreact and drive my feelings to higher levels. I also want to see big problems as big problems, so I do enough to fix them.

 Ignoring problems can make problems bigger and feelings stronger.

6. PROBLEM SOLVING

Name: _Bill_   Date: _____

🖥 Clear Picture of the Problem

★   What is my goal in the situation?

To get my new sneakers today.

_____

🚫   What is keeping me from my goal?

I only have $25 and the ones I want are $75.

_____

🖥   What do I want to fix?

I need to go to the mall to buy new sneakers, and I need $50

more to buy the ones I want.

_____

Size of the problem (circle):   (Small)   Medium   Large

Name: _____   Date: _____

🖥 Clear Picture of the Problem

⭐ What is my goal in the situation?

_____

_____

🚫 What is keeping me from my goal?

_____

_____

🖥 What do I want to fix?

_____

_____

Size of the problem (circle):   Small   Medium   Large

Name: _Bill_ _____   Date: _____

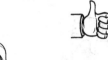 Check All Options

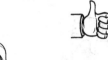 I think of lots of ways to fix my problem and Fast Forward to see how they will work.

Check the pros 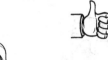 and cons for each option.

1. _I can steal $50 from work._
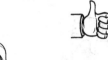 Results: _I will get the $50 and my sneakers._
 Results: _I will get fired and arrested if I get caught._

2. _I can call my sister to see if she will loan me the money._
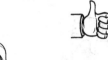 Results: _I might not have to pay my sister back._
 Results: _She will have to send it, and I won't get the money until next week._

3. _I can save my work money and go next week._
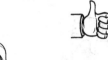 Results: _I should be able to save $50 out of my check._
 Results: _I might have to spend the $50 on other things._

4. _I can buy a less expensive pair of sneakers._
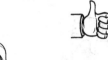 Results: _I will get new sneakers today._
 Results: _I will not be buying my favorite sneakers._

Which is the best fit? _Save my work money._

Name: _____   Date: _____

👍 Check All Options 👎

I think of lots of ways to fix my problem and Fast Forward to see how they will work.

Check the pros 👍 and cons 👎 for each option.

1. _____
👍 Results: _____
👎 Results: _____

2. _____
👍 Results: _____
👎 Results: _____

3. _____
👍 Results: _____
👎 Results: _____

4. _____
👍 Results: _____
👎 Results: _____

👍👎 Which is the best fit? _____

6. PROBLEM SOLVING

Name: _Bill_ Date: _____

 # Make Plans A, B, and C ★

The plan I think will work best is Plan A.

I list the steps I will take to make Plan A work.

A

Plan A: _I will save my money and get new sneakers next week._

Steps to Plan A: _Next Friday I will cash my check._

I will take the bus to the mall.

I will buy my favorite sneakers.

I make Plan B in case Plan A does not work out.

Plan B is my second best option.

B

Plan B: _If I don't have enough money next week, I will save as much as I can and buy them in 2 weeks._

Just in case Plan A and Plan B do not work, I will make Plan C.

Plan C may be to Make Lemonade out of lemons!

C

Plan C: _I will do Problem Solving again in 2 weeks to get new sneakers. I still don't have the money._

 Accept what I can't change.

Name: _____   Date: _____

Make Plans A, B, and C ★

The plan I think will work best is Plan A.

I list the steps I will take to make Plan A work.

A

Plan A: _____

Steps to Plan A: _____

_____

I make Plan B in case Plan A does not work out.

Plan B is my second best option.

B

Plan B: _____

_____

Just in case Plan A and Plan B do not work, I will make Plan C.

Plan C may be to Make Lemonade out of lemons!

C

Plan C: _____

Accept what I can't change.

What's wrong: _____

What do I want? _____

What's in my way? _____

Problem to fix: _____

        Size of the Problem: Small   Medium   Large

Check my options to fix the problem:

1. _____

    Pros: _____

    Cons: _____

2. _____

    Pros: _____

    Cons: _____

3. _____

    Pros: _____

    Cons: _____

4. _____

    Pros: _____

    Cons: _____

What option is the best fit? _____

Plan A: _____

_____

Plan B: _____

Plan C: _____

Expressing Myself is a Calm-Only skill. That means that I can use Expressing Myself only when I am at or below a level 3 emotion. This also means that I can not communicate with another person unless he or she is also below a 3. I Express Myself in Wise Mind; I use 1237 to Express Myself in on-track ways.

What is Expressing Myself? When I Express Myself, I share what is *On My Mind* and *In My Heart.* Thoughts, concerns, and needs are a few things that are On My Mind. Feelings, likes, dislikes, hopes, and dreams are a few things that are In My Heart. I Express Myself by talking. I can talk to someone face-to-face, on the phone, through video, and by sign language. I can Express Myself by writing. If I have trouble reading and writing, someone can help me. I can write letters and e-mails, and use social media and texts. Pictures are also a form of communication. I can make drawings and take photos. I can use body language to Express Myself, such as frowning, smiling, eye rolls, sighs, crossed arms, and eye contact. I also Express Myself when I do New-Me Activities. When I sing, dance, play musical instruments, draw, and act I am Expressing Myself.

Why do I Express Myself? Sharing what is On My Mind and In My Heart can feel great. When I Express Myself through New-Me Activities it makes me feel better about myself and my life. Doing Clear Picture, On-Track Thinking, On-Track Action, New-Me Activities, and Express Myself all together adds joy to my life! I use Expressing Myself with my Calm-Only skills, too. Using Expressing Myself, small issues, concerns, and needs don't grow into big problems. I often have to Express Myself when I do Problem Solving to make a situation better. Expressing Myself is an important part of Getting It Right—Right Words (SEALS). I express respect with Sugar. I talk about what I want in Explain. I make a clear request in Ask. I Express Myself to Seal the Deal. Expressing Myself is used in Relationship Care. I feel better about myself when I can communicate and control my life in an on-track way. I talk and listen and give and take in a Two-Way-Street Relationship. I also Express Myself to Find Middle Ground and do Steps of Responsibility when relationships go off-track.

How do I use Expressing Myself? Talking is one way to communicate. There are pros and cons with talking. Some of the pros are that talking can be a quick, easy, and clear way to make a point. The cons are that there can be miscommunication if I don't choose words carefully. Speech and language differences between people can make it more difficult to understand each other. Communicating through writing also has pros and cons. One pro is that when I write, I can make my whole point without interruption. I can also say things that are hard to say face-to-face. I have to be careful not to write things or send pictures I will regret, because the person can look at them over and over again. I am careful not to just communicate with body language. When I try to be a mind reader, or think someone can read my mind, it creates a fuzzy and not a clear picture. Even when I get nervous about Expressing Myself, I do an On-Track Action to share what is On My Mind and In My Heart.

When do I Express Myself? Expressing Myself is a Calm-Only skill. I use Expressing Myself when both the other person and I are at or below level 3 feeling. Expressing Myself can make my emotions go higher. Because of this, it may be best if I start expressing when I am at a 0–2 level feeling, so that when I Express Myself and the emotion goes up, I can still be under a level 3 feeling. If I start at a 3 feeling and it goes up, I will be at a 4! I can't use Calm-Only skills at a level 4 feeling. When I am over a level 3, I have urges to Express Myself. I use my Clear Picture, On-Track Thinking, and On-Track Action (123 Wise Mind) to Switch Tracks to a Safety Plan, if I go over a level 3 feeling. Even under a level 3 emotion, I am careful about venting; it can make my emotions go up. If I want my emotions to go down, I don't vent about things that are annoying me. It can help to talk with a friend to get a clear picture of the problem or find a solution, but just venting isn't always helpful.

I have to balance Expressing Myself. Overexpressing myself can get my relationship with others out of balance. People's ability to listen to me changes; I may have to ask if this is an OK time to talk. If they say "no," I have to Accept the Situation (or use Finding Middle Ground if it turns into a relationship problem). Otherwise, the person may need to get distance from me. I need to be careful not to underexpress either. This is when I shut down and don't Express Myself when it would be on-track to communicate. Sometimes I am afraid and worry that people won't like me or what I say. I may have to do an On-Track Action—Jump in with Both Feet or Opposite Action—to make myself share what is On My Mind or In My Heart. Do what works!

What Is Expressing Myself?

When I Express Myself, I share things that are
On My Mind and **In My Heart:**

  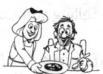

Thoughts   Concerns   Needs   Feelings   Likes and   Hopes and
                                                      dislikes   dreams

I Express Myself through:

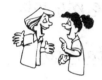

Talking   Writing   Pictures   Body language
(in person, phone, (letter, e-mail,
video, signing)   texting)

I Express Myself when I do New-Me Activities like:

    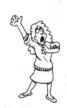

Singing   Dancing   Playing music   Drawing   Acting

Name: _____ Date: _____

Expressing What's On My Mind and In My Heart

Please practice expressing as if you were telling someone.

 Thoughts: I like watching football more than watching baseball.

I think my cat will need medicine.

Concerns: I am concerned about walking outside at night.

I am concerned I might lose my job.

 Needs: I need to have a friend to talk to.

I need to go to the bank.

Feelings: I feel happy that my team won.

I am sad because my cat is sick.

 Likes and dislikes: I like pepperoni pizza.

I don't like the taste of raw onions.

 Hopes and dreams: I hope to work full time in the future.

Someday I want to buy a car.

Name: _____   Date: _____

Expressing What's On My Mind
and In My Heart

Please practice expressing as if you were telling someone.

Thoughts: _____
_____

Concerns: _____
_____

Needs: _____
_____

Feelings: _____
_____

Likes and dislikes: _____
_____

Hopes and dreams: _____
_____

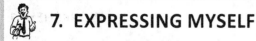

Why Do I Express Myself?

 Expressing Myself can feel great.

Sharing what is on my mind and in my heart with someone who listens and cares is a great feeling. Expressing through New-Me Activities can increase happiness and joy.

 Expressing Myself can help with Problem Solving.

If I Express Myself about what's on my mind when the issues are small, I can keep problems from growing larger!

 Expressing Myself can help with Getting It Right.

Expressing Myself is important when I try to get what I need from people. I Express Myself when I use the Right Words (SEALS) in Getting It Right. I express feelings of respect when I use Sugar. I express my needs when I Explain and Ask for what I want. Expressing Myself helps me Seal the Deal!

 Expressing Myself can help my Relationship Care.

When I Express Myself in on-track ways I build a stronger connection with myself. I am self-aware, self-accepting, self-valuing, and self-trusting. When I Express Myself with others in on-track ways, it helps me have control in my life. It also can help me feel more connected to people in my life. In Two-Way-Street relationships we both have a chance to express and listen, which make both of us happy. I Express Myself to change off-track relationships when I Find Middle Ground and take the Steps of Responsibility.

How Do I Use Expressing Myself?

 Use 1237 to balance Expressing Myself.

Expressing Myself can go off-track quickly. For example, I can say too little or too much. I can be too quiet or too loud. I can be too honest or not honest enough. Using 1237 helps me balance my expressing. 1237 means that I use Clear Picture (1), On-Track Thinking (2), and On-Track Action (3) when I Express Myself (7). Wise Mind expressing (1237) helps me be aware and make changes in how and what I am saying to fit the situation.

 Talking is one way to Express Myself.

Talking can be a good way to communicate, but it isn't the only way. It can be a fast, easy, and clear way to make a point. Unfortunately, speech and language differences can make it more challenging to understand each other. Keep trying!

 Writing to Express Myself can be helpful.

Writing can get my point across in detail and I don't get interrupted. I can also write things that are hard to say face-to-face. Unfortunately, if I write something snarky, the person can read it over and over again. It is helpful to review anything I write to be sure that it is what I want to say and how I want to say it.

 Mind Reading gives a fuzzy picture.

Sometimes I think other people already know what I am thinking or need without me telling them. Other times I think I know what others are thinking without them telling me. Instead, I have to Express Myself in a clear way to be on the same page with people. Fuzzy messages can make my feelings level go up and problems grow.

When Do I Use Expressing Myself?

Calm-Only Skill

 I Express Myself when it will help.

I express my feelings, thoughts, likes, dislikes, needs, concerns, hopes, and dreams when it will be helpful for me, another person, or our relationship. If it is not going to help, I wait until I am clear that Expressing Myself is an On-Track Action.

 Start at a 1–2 level because feelings go up!

Expressing Myself can increase feelings. I start Expressing Myself at level 1 or 2, because when I go into a topic, my feelings can go up. If I start expressing at a level 3 feeling, it may go up to a level 4, which is too high for a Calm-Only skill. Doing 1237 helps me know when to stop expressing and Switch Tracks to a Safety Plan and New-Me Activity to help my feelings go down.

 The difference between waiting and avoiding.

If Expressing Myself drives feelings up, it means that whatever is on my mind could be important. Instead of avoiding it, it may be on-track to wait to express it in a more helpful way. Just waiting until I am calmer may work. Writing a letter or having a friend be with me when I am talking to the person can keep the situation cooler. Avoiding expressing important things may make me feel stuck in a bad situation and can drive my feelings higher.

 Be careful of venting.

Venting with friends about people or situations can feel good, but it actually drives feelings higher. If I want to bring feelings down, I won't vent. If I want them to go up, then I'll vent. Venting can lead to a more negative attitude or it can help me get a clearer picture of the situation. I need to do what works!

Name: _____ Date: _____

Expressing Myself Plan

What is something that is On My Mind or In My Heart?

I want to tell my friend something about her boyfriend.

It is a: Thought   (Concern)   Need   Feeling   Like/dislike   Hope/dream

Other: _____

Who do I need to Express Myself to?

My friend Carol

Why is it important to express this?

I am worried for her safety.

How can I best Express Myself?

(Talk in person)   Phone call   Video   Signing   Letter   E-mail   Text   Body language

Other: _____

When is it best to Express Myself?

I will talk to her Saturday at my house.

Points I need to express:

I care for her and what's best for her.

I heard at work that her boyfriend hit a girl before.

I think she should be careful.

I don't want her to get hurt.

Name: _____   Date: _____

Expressing Myself Plan

What is something that is On My Mind or In My Heart?

_____

It is a: Thought   Concern   Need   Feeling   Like/dislike   Hope/dream

       Other: _____

Who do I need to Express Myself to?

_____

Why is it important to express this?

_____

How can I best Express Myself?

    Talk in   Phone   Video   Signing   Letter   E-mail   Text   Body
    person   call   language

    Other: _____

When is it best to Express Myself?

_____

Points I need to express:

_____

_____

_____

_____

Getting It Right is a Calm-Only skill. That means that I can use Getting It Right only when I am at or below a level 3 emotion. It also means that the person with whom I do Getting It Right must also be at or below a level 3 emotion. I use Getting It Right in Wise Mind; I use skills 1238 to be sure I am Getting It Right in an on-track way.

I use Getting It Right to get things that I want from people.

- First, I make sure I am in the **Right Mind.** I have to be prepared and focused. I have to have a Getting It Right Plan. If my mind is fuzzy instead of clear, I may forget important steps in Getting It Right. In Fuzzy Mind, I might Get It Wrong.

- Then I have to choose the **Right Person** with whom to talk. In some situations, I may have to call that person to set up a time to talk. I have to use my other skills, such as On-Track Action and New-Me Activities, while I am waiting to talk to the Right Person. Learning how to wait without losing focus or getting more upset will help me stay on-track to my goal.

- Choosing the **Right Time and Place** is important. I want the person to be able to focus on me, my needs, and how he can help me. Talking to the person when he is too busy lowers my chance of getting what I want. I DO WHAT WORKS, so waiting for the best time may increase my chances of being successful.

- Using the **Right Tone** is also a must! I use Clear Picture and On-Track Thinking to decide what tone will work. Usually being wimpy makes the person not take me seriously. Often, being demanding makes him pull away, stop listening, and think that I am not skillful. When I have an aggressive tone, it may stress the relationship so much that the person will never want to help me again, or he will make things more difficult for me. If I notice my tone changing, I need to be sure I am still on-track to my goal. It is often best to step back and wait until another time if I am not able to keep the Right Tone the whole time.

- Finally, I have to use the **Right Words: SEALS**

  - *Sugar*: Using Sugar means I am nice and polite to the person; I make him want to help me. Saying "please," "thank you," and "excuse me, do you have a moment?" makes the person feel like I am giving him respect. I say things that I know will make the person happy about helping me.

  - *Explain the Situation*: I clearly explain why it is important that the person help me. When helping me makes the other person feel good, he is more likely to help me.

  - *Ask for What I Want*: I ask for what I want in a clear and direct way, AFTER using Sugar and Explaining the situation!

  - *Listen*: I listen carefully to what the other person says, so that I can figure out how to Seal a Deal. If he is saying "no," "maybe," or "I don't know," I breathe and focus. If I am going over a level 3 feeling, it is best to Switch Tracks, stop Getting It Right, and do a Safety Plan.

  - *Seal a Deal*: If the person agrees to help me, then I Seal a Deal and talk about the details. I make sure the person will follow through on what he offered to do. If the person does not agree, I try to either go to Plan B or step back from the situation and rethink the Getting It Right plan.

Getting What I Want!

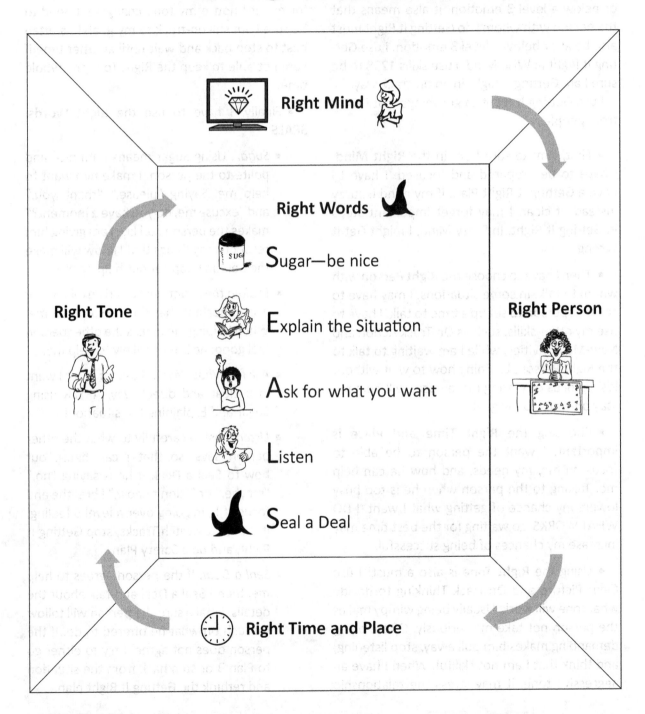

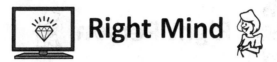 **Right Mind**

Getting It Right is a Calm-Only skill. This means that I can use Getting It Right when I am at a 0–3 emotion. When I am over a level 3, I may have strong urges to get what I want—RIGHT NOW. It is hard to get what I want if am scattered and unfocused. Getting It Right takes lots of focus to do well. There are many steps in Getting It Right. I have to wait until I am in the Right Mind to Get It Right!

 Right Mind means:

I know what I want.

I am aware of the obstacles to getting it.

I am able to make a Getting It Right plan.

I identify who I need to talk to.

I choose the right time and place.

I think about what tone and words will work best.

I am able to be polite and nice—even if I am a little nervous.

I am able to explain the situation clearly.

I am able to ask for what I want.

I am able to listen to other people.

I am able to work with another person to Seal a Deal.

I am able to DO WHAT WORKS in Wise Mind!

Right Person

I have to choose the Right Person to talk to when I use Getting It Right. I pick the person who can best get me what I want. It is usually worth waiting to talk to the Right Person. Talking to the wrong person can keep me from getting what I want. Each situation is different; I use Clear Picture and On-Track Thinking to help me choose the Right Person.

The Right Person is usually the person who is in control of what I want:

 If I want a raise, I usually talk to my boss.

 If I want to change my medications, usually I speak to my doctor.

 If I want my housemate to turn down her music, usually I speak to my housemate.

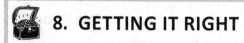

 # Right Time and Place

Choosing the Right Time and Place is important. I want the person to be able to focus on me, my needs, and how she can help me. If the person is busy or distracted, she will not be 100% focused. I want to DO WHAT WORKS so that waiting for the BEST time may increase my chances of being successful. While I am waiting, I need to use my other skills to stay on-track.

  Choosing the Right Time and Place:

Speaking to the person in a quiet and private area
can help me focus my attention.

I have to be able to focus on using the Right Tone and Right Words.

It may work best if the person is able to focus on what I am saying.

If the person is distracted by something else, it may affect her decisions.

Right Tone

Using the Right Tone is very important! Each situation is different; I use Clear Picture and On-Track Thinking to decide what tone will work best. Sometimes I want to be gentle; at other times it is best to be firm. I have to think about what tone will make the person hear what I am saying. I want to use a tone that makes the person want to help me.

Choose the Right Tone:

 Being wimpy can make people not take me seriously.

When I have respect and need in my voice,
the person can feel how important the issue is to me.

I respect you.   You respect me.

 Being demanding can make the person pull away.
Having an aggressive tone can make the person
want to work against me!

Right Words—SEALS

Using the Right Words is important too! I might be nervous when I am Getting It Right, so I plan ahead and practice so that my words come out smoothly.

 I use **S**UGAR to help the person want to help me.

 I **E**XPLAIN THE SITUATION so that the person knows why I need help.

 Then I **A**SK FOR WHAT I WANT in a direct and clear way.

 Then I **L**ISTEN carefully so that I clearly understand what the person is saying.

 I **S**EAL A DEAL to get what I want!

 If the person says "no," I do Clear Picture and On-Track Thinking to figure out how to deal with my emotions and to get my needs met.

Name: _____ Date: _____

Getting It Right Plan

What do I want? _I would like more hours at work._

Whom will I talk to? _My boss_

When and where will I talk to him or her? _I will ask her to meet. I think we will meet in her office, but I will let her decide._

What kind of tone will I use? _Polite, serious, and like I care_

What will I say to use **S**UGAR? _"Please," "thank you," "I appreciate the time you are taking to meet with me."_

How will I **E**XPLAIN my situation? _I really like my job. I have been here a year and I want to move ahead._

How will I **A**SK for what I want? _I would like to increase my hours._

Will I **L**ISTEN to what he or she says? __X__ Yes _____ No

What is the deal I want? _I am working 2 days a week now, and I would like to increase to working 3 days per week._

How will I **S**EAL a DEAL? _If "yes," I will ask, "When can I start?" If "no," I will ask, "What do I need to do to increase my hours?"_

Name: _____ Date: _____

Getting It Right Plan

What do I want? _____

Whom will I talk to? _____

When and where will I talk to him or her? _____

_____

What kind of tone will I use? _____

What will I say to use **S**UGAR? _____

_____

How will I **E**XPLAIN my situation? _____

_____

How will I **A**SK for what I want? _____

_____

Will I **L**ISTEN to what he or she says?   _____ Yes   _____ No

What is the deal I want? _____

_____

How will I **S**EAL a DEAL? _____

_____

Relationship Care is a Calm-Only skill. That means that I can use Relationship Care only when I am at or below a level 3 emotion. It also means that the person I am talking with must also be at or below a level 3 emotion. Building On-Track Relationships, Balancing On-Track Relationships, and Changing Off-Track Relationships are aspects of Relationship Care. I use Relationship Care in Wise Mind; I use skills 1239 to do it in on-track ways.

I use Relationship Care to Build On-Track Relationships with myself and other people.

An On-Track relationship with myself means that I am getting a stronger Core Self. There are four parts:

1. *Self-awareness*: I use Clear Picture to be aware of this moment. I see myself and my life *as it is right now*. I also pay attention to my goals. When I know what I want it is much easier to make a Skills Plan to reach my goals. Sometimes it is hard to see situations clearly, but in the long run, it helps me stay on-track and feel better about myself. As I learn to see myself clearly, I can see others more clearly as well.

2. *Self-Acceptance*: When I see situations and handle my emotions, it is easier to accept myself and other people. As I interact with others, I see that we are all different and that is OK! That's what makes life interesting! When I notice my thoughts and urges to put myself down, I Turn It Up to On-Track Thinking instead.

3. *Self-Value*: As I use my skills to reach goals, I get more of what I want. I feel good about my abilities to handle my emotions, my relationships, and my life. I manipulate things in a good way! Doing what works makes me feel better about myself. When I value me, it is easier to value other people.

4. *Self-Trust*: Using my skills, I am able to stay on-track in more challenging situations. I try new things, which makes me happier. I know I can handle anything that comes my way! As I trust myself, I am more able to trust other people. A stronger relationship with myself, helps me have better relationships with others.

I use Relationship Care to *Balance My On-Track Relationships* with myself and other people.

- There are many different types of relationships in my life. I use Clear Picture, On-Track Thinking, On-Track Action, and my other skills to make on-track choices to keep all my different relationships in balance.

- Keeping Relationships On-Track: I take certain On-Track Actions to make the relationship closer when I want to have a stronger connection with someone. I take different On-Track Actions to get distance in the relationship. I use all of these actions to balance my relationships as I, others, and relationships change.

- A *Two-Way-Street Relationship* occurs when there is an equal give and take between me and another person. Both of us Talk and Listen, Give and Take. We work together. Respect flows back and forth between us. Two-Way-Street Relationships take a lot of attention to keep in balance. Even when I try sometimes, relationships get out of balance. Using other skills such as Expressing Myself can keep the Two-Way-Street Relationship working.

- A *One-Way-Street Relationship* occurs when one or the other person is not Talking and Listening, Giving and Taking. Perhaps, I feel that I am giving and the other person is not. I may be wanting to have a One-Way-Street Relationship if I do not want to Talk and Listen and Give and Take with the person.

I use many skills together to *Change Off-Track Relationships* between myself and other people.

- When I get off-track with myself, I sometimes lose track of my goals, put myself down, and do off-track actions. I get back on-track with myself when I have a Clear Picture of my goals, do On-Track Thinking about myself, and take On-Track Actions. Having and following my On-Track Action Plan helps.

- When my relationship with another person goes off-track I can use *Finding Middle Ground* and/or *Steps of Responsibility* to get it back on-track.

- *Finding Middle Ground*: First I do Problem Solving to get a clear picture of the rela-

tionship problem and decide that talking things out is a helpful option. I decide how to Express Myself (e.g., in person, on the phone, or writing). When I do get together (or write), I use Getting It Right to explain my concerns and ask for what I want to change. I listen to the other person's side of the story. We Find Middle Ground when we can find a solution that is good for both of us. I may need to use a 1236789 skills chain to Find Middle Ground! If feelings go up over a level 3, it is important to Switch Tracks and do a Safety Plan. It may be possible to do Finding Middle Ground at a later time, in a different place, or with other people there to help. When I have tried Finding Middle Ground and serious relationship problems remain, I may have to Accept the Situation as it is, change how I feel about it, or end the off-track relationship.

- *Steps of Responsibility*: When I have done something to hurt another person, I do the Steps of Responsibility. I clearly Admit the Problem, Apologize for what I regret doing, commit to change, and take an On-Track Action that fits for me and makes the relationship better. Taking responsibility can be difficult; I use "1239" to stay on-track.

Relationship Care is a Calm-Only skill. This means that I can only use Relationship Care when I and the other person are at a 0–3 level of emotion. When either person is over a 3, he or she may not be thinking clearly enough to manage relationships well. I use Clear Picture and On-Track Thinking to build, balance, and change my relationships.

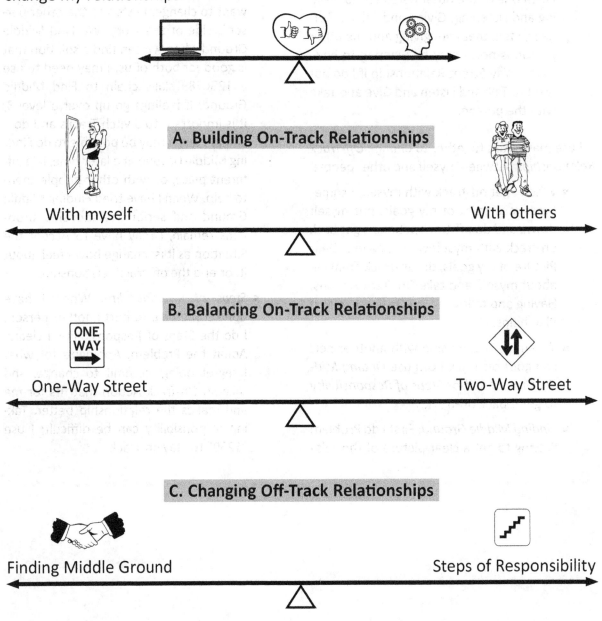

A. Building On-Track Relationships

With myself   With others

B. Balancing On-Track Relationships

ONE WAY →   ⬍

One-Way Street   Two-Way Street

C. Changing Off-Track Relationships

Finding Middle Ground   Steps of Responsibility

A. Building On-Track Relationships

Building an On-Track Relationship with Myself

A stronger core self:

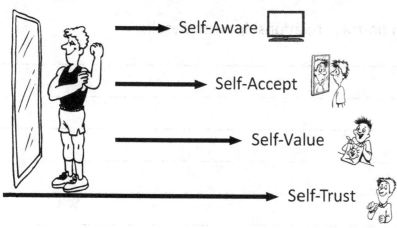

Self-Aware

Self-Accept

Self-Value

Self-Trust

and . . .

Building an On-Track Relationship with Other People

Be aware of, accept, value, and trust

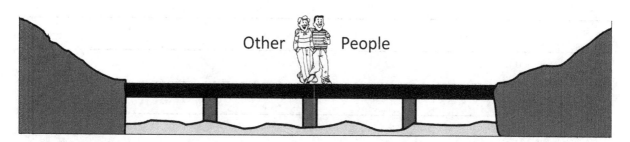

Other People

Name: _____   Date: _____

A. Building On-Track Relationships

Things I do to build an on-track relationship with myself:

_____

_____

_____

_____

_____

and . . .

How do I find new friends and build an on-track relationship with them:

_____

_____

_____

_____

_____

A. Building On-Track Relationships

Different Types of Relationships

Coworkers

Dating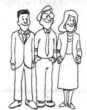

Housemates

Friends

Professionals

Family

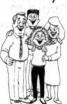

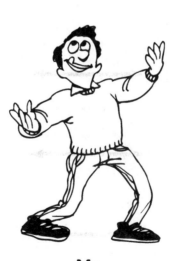

Me

Can you think of others?

B. Balancing On-Track Relationships

Relationships need a lot of CARE.

Keeping Relationship On-Track

Making a closer relationship ⟷ Making a more distant relationship

Act like the person is important.	⟷	Keep conversations short.
Make thoughtful comments.	⟷	Avoid making personal comments.
Call the person/make plans.	⟷	Don't make contact.
Appropriate touch.	⟷	Clear boundaries/keep my space.
Pay compliments/give gifts.	⟷	Focus on what you need to know.
Be flexible.	⟷	Set clear personal limits.

B. Balancing On-Track Relationships

In Two-Way-Street relationships, one or both people try to:

 Talk and listen.

 Give and take

and . . .

 In One-Way-Street relationships, one or both people are:

 Not listening or talking to each other.

Not giving and taking with each other.

Helpful Hints:

Every relationship is different.

> When I have a Two-Way-Street relationship, it is easier to work well with another person.

> In a One-Way-Street relationship, it is harder to work together.

Relationships are tricky sometimes!

> Even when I try to have Two-Way-Street relationships, sometimes One-Way-Street relationships happen because of me or the other person. I use my skills to care for relationships every day.

Name: _____   Date: _____

B. Balancing On-Track Relationships ➡️ONE WAY

List things that you can do to help make Two-Way-Street relationships.

_____

_____

_____

_____

_____

and . . .

List things you do that may lead to One-Way-Street relationships. ➡️ONE WAY

_____

_____

_____

_____

_____

C. Changing Off-Track Relationships

with Myself

Getting on Track with Myself

 Instead of a fuzzy picture about my goals, I get a Clear Picture of my goals.

 Instead of putting myself down, I do On-Track Thinking.

I can do it!

 Instead of Off-Track habits, I take On-Track Actions to care for my body.

Helpful Hints:

Make an On-Track Action plan.

An On-Track Action plan helps me do things each day that keep me in balance. I don't always follow it, so I have to do On-Track Actions to be sure I jump into New-Me Activities with both feet, use Safety Plans, and move away from situations and habits that are off-track for me.

Finding Middle Ground

I use all of my Calm-Only skills to change off-track relationships:

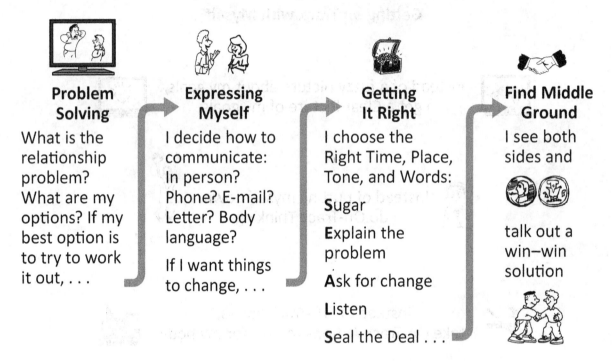

Problem Solving

What is the relationship problem? What are my options? If my best option is to try to work it out, . . .

Expressing Myself

I decide how to communicate: In person? Phone? E-mail? Letter? Body language?

If I want things to change, . . .

Getting It Right

I choose the Right Time, Place, Tone, and Words:

Sugar

Explain the problem

Ask for change

Listen

Seal the Deal . . .

Find Middle Ground

I see both sides and

talk out a win–win solution

Helpful Hints:

Know when to use a Safety Plan.

> If feelings go over a level 3, a Safety Plan may be a good option.

End Off-Track relationships.

> If I have tried to find middle ground and the relationship problems are not better, I may have to end the relationship. I should not be in a situation that is off-track for me.

Finding Middle Ground Plan

Name: _____   Date: _____

What is the relationship problem?
Cindy was rude to my boyfriend.

Planning

How will I communicate: (In person?) Phone?   Writing?
Am I in the Right Mind? (YES) or NO
When is the Right Time? _Friday afternoon_
What is the Right Tone? _Friendly but serious_
Should I use Sugar? (YES) or NO

How will I Explain my side? _____
It upsets me when you are rude to my boyfriend.
I am nice to your friends.

To get to know the other side I will ask: _____
Why don't you like him?

How will I ask for what I want? _Cindy, please be nicer_
to my boyfriend. Talk to me about what is wrong
rather than being rude.

Finding Middle Ground

Will I talk and Listen? (YES) or NO
Will I use a Safety Plan if necessary? (YES) or NO
Will I try to find a win–win solution? (YES) or NO
Will I use skills 123 to help guide my actions? (YES) or NO

Finding Middle Ground Plan

Name: _____   Date: _____

What is the relationship problem?
_____

Planning

How will I communicate: In person?   Phone?   Writing?

Am I in the Right Mind?   YES   or   NO

When is the Right Time? _____

What is the Right Tone? _____

Should I use Sugar?   YES   or   NO

How will I Explain my side? _____
_____
_____

To get to know the other side I will ask: _____
_____

How will I ask for what I want? _____
_____
_____

Finding Middle Ground

Will I talk and Listen?   YES   or   NO

Will I use a Safety Plan if necessary?   YES   or   NO

Will I try to find a win–win solution?   YES   or   NO

Will I use skills 123 to help guide my actions?   YES   or   NO

C. Changing Off-Track Relationships

with Myself

and with Others

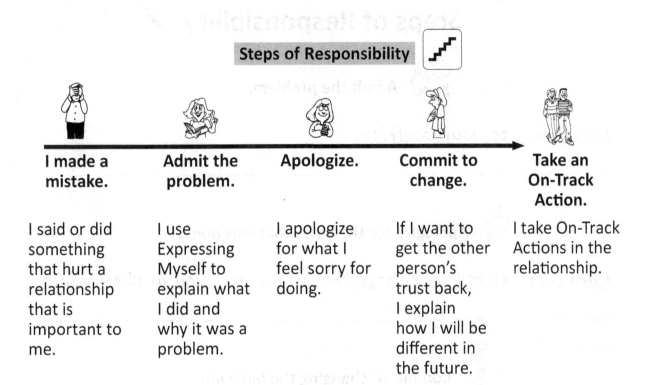

Steps of Responsibility

I made a mistake.	Admit the problem.	Apologize.	Commit to change.	Take an On-Track Action.
I said or did something that hurt a relationship that is important to me.	I use Expressing Myself to explain what I did and why it was a problem.	I apologize for what I feel sorry for doing.	If I want to get the other person's trust back, I explain how I will be different in the future.	I take On-Track Actions in the relationship.

Helpful Hints:

Taking responsibility can increase feelings.

Relationships can be confusing. I sometimes don't even know when I have hurt another person. Finding out about my mistakes can make me feel guilty, ashamed, and even angry. I use Clear Picture and lots of On-Track Thinking to be sure that Relationship Care is an On-Track Action at that time. I want to help the relationship rather than make things worse! I do a Safety Plan and stop doing the steps, if I go over a level 3.

Name: _____   Date: _____

Steps of Responsibility

 <u>**Admit the problem.**</u>

I was rude to your boyfriend.

_____

 <u>**Apologize for the harm that was done.**</u>

I am sorry that I said those things and put you in the middle.

_____

 <u>**Commit to changing the behavior.**</u>

I will talk to you in private next time when I have concerns.

_____

 <u>**Take an On-Track Action.**</u>

I will tell her, "Thanks for being such a good friend."

_____

Name: _____ Date: _____

Steps of Responsibility ▱

Admit the problem.

_____

_____

Apologize for the harm that was done.

_____

_____

Commit to changing the behavior.

_____

_____

Take an On-Track Action.

_____

_____

Name: _____   Date: _____

1. What skill helps me see the moment? _____

2. What skill do I always use after Clear Picture?

   _____

3. What are the numbers of the three skills I use first in all situations?

   _____, _____, and _____

4. What is the skill I use when I do something positive to step toward my goals?

   _____

5. What skill helps me handle risky situations?

   _____

6. What skill helps me focus, feel better, distract myself, and to have fun?

   _____

7. What skill helps me fix situations?

   _____

8. What skill helps me communicate with people?

   _____

9. What skill helps me get what I want from people?

   _____

10. What skill helps me have a positive relationship with myself?

    _____

11. What skill helps me have positive relationships with other people?

    _____

Name: _____   Date: _____

1. What skill helps me see the moment? _Clear Picture_ _____

2. What skill do I always use after Clear Picture?
    On-Track Thinking _____

3. What are the numbers of the three skills I use first in all situations?
    __1__ , __2__ , and __3__

4. What is the skill I use when I do something positive to step toward my goals?
    On-Track Action _____

5. What skill helps me handle risky situations?
    Safety Plan _____

6. What skill helps me focus, feel better, distract myself, and have fun?
    New-Me Activity _____

7. What skill helps me fix situations?
    Problem Solving _____

8. What skill helps me communicate with people?
    Expressing Myself _____

9. What skill helps me get what I want from people?
    Getting It Right _____

10. What skill helps me have a positive relationship with myself?
    Relationship Care _____

11. What skill helps me have positive relationships with other people?
    Relationship Care _____

Skill Master: _____

Cycle #: _____ Date: _____

Group Leader: _____

APPENDIX B

Skills Plan Map

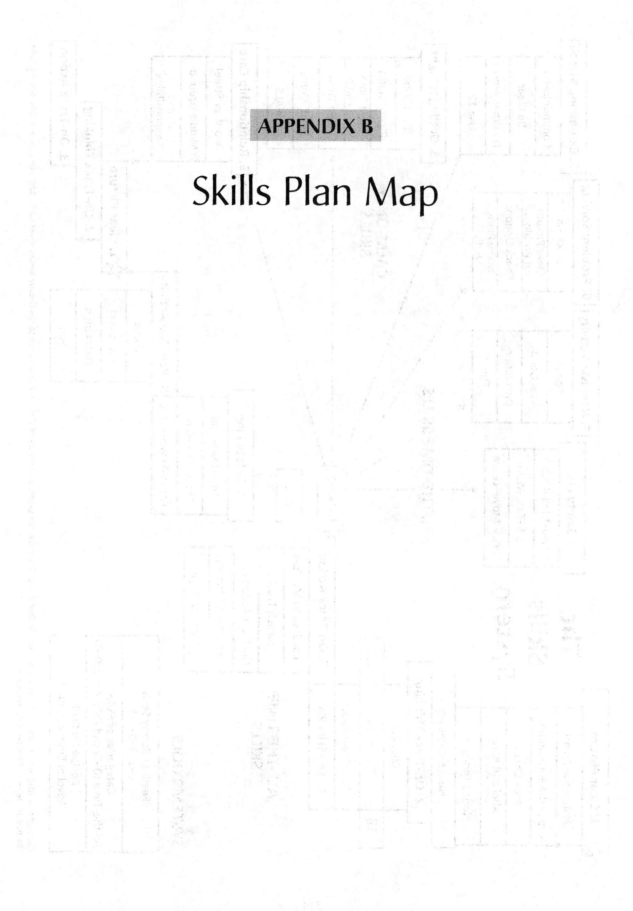

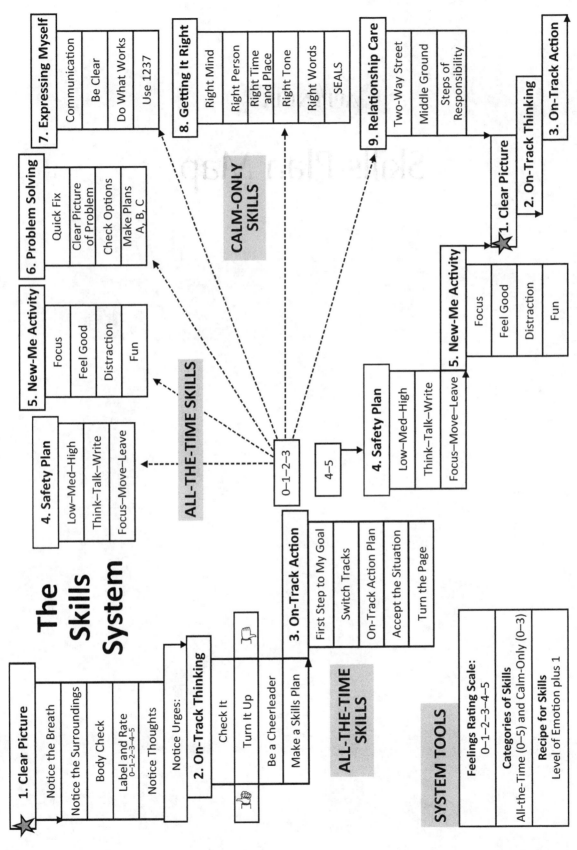

The Skills System

1. Clear Picture
- Notice the Breath
- Notice the Surroundings
- Body Check
- Label and Rate 0–1–2–3–4–5
- Notice Thoughts
- Notice Urges:

2. On-Track Thinking
- Check It
- Turn It Up
- Be a Cheerleader
- Make a Skills Plan

3. On-Track Action
- First Step to My Goal
- Switch Tracks
- On-Track Action Plan
- Accept the Situation
- Turn the Page

ALL-THE-TIME SKILLS

4. Safety Plan
- Low–Med–High
- Think–Talk–Write
- Focus–Move–Leave

5. New-Me Activity
- Focus
- Feel Good
- Distraction
- Fun

6. Problem Solving
- Quick Fix
- Clear Picture of Problem
- Check Options
- Make Plans A, B, C

7. Expressing Myself
- Communication
- Be Clear
- Do What Works
- Use 1237

8. Getting It Right
- Right Mind
- Right Person
- Right Time and Place
- Right Tone
- Right Words
- SEALS

9. Relationship Care
- Two-Way Street
- Middle Ground
- Steps of Responsibility

ALL-THE-TIME SKILLS

CALM-ONLY SKILLS

0–1–2–3

4–5

4. Safety Plan
- Low–Med–High
- Think–Talk–Write
- Focus–Move–Leave

5. New-Me Activity
- Focus
- Feel Good
- Distraction
- Fun

1. Clear Picture
2. On-Track Thinking
3. On-Track Action

SYSTEM TOOLS

Feelings Rating Scale:
0–1–2–3–4–5

Categories of Skills
All-the-Time (0–5) and Calm-Only (0–3)

Recipe for Skills
Level of Emotion plus 1

Skills Coaching Worksheets

Name: _____   Date: _____

1. Clear Picture

→ Breathe ☐ Yes ☐ No

→ Surroundings: _____

→ Body check: _____

→ Feeling: _____ Rating: 0–1–2–3–4–5

→ Thought: _____

→ Urge: _____

2. On-Track Thinking

♡ **Check It** ☐ 👍 Helpful urge ☐ 👎 Not helpful urge

👎 **Turn It Up** 👍 thinking: _____

Cheerleading: _____

_____

Make a Skills Plan: My level of emotion RIGHT NOW: _____

How many skills do I need? _____

What Category of Skills can I use:

All-the-Time skills 0–5 emotion: ☐ Yes ☐ No

Calm-Only skills 0–3 emotion: ☐ Yes ☐ No

Have I used Clear Picture? ☐ Yes ☐ No

Am I using On-Track Thinking right now? ☐ Yes ☐ No

Should I take an On-Track Action? ☐ Yes ☐ No

(continued)

Should I use a Safety Plan? Is there any risk?   ☐ Yes   ☐ No

    ☐ Thinking   ☐ Talking   ☐ Written
    ☐ Low risk   ☐ Medium risk   ☐ High risk
    ☐ Refocus   ☐ Move Away   ☐ Leave area entirely
    I will go: _____

Should I do New-Me Activities?   ☐ Yes   ☐ No

    Focus: _____
    Feel Good: _____
    Distraction: _____
    Fun: _____

Should I do Problem Solving?   ☐ Yes   ☐ No   ☐ Yes, when I am calmer

    Clear Picture of my problem: _____

    Size of the problem: Small   Medium   Large

                   Is it a Quick Fix?   ☐ Yes   ☐ No

    Check all options:
       Option: _____   👍 👍
       Option: _____   👍 👍
       Option: _____   👎 👎
    Plan A: _____
    Plan B: _____
    Plan C: _____

Should I use Expressing Myself?   ☐ Yes   ☐ No   ☐ Yes, when I am calmer

    What do I need to share: _____
    Who do I need to share with: _____
    How will I share it: _____

(continued)

Should I use Getting It Right? ☐ Yes ☐ No ☐ Yes, when I am calmer

Right Mind: _____

Right Person: _____

Right Time and Place: _____

Right Tone: _____

Right Words—Sugar: _____

Explain: _____

Ask: _____

Listen: _____

Seal a Deal: _____

Should I use Relationship Care? ☐ Yes ☐ No ☐ Yes, when I am calmer

Relationship Care with myself: _____

Relationship Care with others: _____

Should I have a Two-Way-Street relationship by listening and talking? ☐ Yes ☐ No

Should I Find Middle Ground? ☐ Yes ☐ No

Should I do the Steps of Responsibility? ☐ Yes ☐ No

Thumbs-Up Thinking: _____

★ What is my goal: _____

Do I have a Skills Plan? ☐ Yes ☐ No

What will my On-Track Action be: _____

Cheer myself on: _____

USING MY SKILLS
(when over a 3 emotion)

Name: _____ Date: _____

1. Clear Picture

→ Breathe ☐ Yes ☐ No

→ Surroundings: _____

→ Body check: _____

→ Feeling: _____ Rating: 0–1–2–3–4–5

→ Thought: _____

→ Urge: _____

2. On-Track Thinking

♡ **Check It** ☐ 👍 Helpful urge ☐ 👎 Not helpful urge

👎 **Turn It Up** 👍 thinking: _____

Cheerleading: _____

_____

🔗 **Make a Skills Plan**: My level of emotion RIGHT NOW: _____

How many skills do I need? _____

What Category of Skills can I use:

All-the-Time skills 0–5 emotion: ☐ Yes ☐ No

Calm-Only skills 0–3 emotion: ☐ Yes ☐ No

(continued)

Should I use a Safety Plan? Is there any risk?   ☐ Yes   ☐ No

☐ Thinking   ☐ Talking   ☐ Written
☐ Low risk   ☐ Medium risk   ☐ High risk
☐ Refocus   ☐ Move Away   ☐ Leave area entirely
I will go: _____

Should I do New-Me Activities?   ☐ Yes   ☐ No

Focus: _____
Feel Good: _____
Distraction: _____
Fun: _____

Skills Plan I will use:

Is that enough?   ☐ Yes   ☐ No

3. On-Track Action: _____

References

Ali, A., Scior, K., Ratti, V., Strydom, A., King, M., & Hassiotis, A. (2013). Discrimination and other barriers to assessing health care: Perspectives of patients with mild and moderate intellectual disability and their carers. *PLoS ONE, 8*(8), 1–13.

American Psychiatric Association. (2013). *Diagnostic and statistical manual of mental disorders* (5th ed.). Arlington, VA: Author.

American Psychological Association. (2007). *APA dictionary of psychology.* Washington, DC: Author.

Ayres, P., & Paas, F. (2012). Cognitive load theory: New directions and challenges. *Applied Cognitive Psychology, 26*(6), 827–832.

Beadle-Brown, J., Mansell, J., Cambridge, P., Milne, A., & Whelton, B. (2010). Adult protection of people with intellectual disabilities: Incidence, nature and responses. *Journal of Applied Research in Intellectual Disabilities, 23*(6), 573–584.

Beckes, L., & Coan, J. (2011). Social baseline theory: The role of social proximity in emotion and economy of action. *Social and Personality Psychology Compass, 5*, 976–988.

Bhaumik, S., Tyrer, F. C., McGrother, C., & Ganghadaran, S. K. (2008). Psychiatric service use and psychiatric disorders in adults with intellectual disability. *Journal of Intellectual Disability Research, 52*(11), 986–995.

Bloom, B. S. (1956). *Taxonomy of educational objectives: Handbook I. The cognitive domain.* New York: David McKay.

Brown, J. F., Brown, M. Z., & Dibiasio, P. (2013). Treating individuals with intellectual disabilities and challenging behaviors with adapted dialectical behavior therapy. *Journal of Mental Health Research in Intellectual Disabilities, 6*(4), 280–303.

Carlin, M. T., Soraci, S. A., Dennis, N. A., Chechile, N. A., & Loiselle, R. C. (2001). Enhancing free recall rates of individuals with mental retardation. *America Journal on Mental Retardation, 106*, 314–326.

Crocker, A. G., Mercier, C., Allaire, J. F., & Roy, M. E. (2007). Profiles and correlates of aggressive behaviour among adults with intellectual disabilities. *Journal of Intellectual Disability Research, 51*(10), 786–801.

Ditchman, N., Werner, S., Kosyluk, K., Jones, N., Elg, B., & Corrigan, P. (2013). Stigma and intellectual disability: Potential application of mental illness research. *Rehabilitation Psychology, 58*(2), 206–216.

Emerson, E., Kiernan, C., Alborz, A., Reeves, D., Mason, H., Swarbrick, R., et al. (2001).

The prevalence of challenging behaviors: A total population study. *Research in Developmental Disabilities, 22,* 77–93.

Feigenbaum, J. D., Fonagy, P., Pilling, S., Jones, A., Wildgoose, A., & Bebbington, P. E. (2012). A real-world study of the effectiveness of DBT in the UK National Health Service. *British Journal of Clinical Psychology, 51*(2), 121–141.

Forte, M., Jahoda, A., & Dagnan, D. (2011). An anxious time?: Exploring the nature of worries experienced by young people with a mild to moderate intellectual disability as they make the transition to adulthood. *British Journal of Clinical Psychology, 50*(4), 398–411.

Glaesser, R. S., & Perkins, E. A. (2013). Self-injurious behavior in older adults with intellectual disabilities. *Social Work, 58*(3), 213–221.

Gold, M. W. (1972). Stimulus factors in skills training of retarded adolescents on a complex assembly task: Acquisition, transfer, and retention. *American Journal on Mental Retardation, 76*(5), 517–526.

Grey, I., Pollard, J., McClean, B., MacAuley, N., & Hastings, R. (2010). Prevalence of psychiatric diagnoses and challenging behaviors in a community-based population of adults with intellectual disabilities. *Journal of Mental Health Research in Intellectual Disabilities, 3*(4), 210–222.

Gross, J. J. (2013). Emotion regulation: Taking stock and moving forward. *Emotion, 13*(3), 359–365.

Gross, J. J. (2014a). Emotion regulation: Conceptual and empirical foundations. In J. J. Gross (Ed.), *Handbook of emotion regulation* (2nd ed., pp. 3–22). New York: Guilford Press.

Gross, J. J. (Ed.). (2014b). *Handbook of emotion regulation* (2nd ed.). New York: Guilford Press.

Gross, J. J., & Thompson, R. A. (2009). Emotion regulation: Conceptual foundations. In J. J. Gross (Ed.), *Handbook of emotion regulation* (pp. 3–26). New York: Guilford Press.

Haaven, J., Little, R., & Petre-Miller, D. (1989). *Treating intellectually disabled sex offenders: A model residential program.* Brandon, VT: Safer Society Press.

Harned, M. S., Jackson, S. C., Comtois, K. A., & Linehan, M. M. (2010). Dialectical behavior therapy as a precursor to PTSD treatment for suicidal and/or self-injuring women with borderline personality disorder. *Journal of Traumatic Stress, 23*(4), 421–429.

Hess, J., Matson, J., Neal, D., Mahan, S., Fodstad, J., Bamburg, J. A. Y., et al. (2010). A comparison of psychotropic drug side effect profiles in adults diagnosed with intellectual disabilities and autism spectrum disorders. *Journal of Mental Health Research in Intellectual Disabilities, 3*(2), 85–96.

Hill, D. M., Craighead, L. W., & Safer, D. L. (2011). Appetite-focused dialectical behavior therapy for the treatment of binge eating with purging: A preliminary trial. *International Journal of Eating Disorders, 44*(3), 249–261.

Horner-Johnson, W., & Drum, C. E. (2006). Prevalence of maltreatment of people with intellectual disabilities: A review of recently published research. *Mental Retardation and Developmental Disabilities Research Reviews, 12*(1), 57–69.

Hübner, R., Steinhauser, M., & Lehle, C. (2010). A dual-stage two-phase model of selective attention. *Psychological Review, 117*(3), 759–784.

Hurley, A. D. (2008). Depression in adults with intellectual disability: Symptoms and challenging behaviour. *Journal of Intellectual Disability Research, 52*(11), 905–916.

Inam Ul, H. (2013). Dialectical behavior therapy for challenging behavior in patients with learning disabilities. *Journal of Pakistan Psychiatric Society, 10*(1), 51–52.

Janssen, C. G. C., Schuengel, C., & Stolk, J. (2002). Understanding challenging behaviour in people with severe and profound intellectual disability: A stress-attachment model. *Journal of Intellectual Disability Research, 46*(6), 445–453.

Kalyuga, S. (2011). Cognitive load theory: How many types of load does it really need? *Educational Psychology Review, 23*(1), 1–19.

Koons, C. R., Robins, C. J., Tweed, J. L., Lynch, T. R., Gonzalez, A. M., Morse, J. Q., et al. (2001). Efficacy of dialectical behavior therapy in women veterans with borderline personality disorder. *Behavior Therapy, 32*(2), 371–390.

Lew, M., Matta, C., Tripp-Tebo, C., & Watts, D. (2006). DBT for individuals with intellectual disabilities: A program description. *Mental Health Aspects of Developmental Disabilities, 9*(1), 1–13.

Lewis, J. J. (2009). Bernice Johnson Reagon quotes about women's history. Retrieved May 1, 2009, from *http://womenshistory.about.com/od/quotes/a/reagon_quotes.htm*.

Lieberman, M. D., Inagaki, T. K., Tabibnia, G., & Crockett, M. J. (2011). Subjective responses to emotional stimuli during labeling, reappraisal, and distraction. *Emotion, 11*(3), 468–480.

Linehan, M. M. (1993a). *Cognitive-behavioral treatment for borderline personality disorder.* New York: Guilford Press.

Linehan, M. M. (1993b). *Skills training manual for treating borderline personality disorder.* New York: Guilford Press.

Linehan, M. M. (2015a). *DBT skills training manual* (2nd ed.). New York: Guilford Press.

Linehan, M. M. (2015b). *DBT skills training handouts and worksheets* (2nd ed.). New York: Guilford Press.

Linehan, M. M., Armstrong, H. E., Suarez, A., Allmon, D., & Heard, H. I. (1991). Cognitive-behavioral treatment of chronically parasuicidal borderline patients. *Archives of General Psychiatry, 48,* 1060–1064.

Linehan, M. M., Dimeff, L. A., Reynolds, S. K., Comtois, K. A., Welch, S. S., Heagerty, P., et al. (2002). Dialectical behavior therapy versus comprehensive validation plus 12-step for the treatment of opioid dependent women meeting criteria for borderline personality disorder. *Drug and Alcohol Dependence, 67*(1), 13–26.

Linehan, M. M., Schmidt, H., Dimeff, L. A., Craft, J. C., Kanter, J., & Comtois, K. A. (1999). Dialectical behavior therapy for patients with borderline personality disorder and drug-dependence. *American Journal on Addiction, 8*(4), 279–292.

Linehan, M. M., Tutek, D. A., Heard, H. L., & Armstrong, H. E. (1994). Interpersonal outcome of cognitive behavioral treatment for chronically suicidal borderline patients. *American Journal of Psychiatry, 151,* 1771–1776.

Lowe, K., Allen, D., Jones, E., Brophy, S., Moore, K., & James, W. (2007). Challenging behaviors: Prevalence and topographies. *Journal of Intellectual Disabilities, 51*(8), 625–636.

Lynch, T. R., Morse, J. Q., Mendelson, T., & Robins, C. J. (2003). Dialectical behavior therapy for depressed older adults: A randomized pilot study. *American Journal of Geriatric Psychiatry, 11*(1), 33–45.

Mastropieri, M. A., Sweda, J., & Scruggs, T. E. (2000). Putting mnemonic strategies to work in an inclusive classroom. *Learning Disabilities Research and Practice, 15*(2), 69–74.

Matson, J., Rivet, T., & Fodstad, J. (2010). Atypical antipsychotic adjustments and side-effects over time in adults with intellectual disability, tardive dyskinesia, and akathisia. *Journal of Developmental and Physical Disabilities, 22*(5), 447–461.

Matson, J. L., Neal, D., & Kozlowski, A. M. (2012). Treatments for the challenging behaviours of adults with intellectual disabilities. *Canadian Journal of Psychiatry, 57*(10), 587–592.

McClure, K. S., Halpern, J., Wolper, P. A., & Donahue, J. J. (2009). Emotion regulation and intellectual disability. *Journal on Developmental Disabilities, 15,* 38–44.

McGrath, A. (2013). Links between the conduct of carers and clients' challenging behaviour. *Learning Disability Practice, 16*(6), 30–32.

Mevissen, L., Lievegoed, R., Seubert, A., & De Jongh, A. (2011). Do persons with intellectual disability and limited verbal capacities respond to trauma treatment? *Journal of Intellectual and Developmental Disability, 36*(4), 278–283.

Miller, A. L., Rathus, J. H., & Linehan, M. M. (2006). *Dialectical behavior therapy with suicidal adolescents.* New York: Guilford Press.

Mitchell, A., Clegg, J., & Furniss, F. (2006). Exploring the meaning of trauma with adults with intellectual disabilities. *Journal of Applied Research in Intellectual Disabilities, 19*(2), 131–142.

Najjar, L. J. (1996). *The effects of multimedia and elaborative encoding on learning* (Technical Report G-IT-GUU-96-05). Atlanta: Georgia Institute of Technology.

Nezlek, J. B., & Kuppens, P. (2008). Regulating positive and negative emotions in daily life. *Journal of Personality, 76*(3), 561–580.

Paas, F., & Sweller, J. (2012). An evolutionary upgrade of cognitive load theory: Using the human motor system and collaboration to support the learning of complex cognitive tasks. *Educational Psychology Review, 24*(1), 27–45.

Paas, F., Van Gog, T., & Sweller, J. (2010). Cognitive load theory: New conceptualizations, specifications, and integrated research perspectives. *Educational Psychology Review, 22*(2), 115–121.

Phillips, N., & Rose, J. (2010). Predicting placement breakdown: Individual and environmental factors associated with the success or failure of community residential placements for adults with intellectual disabilities. *Journal of Applied Research in Intellectual Disabilities, 23*(3), 201–213.

Poppes, P., van der Putten, A. J. J., & Vlaskamp, C. (2010). Frequency and severity of challenging behavior in people with profound intellectual and multiple disabilities. *Research in Developmental Disabilities, 31,* 1269–1275.

Priebe, S., Bhatti, N., Barnicot, K., Bremner, S., Gaglia, A., Katsakou, C., et al. (2012). Effectiveness and cost-effectiveness of dialectical behavior therapy for self-harming patients with personality disorder: A pragmatic randomised controlled trial. *Psychotherapy and Psychsomatics, 81*(6), 356–365.

Reilly, C., & Holland, N. (2011). Symptoms of attention deficit hyperactivity disorder in children and adults with intellectual disability: A review. *Journal of Applied Research in Intellectual Disabilities, 24*(4), 291–309.

Russell, A. T., Hahn, J. E., & Hayward, K. (2011). Psychiatric services for individuals with intellectual and developmental disabilities: Medication management. *Journal of Mental Health Research in Intellectual Disabilities, 4*(4), 265–289.

Safer, D. L., Telch, C. F., & Agras, W. S. (2001). Dialectical behavior therapy for bulimia nervosa. *American Journal of Psychiatry, 158*(4), 632–634.

Sakdalan, J. A., & Collier, V. (2012). Piloting an evidence-based group treatment programme for high risk sex offenders with intellectual disability in the New Zealand setting. *New Zealand Journal of Psychology, 41*(3), 6–12.

Sappok, T., Budczies, J., Bölte, S., Dziobek, I., Dosen, A., & Diefenbacher, A. (2013). Emotional development in adults with autism and intellectual disabilities: A retrospective, clinical analysis. *PLoS ONE, 8*(9), 1–13.

Scott, P. H., Asoko, H. M., & Driver, R. H. (1991) *Teaching for conceptual change: A review of strategies.* Leeds, UK: University of Leeds, Children's Learning in Science Research Group.

Sheppes, G., Scheibe, S., Suri, G., Radu, P., Blechert, J., & Gross, J. J. (2014). Emotion regulation choice: A conceptual framework and supporting evidence. *Journal of Experimental Psychology: General, 143*(1), 163–181.

Sweller, J. (1988). Cognitive load during problem solving: Effects on learning. *Cognitive Science, 12*, 257–285.

Sweller, J. (1989). Cognitive technology: Some procedures for facilitating learning and problem solving in mathematics and science. *Journal of Educational Psychology, 81*(4), 457–466.

Sweller, J. (2010). Element interactivity and intrinsic, extraneous, and germane cognitive load. *Educational Psychology Review, 22*(2), 123–138.

Sweller, J., van Merrienboer, J. J. G., & Paas, F. G. W. C. (1998). Cognitive architecture and instructional design. *Educational Psychology Review, 10*(3), 251–296.

Telch, C. F., Agras, W. S., & Linehan, M. M. (2001). Dialectical behavior therapy for binge eating disorder. *Journal of Consulting and Clinical Psychology, 69*(6), 1061–1065.

Tomasulo, D. (2005) The interactive–behavioral model of group counseling for people with mental retardation and chronic psychiatric illness. *NADD Bulletin, III*(6), Article 3.

Turk, J., Robbins, I., & Woodhead, M. (2005). Post-traumatic stress disorder in young people with intellectual disability. *Journal of Intellectual Disability Research, 49*(11), 872–875.

Tyrer, F., McGrother, C. W., Thorp, C. F., Donaldson, M., Bhaumik, S., Watson, J. M., et al. (2006). Physical aggression towards others in adults with learning disabilities: Prevalence and associated factors. *Journal of Disabilities Research, 50*, 295–304.

van den Bosch, L. M. C., Verheul, R., Schippers, G. M., & van den Brink, W. (2002). Dialectical behavior therapy of borderline patients with and without substance use problems: Implementation and long-term effects. *Addictive Behaviors, 27*(6), 911–923.

van Gog, T., Paas, F., & Sweller, J. (2010). Cognitive load theory: Advances in research on worked examples, animations, and cognitive load measurement. *Educational Psychology Review, 22*(4), 375–378.

Verheul, R., van den Bosch, L. M. C., Koeter, M. W. J., de Ridder, M. A. J., Stijnen, T., & van den Brink, W. (2003). Dialectical behaviour therapy for women with borderline personality disorder: 12-month, randomized clinical trial in the Netherlands. *British Journal of Psychiatry, 182*, 135–140.

Weiss, J. A. (2012). Mental health care for Canadians with developmental disabilities. *Canadian Psychology, 53*(1), 67–69.

Zaki, J., & Williams, W. C. (2013). Interpersonal emotion regulation. *Emotion, 13*(5), 803–810.

Index

Note: f or t following a page number indicates a figure or a table.

Safety plans (*continued*)
 skills knowledge integration and, 77, 77*f*
 types of, 24
SEALS (Sugar [politeness], Explaining, Asking, Listening, a Seal a deal). *See also* Getting It Right (Skill 8)
 Expressing Myself (Skill 7) and, 31
 Getting It Right session (week 10), 168, 169
 overview, 9, 34–36
 Relationship Care session (week 11), 174
Self-acceptance, 36–37, 92, 172
Self-awareness
 Efficacy phase (4) and, 107–108
 mindfulness activity and, 92
 overview, 11–12
 Relationship Care session (week 11), 172
 Relationship Care (Skill 9) and, 36
Self-care, 26, 36–37
Self-determination, 85
Self-dialogue, 11
Self-efficacy, 52, 57, 99
Self-monitoring, 188
Self-soothing activities, 26, 64
Self-talk, 11, 18
Self-trust, 37, 92, 172
Self-value, 92, 172
Shaping technique, 86
Shifting from topic to topic, 61–62, 84–85, 95
Short-term memory, 56*t*
Sight, 26
Simplification, 83
Simultaneous processing of information, 61
Situation, 48, 50, 51
Skills acquisition, 54
Skills cards, 107
Skills chains
 coaching techniques and, 187*f*, 192, 193, 194*t*–195*t*
 managing risk and, 24
 process model of emotion regulation and, 51
 Recipe for Skills and, 19–20, 45–46
 On-Track Action session (week 5), 141
Skills coaching. *See also* Coaching techniques
 coaching relationship and, 193
 contingency management and, 87–88
 Efficacy phase (4) and, 108
 emotion regulation and, 182–183
 handouts and worksheets for, 346–350
Skills Diary Card, 93, 222
Skills games, 107, 154–155

Skills instruction, 54
Skills journaling, 107–108
Skills knowledge, 93, 114, 119–120
Skills List, 4, 5–9, 6*t*, 13–41, 37, 114. *See also* Clear Picture (Skill 1); Expressing Myself (Skill 7); Getting It Right (Skill 8); New-Me Activities (Skill 5); On-Track Action (Skill 3); On-Track Thinking (Skill 2); Problem Solving (Skill 6); Relationship Care (Skill 9); Safety Plan (Skill 4)
Skills List session (week 1). *See also* Skills System
 12-week cycle curriculum and, 73
 Efficacy phase (4) and, 116–118
 Elaboration phase (3) and, 115–116
 Encoding phase (2), 114–115
 Exploring Existing Knowledge Base phase (1) and, 111–114
 handouts and worksheets for, 111, 114, 115–116, 199–204
 overview, 111–118
Skills notebooks, 92–93, 106. *See also* Handouts and worksheets; Homework
Skills Plan, 5, 13, 128–129, 144. *See also* Make a Skills Plan task (4)
Skills Plan Map, 92–93, 344
Skills Review session (week 12). *See also* Skills System
 12-week cycle curriculum and, 73
 Efficacy phase (4) and, 179–180
 Elaboration phase (3) and, 178–179
 Encoding phase (2) and, 178
 Exploring Existing Knowledge Base phase (1) and, 177–178
 handouts and worksheets for, 178, 180, 340–349
 overview, 177–180
Skills surfing, 74–76. *See also* Alternative teaching methods; Teaching methods and strategies
Skills System. *See also* Teaching methods and strategies
 12-week cycle curriculum, 72–74
 alternative teaching methods and, 74–77
 applications of, 3–4
 behavioral regulation and, 57
 benefits of, 71
 coaching techniques and, 188–189, 193
 dialectical behavior therapy (DBT) and, 63–65
 E-Spiral framework and, 70–74, 71*f*, 72*t*
 group skills training and, 67–70
 handouts and worksheets for, 199–204, 340–349

intellectual disability and, 62–63
 overview, 1–3, 4–5, 11–12, 13, 47–48, 66, 109–111
 preparing for a skills training session, 89–90
 process model of emotion regulation and, 50–54, 50*f*
 progressing through the material, 90
 situation–attention–appraisal–response sequence and, 48
 skills acquisition and, 78, 78*t*–79*t*
 skills knowledge integration and, 77, 77*f*
 Skills Plan Map, 344
 subsequent cycles through, 180–181
Skills System Review
 Clear Picture session (week 3), 127
 Exploring Existing Knowledge Base phase (1) and, 92–93
 Expressing Myself session (week 9), 162
 Getting It Right session (week 10), 166
 handouts and worksheets for, 222
 New-Me Activities session (week 7), 151
 Problem Solving session (week 8), 157
 Relationship Care session (week 11), 171
 Skills List session (week 1), 113
 Skills Review session (week 12), 177
 System Tools session (week 2), 119
 On-Track Action session (week 5), 140
 On-Track Thinking session (week 4), 135
Skills System Review Questions
 Clear Picture session (week 3), 127
 handouts and worksheets for, 222
 overview, 92–93
 Skills List session (week 1), 113, 118
Skills System Worksheets, 118
Skills training. *See* Curriculum cycle; Group skills training; Skills System
Smell, 26
Social stigma, 57
Solitary skills, 5. *See also* Clear Picture (Skill 1); New-Me Activities (Skill 5); On-Track Action (Skill 3); On-Track Thinking (Skill 2); Safety Plan (Skill 4)
Soothing the Senses activities, 26
Sorting activities, 26
Steps of Responsibility, 40, 174, 187*f*. *See also* Relationship Care (Skill 9)